WHY GEORGE SHOULD EAT BROCCOLI

BY PAUL A. STITT

Research Director,
Essential Nutrient Research Company, Inc.
Manitowoc, Wisconsin
U.S.A.

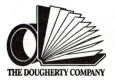

THE DOUGHERTY COMPANY

Development Editor:	*Terry L. Firkins, Ph.D.*
Assistant Editor:	*Barbara Reed Stitt*
Typography:	*Paula Fredrick*
	Sharon Stevens
Cover Design:	*Betsy Svatek*
Lithography:	*Banta Publications Group*

For information concerning special bulk purchases or special editions for educational, promotional, and similar uses, contact the Special Sales Division of the publisher at the address below.

To purchase single copies or small quantities, contact your local bookseller with title, name of author, and ISBN number indicated below. To purchase by mail, send $12.95 plus $1.00 for shipping and handling per copy to Natural Press, *Why George Should Eat Broccoli*, P.O. Box 730, Manitowoc, WI 54221-0730. Allow 6 to 8 weeks for delivery.

Published by:	The Dougherty Company
	A Division of Dougherty
	Publishing Associates, Inc.
	12000 West Park Place
	Milwaukee, Wisconsin 53224-3002

Library of Congress Catalog Card Number: 90-71013

ISBN: 1-878150-00-6

0 9 8 7 6 5 4 3 2 1

ACKNOWLEDGEMENTS

I am deeply grateful to Dr. Chris Beecher, Professor of Medicinal Chemistry at the University of Illinois, Chicago, for collecting the scientific information on the compounds in foods that prevent cancer . Also, Dr. Herbert Pierson, of the Diet and Cancer Branch of the National Cancer Institute, for asking me to become a member of his team.

I am very grateful to my wife Barbara Reed Stitt, who rescued me from poor health in 1982 and also rescued the bakery. Barbara has strongly encouraged me to pursue my scientific interest in finding ways to dramatically improve the nutritional values of the foods Natural Ovens produces.

I am grateful to my son, Todd, and two daughters Anna and Michelle, who have supported me throughout. And to Trace and Lauren Reed, who, with their 3 children, Tyler, Nikolas and Samuel, have proven that the principles of this book really work.

I am also very grateful to all of the 150 men and women with Natural Ovens who have shared in our successes and given so much of their lives to make these successes possible. To name just a few, they are: Glen Hietpas, production manager; Beverly Danay, office manager; Dale Kopidlansky, chief maintenance engineer; Betsy Svatek, graphic artist; Brenda Brogan, packaging supervisor; Barbara Taylor, loading supervisor; Al Holtz, John Ruminski and Joe Scoles, semi-drivers; Paula Fredrick, my personal secretary; Marie O'Grady and Shawn Nelson, Chicago sales supervisors; John Bialozynski, Milwaukee sales supervisor; Dave Vandervieren, Minneapolis sales supervisor, and all of the rest of the employees at Natural Ovens.

I am deeply indebted to all of the customers who have supported Natural Ovens through the years.

I also owe a great deal to a number of people in the media who have supported my cause in helping people and who helped make my first book a success. I wish to thank Roy Leonard at WGN, Phil Donahue, Eddie Jason at WGEE, Ron Zimmerman at WOMT, Jane Brody at the New York Times, and many others who have helped spread the word about the benefits of good nutrition.

My deep appreciation to Terry Firkins of The Dougherty Company for his masterful job of taking my scientific ideas and turning them into words that everyone can understand.

CONTENTS

FOREWORD

Let's pause a moment to talk about a very serious subject. Your body produces over 1000 new cancer cells each and every day, no matter who you are, where you live or what you eat. If not defended against, these cells can, and will, kill you. There's simply no way around it.

The reason I have written this book is to help you fight back. By learning how to strengthen your immune system, you can literally put an end to threats of cancer, heart disease, diabetes, arthritis, and a number of other degenerative diseases, all linked by the most current scientific research to dietary excesses and deficiencies.

My desire is to make this an uplifting as well as an informative book. To do this I have focused on how easy it is to make positive changes in lifestyle, changes that can help you release the champion within. I have also focused on our obligations to our children, so that they may grow up with the strength, happiness, and positive outlook we so dearly wish them to have.

If this book does nothing more than "get you thinking," then it will have accomplished its objective. Hopefully you will go beyond the thinking stage and learn how to feel great and enjoy life to its fullest, free from the worry and fear caused by threats of degenerative diseases. Feeling great is what life is all about!

With Healthful Wishes,

Paul A. Stitt

Paul A. Stitt, M.S. (Biochemistry)

1

WHY GEORGE SHOULD EAT BROCCOLI

When George Bush was growing up, his mother did not know, scientists did not know, in fact no one knew broccoli contained 33 compounds that help prevent cancer. Nor did anyone know that a cigarette after dinner caused heart disease and lung cancer more than it aided digestion, as tobacco advertising of those days claimed.

But today we know a lot more than we did back in the days when George was a boy. Or do we? When George was born, only one out of ten people were expected to die of cancer. Today the ratio is one out of three.

Our nationwide campaign against cigarette smoking has essentially had no effect on the incidence of lung cancer in this country. 21% of all American men with cancer die of lung cancer. That figure has not changed in recent years, and projections see it only increasing.

According to the American Cancer Society, one out of ten American women will develop breast cancer in their lifetime.

26% of all American women dying of cancer are dying of breast cancer. This figure is not expected to decrease but rather to increase in the future. What a horrible, debilitating way to die!

In fact, on the cancer front, we seem to be steadily losing ground despite dramatically increased efforts in man hours and research dollars spent over the past 20 years to find "the cancer cure."

As late as 1984, the number of deaths attributable to cancer was an astounding 450,000 per year. In 1988, the figure was 494,000. Of course, that's not big news. We've been hovering around that figure longer than any of us care to admit. What is big news, however, is that the American Cancer Society has projected that this year the total number of cancer-related deaths in this country will rise to 502,000 per year. This amounts to 1,375 per day, or one every 63 seconds.

The September 20, 1990, issue of *The New England Journal of Medicine* stated, "Cancer will emerge soon after the year 2000 with the *dubious distinction* of being the leading cause of death in the United States."

So, do we really know more about cancer and degenerative diseases than people knew back in the days when George was a boy? Our national health statistics would indicate just the opposite.

In my over 21 years as a biochemist involved with food science and the food industry, it has become increasingly clear to me that America is in fact going backwards in terms of what the average person knows or understands about our single most important source of good health, **fresh whole foods.**

What seems to be missing is a national awareness of the **total benefit**, an across-the-board concentration on those foods which work together to strengthen our immune system, prevent degenerative diseases such as cancer, give our bodies rejuvenative powers, and allow us to achieve peak mental and physical performance in our personal and professional lives. To grasp this **total benefit** requires a thorough knowledge and understanding of **whole foods**.

Simply, **whole foods** are fresh, natural foods—not foods processed to death. They don't have virtually every important nutrient refined or "cooked and canned" out of them under high heat and pressure. They aren't flavor-enhanced or artificially-colored. They don't come swimming in syrup, oil, or grease. Instead they arrive just as Mother Nature herself intended them for human consumption—with **real** color and full of **real** nutrients crucial for maintaining healthy bodies and healthy minds.

When George Bush was a boy, mothers of America knew all of this. True, their pantries weren't filled with processed foods, but they instinctively knew of the **total food benefit.** It would seem, however, their children weren't impressed with this knowledge. Why else would George, as an adult, make a Presidential announcement that he won't eat broccoli? Whatever the reason, it's likely he hasn't been briefed on the following:

> **In addition to its thirty-one other cancer-preventive compounds, broccoli has two compounds known as beta-carotene and indole-3-carbinol. One of the many properties of these very potent biochemical compounds is their ability to counteract nitrosoamines, which are**

known carcinogens, and steroids that cause breast cancer. In scientific terms, nitrosoamines are created when nitrites, used for color enhancement and as a preservative in meat, are exposed to very high temperatures, such as those from burning charcoal. If you're wondering whether cancer can be caused by eating charcoal-grilled meat, the answer is a definite "yes." The beauty of broccoli (specifically beta-carotene) is that it reduces the risk. Also, eating 8 ounces of broccoli with a 6-ounce steak can cut the fat content of the meal by 50%. Hopefully, the President will consider these factors the next time he's flipping a couple of steaks on the grill some summer evening in Kennebunkport.

While he's at it, he should think about a recent Tufts University Diet and Nutrition newsletter, which stated that 1 cup of broccoli has 165% of the recommended dietary allowance (RDA) for vitamin C, 40% for vitamin A, and 20% for calcium. All in 45 calories, with negligible fat or sodium!

It's also nice to know that this same serving of broccoli provides more usable energy than former President Reagan's jelly beans. Sorry, but jelly beans just don't cut it for providing strength and endurance. If anything, they do just the opposite. According to the American Dietetic Association, "high sugar foods cause lethargy." In other words, if you want to mope, eat a lot of jelly beans. In the process, you may even get ulcers as a result of continually loading up on junk food, something that can't be said about eating broccoli. Scientists have known for some time that broccoli is an ulcer preventative, a bit of nutrition "trivia" that may come in handy when in the heat of a budget battle with the U.S. Congress.

I admit to being a little sarcastic. But it's difficult to understand how a person with so much information available can appear so thoroughly uninformed about the vital, yet simple science of whole foods. If the President of the United States is

9

getting low marks in this area, what does that say for the rest of us who are ignoring nutrition and letting habits, speed, convenience and taste dictate our diets?

One of my great hopes in writing this book is that it will lead today's parents to hasten to teach their children the basics of good nutrition. With such an education, perhaps a future president will not unwittingly set such a poor example for our children, who are presently in need of sound nutritional guidance more than any previous generation.

When news broke of President Bush's announcement that he wouldn't eat broccoli, I was engaged with the National Cancer Institute (NCI) in the development of specialized foods (termed Designer Foods) whose primary function is the nutritional prevention of cancer. An evaluation of research made at that time provided proof that there are over 900 compounds in whole foods with the ability to prevent cancer. The tragedy is that the vast majority of people in our country are unaware of this fact!

If you find that distressing, then consider this. According to a national survey done by the National Cancer Institute, only 9% of all Americans eat enough vegetables to qualify as having balanced diets. As vegetables are one of Nature's premium cancer fighters, this means that 91% of us are simply asking to die a slow, agonizing death.

In terms of proper diet and nutrition, it can easily be argued that America is a starving nation. Don't you find that ironic, given our national problem with obesity and weight control, not to mention our ongoing battles with cancer, heart disease, osteoporosis, arthritis, diabetes and a host of other

10

degenerative diseases? The question is: is there a connection between our poor health and our rotten diet?

Well, of course there is a connection. It is called **unintelligent eating habits.** Nibbling on junk food. Feasting on processed food. Reconstituted food. Car-lunching on fast food. Everything but eating the simple, whole foods—fresh fruit, vegetables, and whole grains—given to us by Nature for good health.

How did our fall from proper nutrition begin? How, in a matter of less than fifty years, has America totally "unlearned" what it once knew instinctively about the long-term benefit of whole food?

Some might claim we don't have time to eat right. Who in the world is going to spend two or three hours cooking a balanced meal when he or she has only fifteen minutes to eat it? Mothers are working. Fathers are working. Latch-key kids are coming home to empty houses. To make ends meet means making sacrifices, one of which involves eating out of the can or off a styrofoam plate.

Others might claim we are giving in to convenience and becoming progressively lazy in all of our habits, including our eating habits. When was the last time you walked to the market? Or baked a loaf of bread from scratch? Planted a vegetable garden? Munched on carrot sticks? If you don't feel a tinge of guilt when answering these questions, then you're likely one of the very few who is not swimming in today's sea of convenience.

A final argument might be made that our poor eating habits are a result of misguidance and lack of leadership by the food conglomerates. Those more polarized might go so far as to blame food advertisers and a commitment to maximize profit regardless of what happens to the nation's attitude toward nutrition.

In some ways, speculating about the causes of our nationwide nutrition problem is a misuse of effort and time. What is more important is for each of us to recognize there are vital choices to be made regarding life style, diet, and health. The three are inseparable. One of the objectives of this book is to study their close association so that your choices about how you eat and live may become more educated ones.

Reaching this objective is facilitated by the wealth of scientific data and information regarding the disease-preventive and rejuvenating powers of whole foods. Some of this information will be made available to you for the first time. Other information has been common knowledge among food scientists, nutritionists, and various medical communities for some time, but has not been highly publicized. One thing is clear, however. All of it is critical to an understanding of how each one of us can take personal control of our health needs.

Did you know, for instance, that biochemical compounds in carrots have the power to ward off lung cancer, even among heavy smokers? Did you know that various compounds in flax and other whole grains reduce chances of breast cancer among women? Peppers of every kind contain a compound which dissolves blood clots and also provides one of the strongest cancer preventatives known to science.

Perhaps knowing these and many other facts just like them will be what it takes to turn your life around. In the long run, maybe you'll continue to turn up your nose at beets or lima beans, but at least you'll know what you're missing. Who knows, for the thirty-three reasons which appear below, President Bush might even go back to eating just a little bit of broccoli.

NUMBER OF CANCER-PREVENTIVE COMPOUNDS IN
BROCCOLI...33

BENZOIC ACID,
   PARA-HYDROXY:
BRASSICA,OLERACEA
   DEMUTAGENIC FACTOR
CAFFEIC ACID
CAROTENE,BETA:
CHLOROGENIC ACID
CHLOROPHYLL
CINNAMIC ACID
COUMARIC ACID,PARA:
CYCLOARTANOL,
   24-METHYLENE:
FERULIC ACID

FERULIC ACID,TRANS:
INDOLE-3-ACETONITRILE
INDOLE-3-CARBINOL
INDOLYL,3-3'-DI:METHANE
KAEMPFEROL
LINOLENIC ACID
OLEIC ACID
PHYTIC ACID
PROTEIN
   (BRASSICA OLERACEA)
QUERCETIN
QUERCITRIN
RUTIN

SALICYLIC ACID
SINAPIC ACID
SINIGRIN
SITOSTEROL,BETA:
SQUALENE
STIGMASTEROL
SUCCINIC ACID
THIOCYANATE,ISO:ALLYL:
THIOCYANATE,ISO:
   PHENYL-ETHYL:
VANILLIC ACID
VITAMIN C

(Appendix B contains the scientific research which served as the basis for the above list. There you will also find many other studies of the brassica family, to which broccoli belongs.)

2

IF NOT BROCCOLI, MR. PRESIDENT, HOW ABOUT FLAX?

If President Bush continues to push aside the broccoli, he would be well advised to fill the empty spot on his plate with something equally nutritious. While stabilized, fortified flax may not appear the most appetizing in and of itself, it's still an excellent place to begin rebuilding the broccoli-free diet. Present in a variety of baked goods and high-fiber foods, flax contains a total of 27 cancer-preventive compounds. Two of these, linolenic acid and lignan, rank in the top ten among all known natural anti-carcinogens. That's a pretty impressive record for a single food source.

Here is a complete list of cancer-preventive compounds in flax, prepared by Dr. James Duke of the United States Department of Agriculture and provided by the Napralert Data Base at the University of Illinois. As you read through similar lists in later chapters, you'll undoubtedly become quite familiar with various compounds in whole foods which can keep you off the cancer roster.

NUMBER OF CANCER-PREVENTIVE COMPOUNDS IN
FLAX...**27**

APIGENIN	LINOLENIC ACID	PECTIN
CAFFEIC ACID ESTER	LIGNAN	PHYTIN
BETA CAROTENE	LUTEOLIN	PHYTOL
CHLOROGENIC ACID	METHIONINE	SECOISOLARICIRESINOL
P-COUMARIC ACID ESTER	MUCILAGE	SINAPIC ACID ESTER
EICOSANOL	MYRISTIC ACID	SITOSTEROL
FERULIC ACID ESTER	NIACIN	STIGMASTEROL
FIBER	OLEIC ACID	TOCOPHEROL
GERANYL GERANIOL		VITEXIN
O -GLYCOFLAVONE - C-GLYCOSIDE		

The unique thing about fortified flax is that it contains some of the above compounds at levels of concentration much, much higher than those found in nearly any other food. Many foods don't even contain these compounds. Moreover, stabilized, fortified flax seed is a superior source of dietary fiber. For these reasons, flax is one of the fastest rising stars among today's food scientists and health nutritionists.

While it would appear that fortified flax is a relatively recent discovery, its value as a foodstuff has actually been known for centuries, certainly as long as wheat and barley. 8500 years ago, people were consuming flax along with other wild cereal grasses in the southern part of what is now Turkey, along the Nile Valley, and on the coasts of Greece and Africa. Also oil pressed from flax seed was used in cooking and making paints. Whole seed served as a food in itself. Even fiber from the stalk was used for making rope, cloth, and materials for shelter.

Because of its obvious versatility, flax was a staple in many ancient civilizations.

Today the flax plant is still being used in a variety of ways, among them to make rope, linen, and paper. It's importance as a food source is vastly evident in China, which remains the world's largest grower and consumer of flax. In Russia and various Slavic countries, flax seed is used in making bread and as a condiment. In the U.S., stabilized, fortified, ground flax is rapidly gaining popularity in bread making and in producing energy supplements for athletes. Though flax has never fallen totally into disuse, what we are discovering about its nutritional value is in fact causing a large-scale revival of it as a food.

It's also very exciting that biochemists and nutritional experts are becoming increasingly intrigued with medical applications for fortified flax. Under the direction of Branch Chief, Dr. Ritva Butrum, and Dr. Herb Pierson, the National Cancer Institute, Dietary Prevention Branch, has focused on the properties of stabilized, fortified flax as a cancer preventative. Fortified flax is one of five anti-carcinogenic food types currently under study by the Institute. To demonstrate the level of interest in the disease-prevention potential of these foods, the Institute has budgeted $20.5 million to this one program alone. Fortified flax, interestingly enough, heads the list. The other four are garlic, citrus, licorice root and the parsley family vegetables.

Compounds in stabilized flax receiving the greatest amount of attention among researchers and food scientists are lignans and linolenic acid, as we have already pointed out. Lignans have become particularly well known for their role in the prevention

16

of breast cancer. How this was discovered is certainly quite interesting.

For a number of years scientists believed that a low-fat/high-fiber diet was influential in preventing breast cancer. They were continually troubled, however, by a series of cases which did not fit the theory. Some cases involved countries where breast cancer rates remained low despite prevalently high-fat diets. Other countries continued to show low rates while consuming very little fiber.

Efforts to find a more scientific explanation resulted in confirmation of a high lignan level as common to all diets which produced low incidences of breast cancer, including even high-fat and low-fiber diets. Since that time, studies around the world have added further proof of the dramatic role lignans play in the prevention of cancer.

Dr. H. Setchell at the Karolinska Institute of Finland and Dr. Axelson at the University Hospital in Middlesex, England, found that both colon and breast cancer occur far less frequently among women who consume high levels of lignans. Making their independent findings even more convincing was the generally high occurence of both types of cancer among women with very little or no intake of lignans.

What was the reason for this nutritional deficiency? Those with breast and colon cancer generally didn't like the taste or texture of whole grain foods and therefore wouldn't eat them. Doesn't this explanation sound disturbingly similar to President Bush's refusal to eat broccoli? Unfortunately, it's an explanation heard all too frequently among those with poor nutrition. That is why the message is being put out on flax and many other whole foods just like it.

For instance, in addition to knowing without question that flax is anti-mutagenic (which means it prevents the type of cellular mutations connected with cancer), we have recently learned that flax has a powerful anti-estrogenic property. Because of the molecular shape they share with estrogen, lignans from flax can slow down the action of excess estrogen in women. It is this excess, caused by a host of possible biological and nutritional imbalances, which can lead to various types of female cancer. Now, that is something to give very serious thought to if you are one of America's many women who are neglectful of nutrition!

To take a complete look at the disease-preventive and rejuvenating powers of the many biochemical compounds in flax would mean talking about nothing else for the rest of this book. Personally, I wouldn't object, considering my level of excitement for this marvelous food. However, you as my reader might feel a little cheated if your interest is in becoming more thoroughly rounded in the subject of wellness and whole foods. For the sake of convenience, let's simply take a brief look at some of the many splendid studies done of late on flax and compounds found in flax.

> • **In 1984, Dr. H. M. Sinclair of Great Britain published in the *Journal of Nutrition, Growth, and Cancer* that a deficiency of essential fatty acids , acids found in abundance in flax, causes: lesions of the skin, kidney, and connective body tissues; impaired growth; erythrocyte fragility; and reduced fertility. Dr. Sinclair**

also found this particular deficiency to be common in the diets of Western countries, which accounts for their higher rates of atherosclerosis, coronary thrombosis, multiple sclerosis, diabetes mellitus and hypertension.

• Dr. Terry Schultz of Washington State University, recently fed the equivalent of two tablespoons a day of fortified flax to human subjects. In six weeks, he found a ten to thirty fold rise is anti-cancer compounds in the blood and urine of the subjects.

• A group headed by Dr. B. R. Culp at the University of Michigan found that Omega-3 fatty acids play a positive role in preventing myocardial infarction. Working with laboratory dogs, Dr. Culp's group used Omega-3 to cut ectopic beats in experimentally induced myocardial infarction from 80% to 30% and to reduce the size of the infarction from 25% to 3% . Such significant reductions were all accomplished in a matter of only six weeks of "Omega-3 therapy."

• Psychiatrist Dr. Donald Rudin, found that Omega-3 fatty acid deficiency is directly related to mental illness . Such essential fatty acids in flax and other whole grains provide the substrate upon which niacin and other B vitamins act to form the prostaglandin-3 series tissue hormones which regulate neurocircuits throughout the whole body.

• Using Omega-3 fatty acids in a study of 92 heart disease patients, Dr. R. Saynor of Great Britain was able to rapidly reduce serum triglyceride levels, increase high density lipoprotein and significantly increase clotting time .

• Dr. Patricia Johnston of the University of Illinois, Food Science Department, found that a diet containing 10% linseed oil, derived from flax, changed the prostaglandin content of serum and the fatty acid content of human breast milk by a factor of 10 in 5 days. The dosage of linseed oil was 47 grams. Dr. Johnston also found that a high level of flax in the diet had to be supplemented with zinc, iron, and vitamins B-6 and B-12 in order for it's Omega-3 fatty acids to be maximally utilized. These nutrients are not present in flax. Since Omega-3 fatty acids increase the effectiveness of B-complex vitamins, it was determined that mega doses of vitamins should be avoided.

• Drs. Owren, Hellem, and Odegaard of the Institute of Thrombosis Research at University Hospital in Oslo, Norway, proved flax far superior to corn oil, fish oil or safflower oil in the maintenance of healthy platelets. Using linolenic acid from flax, they were able to reduce adhesions of platelets by 50% in the astoundingly short period of three days.

• Along with other Japanese researchers, Dr. Shimokawa closely studied the effects of linolenic acid on blood pressure. Working with a strain of laboratory rats with a genetic high blood pressure problem, Shimokawa was able to dramatically decrease blood pressure. At the same time he found a substantial reduction in the number of high blood pressure related strokes and a significant increase in average longevity. What is amazing about this study is that it proves that food is more powerful than pharmaceutical science. While many drugs for controlling blood pressure are available on the market today, no drug has yet been discovered which can increase longevity .

• Applying their study to humans, Drs. Berry and Hirsch corroborated Shimokawa's findings that linolenic acid is indeed directly connected to blood pressure control.

• Drs. Adam, Wolfram, and Zoelner of Germany and Hwang of Louisiana State University found that linolenic acid, so abundant in flax, decreases the amount of arachidonic acid made from polyunsaturated fats, thus cutting down on production of prostaglandins which cause muscle inflammation and soreness. In a similar study, Hansen and Jensen specifically pinpointed linolenic acid as decreasing PGE-2, the muscle inflamer.

• In a host of studies, the relationship between linolenic acid and the health and wellness of human cells has been clearly established. Dr. Kinsella and others from Cornell University found linolenic acid has a very positive effect on the integrity of cell walls and the enzymes in cellular membranes. Dr. Marshall of the University of Illinois confirmed that linolenic acid can prevent the synthesis of prostaglandins (messenger hormones among cells) from reaching harmful levels.

• The connection between linolenic acid and normal brain function has been clearly established by Dr. Budowski of Israel and in a French study done by Dr. Bjerve. Though working with different laboratory subjects — in Budowski's case chickens and in Bjerve's rats—both men found substantial learning impairment related to linolenic acid deficiency.

• In addition to finding a connection to retinal damage, Drs. Connor and Neuring of Oregan's Health Science University, like Budowski and Bjerve, found a very positive correlation between linolenic acid deficiency and brain damage. Both visual and brain impairment resulted in learning disabilities among laboratory rats . This finding was verified in a separate study by Drs. Yamamoto and Okuyama, along with other researchers in Japan.

• In a truly remarkable study, Dr. Crawford found linolenic acid deficiency directly connected to severe behavioral problems in laboratory monkeys. When deprived of linolenic acid, in addition to developing skin lesions, laboratory monkeys became extremely hostile, fighting and clawing off each other's gonads. Crawford was then able to reverse the process by adding linolenic acid to the monkeys' diet.

• Dr. Wainwright found that linolenic acid supplements lessened the deleterious effects of alcohol on unborn babies.

• Corroborated by other researchers in Australia, Dr. Storlien discovered that linolenic acid has a beneficial effect on diabetics, as it facilitates insulin receptors to respond to insulin in the blood. He also found that excess linolenic acid burns five times more efficiently than saturated fats. This finding has an application for athletes who need long-term energy sources and easy energy conversions, such as long distance runners.

• Dr. Cunnane of Canada found linolenic acid and other compounds from fish oil to be closely allied with weight control. Using laboratory rats with genetic obesity problems, Cunnane was able to prevent obesity by increasing these compounds in the diet.

• In a very enlightening study by Drs. Fritsch and Johnson of the University of Illinois, published as recently as 1989, it was found that linolenic acid fortifies the immune system. Though the study was conducted on laboratory rats, there is no reason to assume that linolenic acid would not have the same effect on humans.

• Dr. H. Okuyama and associates in Nagoya City University, Japan, found that linolenic acid can effectively block the conversion of linoleic acid to arachidonic acid and is effective in suppressing the thrombotic tendency in humans. They proposed "that linolenic acid should be consumed in amounts greater than 4000 miligrams per day and that linoleic acid consumption be cut from the present 24 grams per day because it interferes with the metabolism of linolenic acid. "

• In 1989, Dr. C. Y. Guesennec published in the *International Journal of Sports Medicine* that docosahexaenoic acid (DHA), which is made from linolenic acid in the body, can increase red blood cell flexibility by 53%. This allows the red blood cells to enter much smaller spaces in the lungs to pick up more oxygen faster, and it allows the red blood cells to enter smaller spaces in the muscles, brain and other tissues that use oxygen so that more oxygen is released faster.

• **Finally, in 1987, Dr. Karmali of Rutgers University was able to prove that linolenic acid inhibits the production of arachidonic acid, which is known to promote growth of tumors. This provided a positive link between linolenic acid and cancer prevention.**

The health and wellness benefits of flax and linolenic acid are so clearly apparent in the research literature of recent years that it seems truly odd they have not been acknowledged by American food manufacturers, the medical world, and health insurers everywhere.

Perhaps someone actually stands to profit by the rising health care costs and continued increase in degenerating disease rates across the country. Perhaps the American people are just not ready for a preventive health maintenance philosophy. Whatever the reason, it is clear all of these attitudes will have to change before Americans can stop worrying that, upon the first sign of physical abnormality, they have contracted cancer or are having a stroke or coronary arrest.

With a strong immune system, created by a comprehensive dietary wellness program, which includes eating foods such as fortified flax, we will no longer have to walk the **tightrope of health.**

NOTES ON FLAX

Stabilized, fortified flax can be added to the diet in a variety of ways. It can be added to salads as a topping or to your favorite soup as a thickening agent. You can also use flax when making bread or cookies. To convert recipes to accommodate flax, simply increase the amount of water. Flax also makes an ideal health drink when blended with your favorite juice.

Stabilized, fortified flax can be purchased in health food or natural food sections of grocery stores. Flax breads, cookies and muffins are also available. For an up-to-date list of companies making food with stabilized, fortified flax, send a self-addressed stamped envelope to Essential Nutrient Research Company, P.O. Box 730, Manitowoc, WI 54221-0730.

WARNING

Do not use ordinary flax but rather flax that has been fortified and stabilized. Ordinary flax has a tendency to become rancid and also does not contain zinc and vitamin B-6, nutrients essential to the proper functioning of Omega-3 in the flax.

SUGGESTED FURTHER READING ON THE SUBJECTS OF FLAX, LIGNANS, AND LINOLENIC ACID

Adam, O., Wolfram, G., Zollner, N. "Effect of a-linolenic acid in the human diet on linoleic acid metabolism and prostaglandin biosynthesis." *J Lipid Res*, Vol. 27 (1986), pp. 421-26.

Adlercreutz, H., Fotsis, T., Heikkinen, R., Dwyer, J.T., Goldin, B.R., Gorbach, S.L., Lawson, A.M., Setchell, K.D.R. "Diet and urinary excretion of lignans in female subjects." *Medical Biology*, Vol. 59 (1981), pp. 259-61.

Adlercreutz, H. "Lignans and Phytoestrogens." *Front Gastrointest, Res*, Vol. 14 (Karger, Basel 1987), pp. 00-00.

Aldercreuta, H., Fotsis, T., Bannwart, C., Wahala, K., Makela, T., Brunow, G., Hase, T. "Determination of urinary lignans and phytoestrogen metabolites, potential antiestrogens and anticarcinogens, in urine of women on various habitual diets." *J Steroid Biochem*, Vol. 25, No. 5B (1986), pp. 791-97.

Aldercreutz, H. "Does fiber-rich food containing animal lignan precursors protect against both colon and breast cancer? An extension of the 'fiber hypothesis.'" *Gastroenterology*, Vol. 86 (1984), pp. 761-66.

Axelson, M., Sjovall, J., Gustafsson, B.E., Setchell, K.D.R. "Origin of lignans in mammals and identification of a precursor from plants." *Nature*, Vol. 298 (August 1982), pp. 659-60.

Berry, E.M. and Hirsch, J. "Does dietary linolenic acid influence blood pressure?" *Am J Clin Nutr*, Vol. 44 (September 1986), pp. 336-40.

Bjerve, K.S., Fischer, S., Wammer, F., Egeland, T. "a-Linolenic acid and long-chain w-3 fatty acid supplementation in three patients with w-3 fatty acid deficiency: effect on lymphocyte function, plasma and red cell lipids, and prostanoid formation 1-3." *Am J Clin Nutr*, Vol. 49 (1989), pp. 290-300.

Bjerve, K.S., Mostad, I.L., Thoresen, L. "Alpha-linolenic acid deficiency in patients on long-term gastric-tube feeding: estimation of linolenic acid and long-chain unsaturated n-3 fatty acid requirement in man." *Am J Clin Nutr*, Vol. 45 (1987), pp. 44-77.

Bjerve, K.S., Thoresen. L., Borsting, S. "Linseed and cod liver oil induce rapid growth in a 7-year-old girl with n-3 fatty acid deficiency." *J Par Ent Nutr*, September/October 1988, pp. 521-25.

Bourre, J.M., Durand, G., Pascal, G., Youyou, A. "Brain cell and tissue recovery in rats made deficient in *n*-3 fatty acids by alteration of dietary fat." *Am Inst Nutr*, 1989, pp. 15-22.

Budowski, P. and Crawford, M. "Effect of dietary linoleic and *a*-linolenic acids on the fatty acid composition of brain lipids in the young chick." *Prog Lipid Res*, Vol. 25 (1986), pp. 615-18.

Budowski, P. and Crawford, M.A. "*a*-Linolenic acid as a regulator of the metabolism of arachidonic acid: dietary implications of the ratio, *n*-6:*n*-3 fatty acids." *Proceedings of the Nutr Society*, Vol. 44 (1985), pp. 221-29.

Budowski, P. "Review: Nutritional effects of *w*-3-polyunsaturated fatty acids." *Isr J Med Sci*, Vol. 17 (1981), pp. 223-31.

Clandinin, M.T., Chappell, J.E., Leong, S., Heim, T., Swyer, P.R., Chance, G.W. "Intrauterine fatty acid accretion rates in human brain: implications for fatty acid requirements." *Early Human Devel*, Vol. 4/2 (1980), pp. 121-29.

Connor, W.E., Neuringer, M.,, Barstad L., Lin, D.S. "Dietary deprivation of linolenic acid in rhesus monkeys: effects on plasma and tissue fatty acid composition and on visual function." *Assoc AM Physicians*, Vol. 97 (1989), pp. 1-9.

Crawford, M.A. "Essential fatty acids and brain development." *Lipids in Modern Nutrition*, Vevey/Ravin Press, N.Y., 1987.

Cunnane, S.C., McAdoo, K.R., Horrobin, D.F. "*n*-3 essential fatty acids decrease weight gain in genetically obese mice." *Br J Nutr*, Vol. 56 (1986), pp. 87-95.

Dyerberg, J. "Linolenate-derived polyunsaturated fatty acids and prevention of atherosclerosis." *J Nutr Rev*, Vol. 44 (1986), pp. 124-34.

Emken, E.A., Rohwedder, W.K., Adlof, R.O., Rakoff, H., Gulley, R.M. "Metabolism in Humans of *cis*-12, *trans*-15-octadecadienoic acid relative to palmitic, stearic, oleic and linoleic acids." *Lipids*, Vol. 2, No. 7 (1987), pp. 495-504.

Endres, S., Ghorbani, R., Kelley, V., Georgilis, K., Lonnemann, G., Van Der Meer, J.W., Cannon, J.F., Rogers, T.S., Klempner, M.S., Weber, P.C., Schoeffer, E.J., Wolff, S.M., Dinarello, C.A. "The effect of dietary supplementation with *n*-3 polyunsaturated fatty acids on the synthesis of interleukin-1 and tumor necrosis factor by mononuclear cells." *N Engl J Med*, Vol. 320 (1989), pp. 265-71.

Garg, M.L., Wierzbicki, A.A., Thomson, A.B.R., Clandinin, M.T. "Dietary saturated fat level alters the competition between *a*-linolenic and linoleic acid." *Lipids*, Vol 24, No. 4 (1989), pp. 334-39.

Greenwood, C.E., McGee, C.D., Dyer, J.R. "Influence of dietary fat on brain membrane phospholipid fatty acid composition and neuronal function in mature rats." *Nutrition*, Vol. 5, No. 4, (July/August 1989), pp. 278-81.

Guesennec, C.Y. "Influence of polyunsaturated fatty acid diet on the hemorrheological response to physical exercise in hypxia. *Int J Sports Med*, Vol. 10 (1989), pp. 286-91.

Hansen, H. and Jensen, B. "Urinary prostaglandin E2 and vasopressin excretion in essential fatty acid-deficient rats: effect of linolenic acid supplementation." *Lipids*, Vol, 18, No. 10 (1983), pp. 682-90.

Hargreaves, K.M. and Clandinin, M.T. "Phosphocholinetransferase activity in plasma membrane: effect of diet." *Biochem Biophys Res Comm*, Vol. 1145 (1987), pp. 309-15.

Henderson, D., Black, H.S., Wolf Jr., J.E. "Influence of Omega-3 and Omega-6 fatty acid sources on prostaglandin levels in mice." *Lipids*, Vol. 24 (1989), pp. 502-05.

Hoffman, P. and Forster, W. "Antihypertensive effect of dietary sunflower seed oil and linseed oil in spontaneously hypertensive rats furing a multigeneration study." *Prost Leukotr Med*, Vol. 25 (1986) pp. 65-70.

Holman, R.T., Johnson, S., Hatch, T. "A case of human linolenic acid deficiency involving neurological abnormalities." *Am J Clin Nutr*, Vol. 35 (1982), pp. 617-23.

Hwand, D.H., Boudreau, M., Chanmugam, P. "Dietary linolenic acid and longer-chain *n*-3 fatty acids: comparison of effects on arachidonic acid metabolism in rats." *Am Inst Nutr*, July 1987, pp. 427-37.

Hwang, D.H. and Carroll, A.E. "Decreased formation of prostaglandins derived from arachidonic acid by dietary linolenate in rats." *Am J Clin Nutr*, Vol. 33 (March 1980), pp. 590-97.

Jacotot, B., Lasserre, M., Mendy, F. "Effects of different diets rich in polyunsaturated fatty acids on plasma phospholipids in the human." *Prog Lipid Res*, Vol. 25 (1986), pp. 185-88.

Jones, P.J. and Schoeller, D.A. "Polyunsaturated: saturated ratio of diet fat influences energy substrate utilization in the human." *Metabolism*, Vol. 37 (1988), pp. 145-51.

Kinsella, J.E., Lokesh, B., German, B.J., Swanson, J., Zuniga, M. "Proceedings of the AOCS short course on polyunsaturated fatty acid and eicosanoids. Eicosanoid synthesis and membrane enzymes are affected by dietary fat level and ratios of n-6 and n-3 polyunsaturated fatty acids." *Lipids Research Laboratory Inst of Food Science*, Cornell University, Ithaca, NY 14853, pp. 416-21.

Klosterman, H.J., Lamoureux, G.L., Parsons, J.L. "Isolation, characterization and synthesis of linatine." *Biochem*, Vol. 6 (1967), pp. 170-75.

Lasserre, M., Mendy, F., Spielmann, D., Jacotot, B. "Effects of different dietary intake of essential fatty acids on C20:3w6 and C20:4w6 serum levels in human adults." *Lipids*, Vol. 20, No. 4 (1985), pp. 227-33.

Leat, W.M.F, Northrop, C.A., Harrison, F.A., Cox, R.W. "Effect of dietary linoleic and linolenic acids on testicle development in the rat." *Quarterly J Exp Phy*, Vol. 68 (1983), pp. 221-31.

Lokesh, B.R., Black, J.M., Kinsella, J.E. "The suppression of eicosanoid synthesis by peritoneal macrophages is influenced by the ratio of dietary docosahexaenoic acid to linoleic acid." *Lipids*, Vol. 24, No. 7, pp. 589-93.

MacRae, W.D. and Towers, G.H. "Biological activities of lignans." *Phytochemistry*, Vol. 23, No. 6 (1984), pp. 1207-20.

Marshall, L., Szezesniewski, A., Johnston, P.V. "Dietary a-linolenic acid and prostaglandin synthesis: a time course study 1-3." *Am J Clin Nutr*, Vol. 38 (December 1983), pp. 895-900.

Miles, C.W., Webb, P., Bodwell, C.E. "Metabolizable energy of human mixed diets." *Applied Nutrition*, Vol. 40A (1986), pp. 333-46.

Morson, L.A., Clandinin, M.T. "Diets varying in linoleic and linolenic acid content alter liver plasma membrane lipid composition and glucagon-stimulated adenylate cyclase activity." *J Nutr*, Vol. 116 (1986), pp. 2355-62.

Neuringer, M. and Connor, W.E. "n-3 fatty acids in the brain and retina: evidence for their essentiality." *Nutr Rev*, Vol. 44, No. 9 (September 1986), pp. 285-94.

Olson, R.E. "Combined DFA deficiency in a patient on long-term TPN." *Nutr Rev*, Vol. 44 (1986), pp. 301-05.

Oster, P., Arab, L., Schellenberg, C.C., Heuch, C.C., Mordasini, R., Schlierf, G. "Blood pressure and adipose tissue linoleic acid." *Exp Med (Berl)*, Vol. 175 (1979), pp. 287-91.

Owren, P.A., Hellem, A.J., Odegaard, A. "Linolenic acid for the prevention of thrombosis and myocardial infarction." *Lancet*, November 1964.

Palmer, I.S., Olson, O.E., Halverson, A.W., Miller, R., Smith, C. "Isolation of f acots in linseed oil meal protective against chronic selenosis in rats." *J Nutr*, Vol. 110 (1980), pp. 145-150.

Ramolingaswami, V. and Sinclair, H.M. "The relation of deficiencies of vitamin A and of essential fatty acids to follicular hyperkeratosis in the rat." *Brit J Derm*, Vol. 65 (January 1953), pp. 1-20.

Renaud, S. and Nordoy, A. "'Small is beautiful': *a*-linolenic acid and eicosapentaenoic acid in man." *Lancet*, 1983, pp. 1169.

Riemersma, R.D., Wood, D.A., Butler, S. "Linoleic acid content in adipose tissue and coronary heart disease." *Br Med J*, Vol. 292 (1986), pp. 1423-26.

Rogers, J.B. "Nutritional attributes of fatty acids." *JAOCS*, Vol. 65, No. 1 (Jan 1988).

Rudin, D.O., M.D. "Omega-3 essential fatty acids in medicine." *Yearbook of Nutr Med*, 1984-85, pp. 37-54.

Salonen, J.T., Salonen, R., Ihanainen, M., Parviainen, M., Seppanen, R., Seppanen, K., Rauramaa, R. "Vitamin C deficiency and low linolenate intake associated with elevated blood pressure: The Kuopio Ischaemic heart disease risk factor study." *J Hypertension*, Vol. 5 (1987), pp. 521-23.

Saunders, D. and Sillery, J. "Absorption of triglyceride by human small intestine: dose-response relationships." *Am J Clin Nutr*, Vol. 48 (1988), pp. 988-91.

Schilcher, H., Schulz, V., Nissler, A. "Effectiveness and toxicology of flaxseed." *Z fr Phytotherapie*, Vol. 7 (1986), pp. 113-17.

Setchell, K.D.R, Borriello, S.P., Gordon, H., Lawson, A.M., Harkness, R., Morgan, D.M.L. *Lignan Formation in Man — Microbial Involvement and Possible Roles in Relation to Cancer.*

Setchell, K.D.R., Lawson, A.M., McLaughlin, L.M., Patel, S., Kirk, D.N., Axelson, M. "Measurement of enterolactone and enterodiol. The first mammalian lignans, using stable isotope dilution and gas chromatography mass spectrometry." *Biomedical Mass Spectrometry*, Vol. 10, No. 3 (1983), pp. 227-35.

Shimokawa, T., Moriuchi, A., Hori, T., Saito, M., Naito, Y., Kabasawa, H., Nagae, Y., Matsubara, M., Okuyama, H. "Effect of dietary alpha-linolenate/linoleate balance on mean survival time, incidence of stroke and blood pressure of spontaneously hypertensive rats." *Life Sci*, Vol. 43, pp. 2067-75.

Sinclair, A.J., Fiennes, W., Hay, W.M., Watson, G., Crawford, M.A. "Linolenic acid deprivation in Capuchin monkeys." *J Med Prim*, Vol. 2(1973), pp. 155-69.

Stitt, P. *Nutritional Importance of Flax.* Presented at the 51st Annual Flax Institute of the United States, January 1986.

Stitt, P. *Use of Flax in Foods.* Presented at the 51st Annual Flax Institute of the United States, January 1986.

Storlien, L.H., Jenkins, A.B., Khouri, S., Pascoe, W.S., Chisholm, D.J., Kraegen, E.W. "The type of dietary fat has a profound influence on development of insulin resistance in rats." *Diabetes Res Clin Pract*, Vol. 5(suppl 1): S267(abstr), 1988.

Storlien, L.H. "Not all fats lead to obesity." *Am J Clin Nutr*, Vol. 990, No. 51, pp. 1114.

Thompson, L.U. *Effect of Flaxseed on Breast and Colon Cancer: A Short Term Study. Final Report.* University of Toronto, Toronto, Ontario.

Thomson, A.B.R., Keelan, M., Garg, M.L., Clandinin, M.T. "Influence of dietary fat composition on intestinal absorption in the rat." *Lipids*, Vol. 24, No 6 (1989), pp. 494-501.

Tinoco, J., Babcock, R., Hincenbergs, I., Medwadowski, B., Miljanich, P., Williams, M.A. "Linolenic acid deficiency." *Lipids*, Vol. 14, No. 2, pp. 166-73.

Tinoco, J., Babcock, R., Hincenbergs, I., Medwadowski, B., Miljanich, P. "Linolenic acid deficiency: changes in fatty acid patterns in female and male rats raised on a linolenic acid-deficient diet for two generations." *Lipids*, Vol. 13, No. 1, pp. 6-17.

Tinoco, J. "Dietary requirements and functions of a-linolenic acid in animals." *Prog Lipid Res*, Vol. 21 (1982), pp. 1-45.

Wainwright, P.E., Huang, Y.S., Mills, D.E., Ward, G.R., Ward, R.P., McCutceon. "Interactive effects of prenatal ethanol and n-3 fatty acid supplementation on brain development in mice." *Lipids*, Vol. 24 (1989), pp. 989-97.

Watanabe, S., Suzuki, E., Kojima, N., Kojima, R., Suzuki, Y., Okuyama, H. "Effect of dietary a-linolenate/linoleate balance on collagen-induced platelet aggregation and serotonin release in rats." *Chem Pharm Bull*, Vol. 37(6) (1989), pp. 1572-75.

Wirth, M., Singer, P., Berger, I., Voight, S., Kretschmer, G.U. "Relationship of arachidonic and eicosapentaenoic acids in serum lipids following dietary addition of linoleic and linolenic acids." *Z Klin Med*, Vol. 41 (1986), pp. 2095-98.

Yamamoto, N., Hashimoto, A., Takemoto, Y., Okuyama, H., Nomura, M., Kitajima, R., Togashi, T., Tamai, Y. "Effect of the dietary a-linolenate/linoleate balance on lipid compositions and learning ability of rats. II. Discrimination process, extinction process, and glycolipid compositions." *J Lipid Res*, Vol. 29 (1988), pp. 1013-21.

Zimmerman, D.C. *Flax, Linseed Oil and Human Nutrition.* Presented at the 52nd Annual Flax Institute of the United States, Fargo, North Dakota, January 1988.

3

TASTE THE BENEFIT

While the names of various vegetables, fruits, grains and herbs in this chapter will be immediately recognizable, their constituent compounds will likely mean nothing to you. That's OK. They definitely mean something to your body.

CARROTS

Certainly we must all remember being scolded at the dinner table, "Eat your carrots, they're good for your eyes!" Oh, the pain of these words! Especially when they meant shoveling in a spoonful of those terrible orange things in order to get dessert.

For a moment imagine what we would have thought had our parents pulled out a list such as the one below and given us a periodic eye test with it, followed by, "Eat your carrots, they prevent cancer!" Would it have made that shovel-sized spoonful any easier to swallow? Probably not. But in later life the good eating habits and cancer-free health we'd enjoy would be a very delicious dessert, indeed.

NUMBER OF CANCER-PREVENTIVE COMPOUNDS IN
CARROTS..42

AESCULETIN	FERULIC ACID	PSORALEN
ALANINE	GERANIOL	PSORALEN,5-METHOXY:
APIGENIN	GLYCINE	QUERCETIN-3-0-
ARACHIDONIC ACID	IONONE,BETA:	BETA-GLUCOSICE
BENZOIC ACID,	KAEMPFEROL	QUERCETIN
PARA-HYDROXY:	LIMONENE	QUERCETRIN
CAFFEIC ACID	LINALOOL	SCOPOLELTIN
CAROTENE,BETA:	LINOLENIC ACID	SERINE
CHLOROGENIC ACID	LUTEOLIN	SITOSTEROL,BETA:
CHLOROGENIC ACID,ISO:	LUTEOLIN-7-0-	STIGMASTEROL
CHLOROPHYLL	BETA-GLUCOSIDE	SUCCINIC ACID
CHRYSIN	METHIONINE	TYROSINE
CINNAMIC ACID	MYRISTICIN	UMBELLIFERONE
COUMARIC ACID,PARA:	OLEIC ACID	VANILLIC ACID
EUGENOL	PINENE,ALPHA:	VITAMIN C

The group of compounds of greatest protective potential in carrots are called **carotenes**. One in particular, beta carotene, can be converted to vitamin A by most mammals, including humans. While vitamin A by itself is a relatively weak cancer preventative, various carotenes in combination are powerful cancer-fighting agents.

The direct link between carotene and cancer prevention is well-documented in current medical and nutritional research literature. In his review of over 50 studies, Dr. Richard Peto confirmed that high carotene consumption accounts for lower incidences of lung, prostate, and pancreas cancer.

Research shows, too, the risk of lung cancer for cigarette smokers is lower among those with carotene-rich diets. Dr. Marilyn Menkes found smokers with carotene-poor diets to be four times more likely to develop lung cancer than smokers who ate the equivalent of only one raw carrot a day. For nonsmokers, the cancer protection provided by carotene is simply an added bonus.

In 1981, Dr. Richard Shekelle was able to take Dr. Menkes' research one step further. His investigation confirmed that smokers with carrot-rich diets were eight times less likely to contract lung cancer than those who ate either few or no carrots at all. Beta carotene once again proved to be the critical link.

Lengthening the list of lung cancer fighters, Regina Ziegler found that carotene levels in sweet potatoes and winter squash were on par with that of carrots. What she also found was that all three vegetables not only help prevent lung cancer but also repair lung and throat tissue damaged by smoking. In other words, carotene showed a healing as well as preventive potential — further encouragement to smokers who are not able to "kick the habit." The findings of Ms. Ziegler make it even more clear that the human body's ability to heal itself is in direct proportion to the quality of its nutritional intake.

The beauty of carrots and other members of the parsley family is multifaceted, to say the least. As the previous chart shows, a single carrot contains over 40 protective compounds. Considering that other relatives of the parsley family can supply even further compounds, you can assemble quite a colorful disease-fighting plate of "veggies" for yourself.

As these other compounds will be examined in depth elsewhere in this book, we will conclude our "parental lecture" on carrots with a bit of cooking advice. Because cooking destroys some of the carotene and other cancer-preventive compounds to some degree, carrots should be eaten raw. If you simply can't stand them raw, then eat them steamed, along with generous servings of squash and sweet potatoes. Either way, "they're good for your eyes." Right?

PEPPERS

Peppers have been used as a general medicinal longer than aspirin. For one reason, they've been around a few more centuries. My great uncle, Dr. Bedford, like other old-fashioned country doctors of his day, prescribed them for everything from congestion to the pain of arthritis. As he used to say, "They're sure to cure you if not too much ails you." Were he alive today, Dr. Bedford would likely get drummed out of the American Medical Association for prescribing peppers to cure the common cold.

Imagine paying a physician thirty dollars for an office call, only to be told to go home, drink plenty of fluids, and take three hot peppers. We'd feel robbed. Today we feel a lot better going to the doctor, paying him for a scribbled note we can't even read, then going on to the drugstore and paying the pharmacist for an expensive prescription. Old Dr. Bedford would be horrified. He, like this author, would contend that we can get the job done with those three peppers.

Perhaps what has been forgotten is that much of what is best for us is still free. A flower doesn't charge by the hour. A sunset doesn't bill us a hundred and twenty-five dollars for stress therapy. And a bird doesn't ask to be paid for its morning song.

Another gift of nature, peppers prevent cancer, free of charge, by adding the following preventive compounds to a person's diet:

NUMBER OF CANCER-PREVENTIVE COMPOUNDS IN
PEPPERS & PAPRIKA...............................**20**

ALANINE	CYCLOARTANOL,	PIPERINE
CAFFEIC ACID	24-METHYLENE:	PULEGONE
CAPSAICIN	GLYCINE	SERINE
CAROTENE, BETA:	LANOSTEROL	SITOSTEROL,BETA:
CHLOROGENIC ACID	LINOLENIC ACID	STIGMASTEROL
CINNAMIC ACID	LUTEOLIN-7-0-BETA-	TYROSINE
COUMARIC ACID,PARA:	D-GLUCOSIDE	VITAMIN C
	OLEIC ACID	

All green, red, and yellow peppers contain capsaicin, the compound that gives them their hotness. The "very hot" varieties simply contain more capsaicin. As all peppers stimulate the circulatory system, raise basal metabolic rates (burn fat faster), and provide one of the highest nutritional densities (see *Why Calories Don't Count,* Paul Stitt, 1982), hot peppers do all of these things to a greater degree. In addition, they dissolve blood clots, eliminate pain, kill parasites, and serve as a nasal and lung decongestant. If that's not enough to get you to "pop a few jalapenos," then consider this: a single pepper contains more Vitamin C than an orange. It also contains very high levels of beta carotene, one of Nature's most potent cancer preventatives.

Today a handful of physicians are still relying on the power of the pepper. Dr. Irwin Zimet, a pulmonary expert, prescribes chili peppers for bronchitis and emphysema. Though other doctors may be shocked by this, there's nothing radical or "unscientific" about Dr. Ziment's approach. It's a proven fact that chili peppers increase the flow of fluids in the body, thus thinning lung and throat secretions and making them easier for the body to expel.

Also, inhaling the fumes of hot peppers or gargling with a mixture of water and hot pepper sauce, such as Tabasco, are proven decongestants. The "pepper remedy" (specifically that provided by capsaicin) is in fact identical to modern cold medicines, such as Robitussin. The only difference is, the "pepper remedy" has two advantages. First, it not only cures mucous problems associated with many viral infections, it prevents infections from ever taking a hold in the first place, thus eliminating the need for a cold remedy. Now, if that doesn't talk everybody's language, then perhaps the second advantage will: a pepper is a lot easier on the wallet than an expensive bottle of cold medicine.

Other nutritional benefits of the pepper are leading to a number of very exciting lines of research. One study in particular, done by Dr. Thomas Burks of the University of Arizona Health Sciences Center in Tuscon, has real "breakthrough potential." Dr. Burks found that an ointment made of capsaicin provided long term pain relief in laboratory-tested guinea pigs. From this knowledge may come the discovery of a new pain reliever for arthritis sufferers. Unfortunately when such a medicine is discovered, it will be quickly patented by a pharmaceutical manufacturer, given a lot of advertising hype which will boost the base price of the product, and made to appear as though it's something we can't live without, seeing that it's "proven scientifically effective."

But that's the way it goes. Long gone are the days when we walked into a pharmacy and saw a glass jar filled with something labeled "Capsaicin." It was inexpensive. It worked for a number of ailments, including pain relief and even diminished sexuality. And it consisted of nothing more than powdered peppers straight from Nature. Had my great uncle Dr. Bedford explained this, perhaps we would have gone home to the garden and attempted to grind our own.

One final note: for injesting pepper, Dr. John Christopher, the Master Herbalist, recommends starting gradually with 1/4 teaspoon cayenne pepper in a little cold water 3 times a day. Add 1/4 teaspoon to this dosage every three days until you are taking 1 teaspoon 3 times daily. Warning: until you are used to it, make sure you have plenty of COLD water nearby. It's real hot. The quickest and most effective preparation of cayenne is to make a tea with it. Mix a teaspoon of cayenne in a cup of warm water and drink it. During the first few days of taking the cayenne, it may be hot going in. But after you get accustomed to it, it shouldn't bother you. You may also purchase pepper in capsule form from natural food stores.

CITRUS FRUIT

Certainly we all have heard at one time or another about the discovery of a cure for scurvy? But we probably haven't heard that the role of citrus fruit in scurvy prevention had to be discovered no less than three separate times before the medical communities of the day would acknowledge it.

In 1600, John Hall prescribed juniper berries and lemons to treat scurvy. While his remedy never failed, his credibility as a scientist came under severe attack. He could show results, but he was unable to support them in a "manner befitting a scientist".

In 1753, a Scottish naval surgeon, James Lind, proved in a controlled experiment that citrus fruit cured scurvy. He, too, was discredited when he couldn't provide a scientific explanation. When pressed to identify the compound in citrus fruit which combatted scurvy, he had to admit that he didn't know, and citrus fruit again fell rapidly into disuse.

Necessity eventually overruled the defensive egos of the scientific community and rescued citrus fruit once more from oblivion. By 1795 the British Admiralty was faced with a scurvy problem of epidemic proportions among its long distance sailors. Entire crews of sailors were dying on long voyages, and replacements were impossible to find in exotic lands or in the middle of the ocean. The solution was to lay in large stores of citrus fruit and require sailors to eat them daily while at sea. It worked. The only irony is that 40 years had passed since the first discovery of a cure for scurvy, and 200,000 sailors died in the meantime. So much for the delays of science.

Had John Hull or James Lind been able to produce a chart like the following, history might have taken a slightly different course.

NUMBER OF CANCER-PREVENTIVE COMPOUNDS IN
ORANGES, LEMONS, ETC.........................58

AESCULETIN
ALANINE
ANETHOLE
APIGENIN
CAFFEIC ACID
CAFFEINE
CAROTENE, BETA:
CARVONE
CHLOROPHYLL A
CHLOROPHYLL B
CITRAL
COUMARIC ACID, PARA:
CYCLOARTANOL,
   24-METHYLENE:
DECAN-1-AL
ERIODICTYOL
ESTRAGOLE
FERULIC ACID
FLAVONE,3'-4'-5-6-7-8-
   HEXAMETHOXY:

FLAVONE,4'-5-6-7-8-
   PENTAMETHOXY:
FLAVONE, 5-HYDROXY
-3'-4'-6'-7-8-PENTAMETHOXY:
GERANIOL
GLYCINE
HESPERETIN
IONONE, BETA:
KAEMPFEROL
LIMONENE
LIMONENE,(+):
LINALOOL
LINOLENIC ACID
LUTEOLIN
MENTHONE
METHIONINE
MYRCENE, BETA:
NARINGENIN
NARINGIN
NOBILETIN
OLEIC ACID

PHLOROGLUCINOL
PINENE, ALPHA:
PSORALEN
PSORALEN, 5-METHOXY:
QUERCETIN
RHAMNETIN, ISO:
RUTIN
SCOPOLETIN
SCUTELLAREIN
SERINE
SITOSTEROL, BETA:
STIGMASTEROL
SUCCINIC ACID
SYNEPHRINE
TANGERETIN
TYRAMINE, N-METHYL:
TYROSINE
UMBRELLIFERONE
VITAMIN C
VITEXIN, ISO:
XANTHOTOXOL

Perhaps the very type of scientific censorship and dinosaur mentality that accounted for the death of 200,000 British sailors is being used with the American people of today. Now, as then, economics play a dreadfully significant role in what and how information gets disseminated to the American public. What if we were to stop chasing our tails trying to find a "miracle cure" for cancer and spend more energy, money and time teaching ourselves to eat better? Citrus fruit, like so many of nature's nutritional gifts, is a **proven cancer preventive.** Why isn't each of us aware of this fact? And if we are aware of it, why haven't we been encouraged or taught to act upon it? Do the American Cancer Society, the American Medical Association, and other self-sustaining bureaucratic organizations actually have a vested interest in perpetuating the cancer scare and suppressing the cancer cure?

Here are the facts. Citrus fruit is rich with vitamin C, or ascorbic acid. Ascorbic acid, a powerful anti-oxidant, counteracts carcinogenic compounds such as nitrosoamines which, as we discussed in Chapter 1, are derived from nitrites used to preserve meat. It also works in conjunction with other compounds found in garlic and fortified flax to enhance cancer prevention.

In addition to containing vitamin C, citrus fruit is high in limonene, an oil found in the pulp and rind, as well as in the flesh of the fruit. Limonene is irrefutably one of the most powerful compounds known, natural or synthetic, for not only preventing but *reversing* cancerous growth without causing deleterious side effects.

One of the most exciting articles on limonene research in recent years appeared in the *Journal of the National Cancer Institute* (volume 76, pp. 323-325, 1986.) A study done by Dr. Charles Ellson and others at the University of Wisconsin, McCardle Cancer Research Institute, in conjunction with the Nutritional Science Department, provided the link between limonene and cancer control. An experimental group of female laboratory rats with large, advanced breast tumors was administered a diet of 10% limonene. The control group received a diet without limonene. Within eight weeks, nearly all of the tumors in the experimental group had abated or disappeared; the control group experienced rampant tumor growth.

Remarkably, nearly five years have passed since the publication of Dr. Ellson's research, with little or no follow-up by other cancer researchers or the medical community at large. Even more remarkable is the fact that the limonene level used on Ellson's rats is well within the dosage levels tolerable among humans. Thousands of American women do not have to die of breast cancer yearly. Nor do they need to have radical mastectomies and suffer the long term physical and psychological problems connected with this surgery. None of these things have to happen because limonene is an FDA-approved food product. Women of America just don't know about it or about Dr. Ellson's research and a lot more research just like it.

During 1990, the National Cancer Institute, Dietary Prevention Branch, has committed itself to picking up where the University of Wisconsin left off. Over the next two years, they will be devoting extensive research to the cancer preventive effects of limonene in animals and humans, in pure form and in combination with other food compounds. Hopefully, women of America will hear about the results of this work.

In the meantime, we at Natural Ovens have shown our commitment to this cause by using cancer preventive limonene in our products. We are also in the process of founding and sponsoring the Cancer Prevention Research Foundation, dedicated to the research of dietary cancer prevention and the special study of anti-cancer food compounds, such as limonene, lignans, and linolenic acid. Cancer researchers from across the country are invited to participate. If we work together, we may very well be able to prevent history from repeating itself. This, time, rather than providing a cure for scurvy, citrus fruit will go down as saving us from cancer... that is if we can get the scientific and medical communities of our own day to listen.

BANANAS

There's a very pure logic about bananas. It goes like this. Potassium counteracts the harmful effect of sodium on blood pressure. Bananas are rich with potassium. You draw the conclusion.

Also draw a conclusion from these facts. Americans eat relatively few bananas. The Japanese consume far more sodium than Americans and still maintain a lower national average blood pressure. Why? Because the Japanese consume more bananas and other fruit, vegetables and whole grains which are abundant in potassium.

The following chart may help to explain why the Japanese also get lung cancer less frequently than Americans, despite the fact that the Japanese are much heavier smokers.

NUMBER OF CANCER-PREVENTIVE COMPOUNDS IN
BANANAS...*11*

CYCLOARTANOL, 24- METHYLENE: DELPHINIDIN KAEMPFEROL	LINOLENIC ACID OLEIC ACID QUERCETIN SITOSTEROL, BETA:	STIGMASTEROL SUCCINIC ACID TRYPTAMINE, 5-HYDROXY: VANILLIC ACID

In addition to its cancer-preventive powers, the banana has been found to provide gastro-intestinal benefits. According to Dr. Ralph Best of the Department of Pharmacy at the University of Aston in England, bananas strengthen the stomach lining by creating a coating that serves as a barrier against stomach acids. Dr. Best determined that laboratory rats which had been fed bananas had a *visibly* thicker stomach lining than those which had been fed Tagamet, a common treatment for ulcers. Bananas were also found to increase the manufacture of mucous-producing cells used by the stomach lining as protection against pepsin and hydrochloric stomach acid.

Of the 60 medical and scientific reports and articles consulted for this work, 12 showed bananas are beneficial for ulcers, 4 proved they are cancer preventatives, and over 20 confirmed their ability to kill harmful bacteria, viruses, and fungus. Combine these benefits with what the Japanese have shown us about heart disease and lung cancer control and the evidence is clear. We definitely should be eating more bananas.

APPLES

The ancient Greeks knew apples were nectar for the gods. They didn't write scholarly papers on the subject. Nor did they scramble after government grants to study the effects of apple juice on sick laboratory rats. But they were smart enough to figure out the apple is phenomenal in its ability to cure and prevent disease. They also were smart enough to eat wheat, barley, flax, and lentils in place of coffee, cigarettes, and candy bars. But the ancient Greeks may have been a little ahead of their time, just as the list below may be a little ahead of its time, given the somewhat backward nature of the American diet.

NUMBER OF CANCER-PREVENTIVE COMPOUNDS IN
APPLES..*13*

CATECHIN,(+)	COUMARIC ACID,PARA:	QUERCITRIN,ISO:
CATECHIN,EPI:(-):	ESTRAGOLE	RUTIN
CHLOROGENIC ACID	HYPEROSIDE	URSOLIC ACID
CHLOROGENIC ACID,ISO:	INDOLE-3-ACETIC ACID	VITAMIN C
	QUERCITRIN	

In addition to being anti-carcinogenic, the apple is a superior anti-viral. According to a Canadian study done by Dr. J. Konowalchuk, (*Applied and Environmental Microbiology*, Vol 6, 1978, pp. 798-801), even apple juice, right from the grocer's shelf, is strong enough to eradicate polio virus with 100% effectiveness.

No wonder researchers at Michigan State University deemed the apple Nature's all-round health food. Not only does it counteract throat infections, relieve tension, and generally fortify the human immune system, but it also prevents heart disease. In several corroborative studies, researchers from Italy, Ireland and France found apples to lower cholesterol by as much as 10% when test patients were administered two apples a day for a month. This translates into a 20% reduction in the likelihood of developing heart disease. Out of this research also came the knowledge that whole apples are stronger heart disease preventatives than pure pectin extracted from apples. Active compounds in the fruit's skin and meat make it important to eat the whole apple to get the fullest benefit, which just goes to show how Nature is her own best frugal gourmet. Nothing is wasted.

Because apples stabilize human blood glucose levels, they have an obvious importance for diabetics. Also, people suffering from high blood pressure will be happy to learn that the Psychophysiology Center of Yale University has found in several studies that the aroma of spiced apple juice lowers blood pressure. Given all of the apple's disease-preventive attributes, it should come as no surprise that Michigan State University researchers confirmed that people who regularly eat apples visit their doctors 33% less than those who eat few apples.

In the final analysis, there is only one thing that might be said against this wonderful fruit. Ironically, the fruit itself is not the problem. Recently a heated debate began over the health hazard posed by pesticides used by apple growers. As with most "scares" of this type, the issue has been blown completely out of proportion. First, the threat posed by pesticides is outweighed by the health benefits provided by apples. And second, it has been proven only that extremely high doses of pesticide create dangerous levels of toxicity in laboratory animals. At levels used in growing apples, pesticides of this type pose a health hazard that is very minor, certainly not great enough for you to eliminate apples from your diet entirely. In terms of what you would be denying your body, that would be a big mistake.

CHERRIES

If you like cherry pie, cherry cobbler or cherries jubilee, here are 46 reasons you should prefer natural, whole cherries.

NUMBER OF CANCER-PREVENTIVE COMPOUNDS IN
CHERRIES..**46**

AMYGDALIN
APIGENIN
AROMADENDRIN
BENZOIC ACID ETHYL ESTER
BENZOIC ACID PARA-
   HYDROXY:
CAROTENE, BETA:
CATECHIN,(+):
CATECHIN,EPI:(-):
CHLOROGENIC ACID
CHRYSIN
COUMARIC ACID,PARA:
COUMARIN
COUMARIN,DIHYDRO:
CRESOL,ORTHO:
CRESOL,PARA:

CYCLOARTANOL,
   24-METHYLENE:
DECAN-1-AL
EUGENOL
EUGENOL METHYL
ETHERFRAXINOL
GALLIC ACID
GENISTEIN
HYPEROSIDE
IONONE,BETA:
KAEMPFERIDE
KAMEPFEROL
LINALOON
LINOLENIC ACID
NARINGENIN
OLEANOLIC ACID
OLEIC ACID

QUERCETIN
QUERCETIN,DIHYDRO:
QUERCITRIN-3-D-
   BETA-D-GLUCOSIDE
QUERCITRIN
RUTIN
SALICYLATE,METHYL:
SITOSTEROL,BETA:
SQUALENE
STIGMASTEROL
SUCCINIC ACID
TAXIFOLIC
TECTOCHRYSIN
URSOLIC ACID
VANILLIC ACID
VITAMIN C

According to research conducted by Dr. Chris Beecher at the University of Illinois-Chicago, each of the above compounds has been proven to counteract and prevent cancerous growth in laboratory animals, as well as in humans.

By the way, if you're thinking of getting these compounds in food containing cherry flavoring, think again. Cherry derivatives and artificial substitutes contain none of the above compounds. This simply reaffirms the importance of eating natural, whole foods.

GARLIC

In the folklore of medicine, garlic is a "classic." It has been used throughout the centuries to cure everything from the common cold to more ominous maladies. In addition, it has enjoyed wide acceptance as having the power to ward off all types of physical and psychological infirmities. Though often surrounded by an aura of intrigue and mystery, garlic and its disease-preventive capabilities have recently become the focus of intense scientific study. Hopefully, affirmation will come without the need for a drug manufacturer to patent and market for thousands of dollars what Nature gives us almost free of charge! As you can see from the following chart, garlic has enough cancer-preventive clout that a drug company might certainly want to muscle in on the action.

NUMBER OF CANCER-PREVENTIVE COMPOUNDS IN
GARLIC, ONION..*35*

ALANINE
ARACHIDONIC ACID
BENZOIC ACID,
   PARA-HYDROXY:
CAFFEIC ACID
CHLOROGENIC ACID
CHLOROPHYLL
COUMARIC ACID,PARA:
CYCLOARTANOL,
   24-METHYLENE:
DIALLYL DISULFIDE
DIALLYL SULFIDE
FERULIC ACID

GLYCINE
KAEMPFEROL
LINOLENIC ACID
METHIONINE
OLEANOLIC ACID
OLEIC ACID
PHLOROGLUCINOL
PHYTIC ACID
PROSTAGLANDIN A-1
PROSTAGLANDIN E-1
QUERCETIN
QUERCETIN-3-0-
   BETA-D-GLUCOSIDE

RUTIN
SERINE
SINAPIC ACID
SITOSTEROL,BETA:
STIGMASTEROL
SUCCINIC ACID
TAURINE
TOCOPHEROL,ALPHA:
TOCOPHEROL,BETA:
TYROSINE
VITAMIN A
VITAMIN C

Solid scientific evidence today confirms that, in addition to its role in cancer prevention, garlic destroys harmful bacteria better than penicillin and tetracycline. In China, it has been proven to cure meningitis, a usually fatal inflammation of the meninges of the brain and the spinal cord, caused by bacterial infection. As an anti-infectant, garlic kills fungus, parasites, protozoa and viruses.

And that's not all. The list of healing and disease-preventive credits for garlic is very impressive indeed:

> • Garlic vigorously fortifies the immune system, which means it may very well find its way into the area of AIDS research.

> • Garlic is a wonder drug for the human circulatory system. It reduces cholesterol, thins the blood, and prevents clotting. In fact, simple garlic proved superior to Clofibrate in lowering cholesterol. Clofibrate is the drug most prescribed for patients with problems of high cholesterol. In India, fresh garlic juice lowered human cholesterol counts on the average from 305 to 218 within two months, with no harmful side effects. [When a program of garlic cleansing is first implemented, blood cholesterol levels may rise for a short period and then fall dramatically within a few months. (A.K. Bordia, J.Assoc. Phys. Ind. 22: 267, 1974)]

> • Garlic is a safe and effective natural decongestant.

• Garlic contains an intense anti-oxidant. This means it prevents "free radicals" and "carcinogens" from getting a cancer hold on our bodies. Recognizing this, the National Cancer Institute has placed garlic high on its research list of cancer-preventive foods.

What is somewhat strange about garlic is that its curative applications depend on whether or not it is cooked. When raw, it fortifies the immune system and fights bacteria; when cooked, it lowers blood pressure and acts as a decongestant. Either way, garlic is an excellent all around "natural medicinal."

Of course, you're likely wondering whether you'll have a friend to your name after introducing garlic into your wellness regimen. To set your mind at rest, try this method for "taking" garlic. Press raw garlic in a garlic press. With pulp on the tip of a spoon, place the pressed garlic on the back of your tongue. Swallow and wash down with a large glass of water, much as you would when taking aspirin. Do not chew. Also take garlic just before going to bed. It's important to take it on an empty stomach (2 hours before or after eating).

Of course, garlic can be enjoyed in many types of cuisine, from Italian to Oriental. When cooking with garlic, always use fresh garlic, as garlic salt is a very poor substitute. Also, because fresh onion contains many of the same beneficial compounds, it's good to use both liberally in your cooking.

If none of the above methods work for you, we recommend aged, dry garlic in capsule form. Kyolic and Pure-Gar are two research tested products available at any health food store.

51

BARLEY

Long before Homer ever composed the *Iliad* and the *Odyssey*, barley and flax were the main ingredients in a drink called KYKION, used by ancient Spartans to help sustain warriors in battle. In view of the fact that ancient Greek wars appear to have lasted scores of years, the potency of this drink must have been Herculean, indeed.

Humor aside, as best as can be determined, the use of barley as food dates back 8,000 years, approximately to the time when other grains, such as wheat and flax, were being domesticated for human consumption. Since then a great deal has changed. The Trojan War, fought over the beautiful Helen of Troy, petered out. Empires have risen and crumbled. But through it all, one thing that has remained constant— Nature and her gift of food for wellness. With this in mind, remember that the following cancer-fighting nutrient group may appear to be a scientific discovery of the modern age, when in reality it has been present in barley since its very beginning.

NUMBER OF CANCER-PREVENTIVE COMPOUNDS IN
BARLEY...***15***

CAFFEIC ACID	LINOLENIC ACID	STIGMASTEROL
CALMODULIN	LUTEOLIN-7-O-	TOCOPHEROL,ALPHA:
CHLOROGENIC ACID	BETA-D-GLUCOSIDE	TYRAMINE,N-METHYL:
CITRININ	OLEIC ACID	UMBELLIFERONE
COUMARIC ACID,PARA:	SITOSTEROL,BETA:	VANILLIC ACID
FERULIC ACID,TRANS:		

In addition to its potential as a cancer preventative, barley has been proven to thwart heart disease, along with constipation and other digestive maladies. Experiments on heart bypass patients conducted at the University of Wisconsin School of Medicine showed also that oil from barley can lower blood cholesterol as much as 18%. Barley, like brown rice, contains tocotrienols, which retard the manufacture of HMG reductase enzyme. This in turn inhibits the process of synthesizing LDL cholesterol in the human body. LDL cholesterol is commonly referred to as "bad cholesterol," which has been linked directly to arteriosclerosis, or hardening of the arteries, a number one cause of heart disease. Finally, barley also contains protease inhibitors known to suppress cancer-causing agents in the human intestinal tract. There is strong evidence to believe that it actually may reverse cancerous growth.

Barley can be used a number of different ways, all of which provide excellent nutritional value. When sprouted and reduced to maltose, "malted barley" provides a sweetener. And, of course, pearled barley is great in soups.

While you might expect to find many of the nutritional benefits of barley in beer, quite the opposite is true. If anything, the brewing process seems intentionally designed to remove all of the healthful nutrients from barley. Do you know where these nutrients go? Would you believe they end up in animal feed? True! They are actually extracted from the barley and used in the manufacture of food for livestock. What remains is converted into alcohol, which is toxic to the human brain, liver, and other organs. As with so many processed foods, the best part goes to the animals.

TAKE STOCK OF YOUR DIET

As you browse through the following charts, take a personal inventory. How many ways are you helping yourself prevent cancer on a daily basis by eating these foods?

NUMBER OF CANCER-PREVENTIVE COMPOUNDS IN
BASIL..*34*

ANETHOLE
APIGENIN
CAFFEIC ACID
CAROTENE,BETA:
CARVONE
CEDRENE,
CITRAL
COUMARIC ACID,PARA:
ESTRAGOLE
EUGENOL
EUGENOL METHYL ETHER

EUGENOL,ISO:METHYL
ETHER
GERANIOL
KAEMPFEROL
LIMONENE
LINONENE,(+):
LINALOOL
LINOLENIC ACID
LUTEOLIN
MYRCENE,BETA:
OLEANOLIC ACID
OLEIC ACID

ORIENTIN
PINENE, ALPHA:
QUERCETIN
QUERCITRIN,ISO:
ROSMARINIC ACID
RUTIN
SAFROLE
SITOSTEROL,BETA:
STIGMASTEROL
SUCCINIC ACID
URSOLIC ACID

NUMBER OF CANCER-PREVENTIVE COMPOUNDS IN
BLUEBERRY..*47*

AESCULETIN
BENXOIC ACID,PARA-
    HYDROXY:
CAFFEIC ACID
CAROTENE,BETA:
CATECHIN,(+):
CATECHIN,EPI:(-):
CEDRENE,ALPHA:
CHLOROGENIC ACID
CINNAMALDEHYDE
CINNAMALDEHYDE,TRANS:
CINNAMIC ACID,4-HYDROXY:
COUMARIC ACID,PARA:
CRESOL,PARA:
DECALACTONE,GAMMA:
DELPHINIDIN

ELLAGIC ACID
EUGENOL
EUGENOL,ISO:
FERULIC ACID
GALLIC ACID
GERANIOL
HYPEROSIDE
IONONE,BETA:
LIMONENE
LINALOOL
MYRICETIN
MYRISTICIN
OLEANOLIC ACID
ORIENTIN
PHENOL
PHLOROGLUCINOL
PINENE, ALPHA:

PIPERONAL
PULEGONE
QUERCETIN
QUERCETIN-3-O-BETA-
    D-GLUCOSIDE
QUERCITRIN
QUERCITRIN,ISO:
ROSMARINIC ACID
RUTIN
SCOPOLETIN
SITOSTEROL,BETA:
URSOLIC ACID
VALERIC ACID,ISO: ETHYL
    ESTER
VANILLIC ACID
VANILLIN
VITAMIN C

NUMBER OF CANCER-PREVENTIVE COMPOUNDS IN
BROWN RICE..9

COUMARIC ACID,PARA:	ORYZA SATIVA CYSTEINE	SQUALENE
GLYCINE	PROTEINASE INHIBITOR	STIGMASTEROL
METHIONINE	SERINE	TRYOSINE
	SITOSTEROL,BETA:	

NUMBER OF CANCER-PREVENTIVE COMPOUNDS IN
CELERY...27

CAFFEIC ACID	LUTEOLIN	QUERCITRIN,ISO:
CAROTENE,BETA:	LUTEOLIN-7-0-BETA-	RUTIN
CARVONE	D-GLUCOSIDE	SCOPOLETIN
CHLOROGENIC ACID	MENTHONE	SERINE
CHLOROGENIN ACID,ISO:	MYRISTICIN	SUCCINIC ACID
COUMARIC ACID,PARA:	OLEIC ACID	TOCOPHEROL,ALPHA:
EUGENOL	PINENE,ALPHA:	UMBELLIFERONE
FERULIC ACID	PSORALEN	VALERICACI
LIMONENE,(+)	QUERCETIN-3-0-BETA-D-	D,ISO:ETHYL
LINOLENIC ACID	GLUCOSICE	ESTER
		VITAMIN C

NUMBER OF CANCER-PREVENTIVE COMPOUNDS IN
CORN..37

BENZALDEHYDE PARA-	FERULIC ACID,TRANS:	PELARGONIDIN
HYDROXY	GALLATE,N-PROPYL:	PINENE,ALPHA:
CAFFEIC ACID	GALLIC ACID	QUERCETIN-3-O-BETA-
CAROTENE,BETA:	GERANIOL	D-GLUCOSIDE
CINNAMIC ACID ETHYL	GLUTATHIONE	QUERCITRIN,ISO:
ESTER	INDOLE	SITOSTEROL,BETA:
COUMARIC ACID,PARA:	INDOLE-3-ACETIC ACID	SQUALENE
COUMARIN	IONONE,BETA:	STIGMASTEROL
CYCLOARTANOL,	LIMONENE	SYRINGALDEHYDE
24-METHYLENE:	LINALOOL	TOCOTHEROL,ALPHA:
DECAN-1-AL	LINOLENIC ACID	VANILLIC ACID
EUGENOL	METHIONINE	VANILLIN
FERULIC ACID	OLEIC ACID	VITAMINC
	ORIENTIN	VITEX

NUMBER OF CANCER-PREVENTIVE COMPOUNDS IN
CUCUMBERS...**15**

ALANINE	CURCUMIN	LINOLENIC ACID
CAFFEIC ACID	CYCLOARTANOL,	OLEIC ACID
CAROTENE,BETA:	24-METHYLENE:	SITOSTEROL,B
CHLOROGENIN ACID	FERULIC ACID	SQUALENE
CUCURBITACIN B	GLYCINE	STIGMASTEROL
		TYROSINE

NUMBER OF CANCER-PREVENTIVE COMPOUNDS IN
GINGER...**22**

BENZOIC ACID,	DELPHINIDIN	MYRICETIN
PARA-HYDROXY:	FERULIC ACID	PINENE, ALPHA:
CAFFEIC ACID	GERANIOL	QUERCETIN
CAPSAICIN	GINGEROL	SERINE
CHLOROGENIC ACID	GLYCINE	SITOSTEROL, BETA:
CITRAL	KAEMPFEROL	VANILLIC ACID
COUMARIC ACID,PARA:	LIMONENE	VANILLIN
CURCUMIN	LINALOOL	

NUMBER OF CANCER-PREVENTIVE COMPOUNDS IN
GRAPES, RAISINS..**24**

BENZOIC ACID,PARA-	ELLAGIC ACID	QUERCETIN
HYDROXY:	FERULIC ACID	QUERCITRIN
CAFFEIC ACID	GALLIC ACID	QUERCITRIN,ISO:
CAROTENE,BETA	GERANIOL	RUTIN
CATECHIN, (+)	KAEMPFEROL	SINAPIC ACID
CATECHIN,EPI:(-):	LIMONENE	SITOSTEROL,B:
CATECHIN,EPI:GALLATE(-):	LINALOOL	SQUALENE
CHLOROGENIC ACID	LINOLENIC ACID	STIGMASTEROL
	OLEIC ACID	

NUMBER OF CANCER-PREVENTIVE COMPOUNDS IN
KIWI...**4**

COUMARIC ACID, PARA:	SITOSTEROL,BETA:	VITAMIN C
	SUCCINIC ACID	

NUMBER OF CANCER -PREVENTIVE COMPOUNDS IN
LICORICE..*29*

APIGENIN	GLYCYRRHETINIC ACID	NARINGENIN
BENZOIC ACID, PARA-HYDROXY	GLYCYRRHIZIN	PHENOL
	INDOLE	PHENOL, PARA-METHOXY:
FORMONONETIN	KAEMPFEROL	PHENYLPROPIONIC ACID
GALANGIN	LICOCOUMARONE	QUERCETIN
GENISTEIN	LICOFLAVANONE	QUERCITRIN,ISO:
GERANIOL	LINALOOL	SALICYLIC ACID
GLABRENE	LIQUIRITIGENIN	SITOSTEROL, BETA:
GLABRIDIN	LIQUIRITIGENIN, ISO:	STIGMASTEROL
GLABROL	MALTOL	VITEXIN

NUMBER OF CANCER-PREVENTIVE COMPOUNDS IN
MELONS..*12*

BENZOIC ACID,PARA-HYDROXY:	FERULIC ACID	OLEIC ACID
CAFFEIC ACID	FRAXIDIN,ISO:	RUTIN
CUCURBITACIN B	IONONE,BETA:	STIGMASTEROL
EUGENOL METHYL ETHER	LINOLENIC ACID	VITAMIN C

NUMBER OF CANCER-PREVENTIVE COMPOUNDS IN
MINTS..*39*

ANETHOLE	DELPHINIDIN	OLEANOLIC ACID
APIGENIN	ERIODICTYOL	PELARGONIDIN
CAFFEIC ACID	EUGENOL	PHENOL
CARVONE	FERULIC ACID	PINENE, ALPHA:
CHLOROGENIC ACID	HESPERETIN	PULEGONE
CHLOROGENIC ACID, ISO:	HYMENOXIN	QUERCITRIN
CHLOROPHYLL A	IONONE, BETA:	ROSMARINIC ACID
CHLOROPHYLL B	JASMONE	SALICYLATE, METHYL
CITRAL	LIMONENE	SALICYLIC ACID
COUMARIC ACID, PARA:	LIMONENE, (+):	SITOSTEROL, BETA:
COUMARIN	LINALOOL	STIGMASTEROL
CRESOL, PARA:	LUTEOLIN	URSOLIC ACID
DECALACTONE, GAMMA:	MENTHONE	VANILLIN

NUMBER OF CANCER-PREVENTIVE COMPOUNDS IN
MUNG BEANS..*10*

BIOCHANIN A	DAIDZIN	METHIONINE
COUMARIC ACID,PARA:	FORMONONETIN	NARINGENIN
DAIDZEIN	GENISTEIN	ROBININ
	LINOLENIC ACID	

NUMBER OF CANCER-PREVENTIVE COMPOUNDS IN
OATS...*18*

BENZOIC ACID,PARA-HYDROXY:	FERULIC ACID	STIGMASTEROL
CAFFEIC ACID	IONONE,BETA:	VANILLIC ACID
CHLOROTHYLL A	LINONENE	VANILLIN
CHLOROPHYLL B	QUERCETIN	VITAMIN A
COUMARIC ACID,PARA:	SCOPOLETIN	VITEXIN,ISO:
	SINAPIC ACID	VITEXIN-2"-0-RHAMNOSIDE
	SITOSTEROL,BETA:	

NUMBER OF CANCER-PREVENTIVE COMPOUNDS IN
OREGANO...*26*

ANETHOLE	LIMONENE	PHENYL-BETA-D-GLUCOPYRANOSIDE,4-(3-4 DIHYDROXY-BENZOYL-OXY-METHYL):
APIGENIN	LIMONENE,(+)	
AROMADENDRIN	LINALOOL	
CAFFEIC ACID	LUTEOLIN	
CARVONE	LUTEOLIN-7-0-BETA-D-GLUCOSIDE	PINENE,ALPHA:
COUMARIC ACID,PARA:	NARINGIN	QUERCETIN
DIOSMETIN	OLEANOLIC ACID	ROSMARINIC ACID
ERIODICTYOL	ORIENTIN	RUTIN
GERANIOL		URSOLIC ACID
INDOLE-3-ACETIC ACID		VITEXIN
		VITEXIN,ISO:

NUMBER OF CANCER-PREVENTIVE COMPOUNDS IN
PARSLEY..22

APIGENIN
CAFFEIC ACID
CHLOROGENIC ACID
COUMARIC ACID, PARA:
ERIODICTYOL
KAEMPFEROL
LIMONENE

LIMONENE, (+)
MYRISTICIN
NARINGENIN
NICOTINAMIDE
OLEIC ACID
PINENE,ALPHA:
PSORALEN

PSORALEN,5-METHOXY:
QUERCETIN
ROSMARINIC ACID
RUTIN
SUCCINIC ACID
TAURINE
VITAMIN A
VITAMIN C

NUMBER OF CANCER-PREVENTIVE COMPOUNDS IN
PEAS...19

ALANINE
BENZOIC ACID, PARA-
   HYDROXY:
CAFFEIC ACID
CAROTENE,BETA:
COUMARIC ACID,PARA:
FERULIC ACID

GLYCINE
LINOLENIC ACID
METHIONINE
NICOTINAMIDE
OLEIC ACID
SALICYLIC ACID
SERINE

SITOSTEROL,BETA:
SQUALENE
STIGMASTEROL
TRYPTAMINE,5-HYDROXY:
TYROSINE
VITAMIN C

NUMBER OF CANCER-PREVENTIVE COMPOUNDS IN
POTATOES...14

CAFFEIC ACID
CHLOROGENIC ACID
KAEMPFEROL
LINOLENIC ACID
LUTEOLIN

MYRICETIN
OLEIC ACID
QUERCETIN
QUERCITRIN,ISO:
QUINIC ACID,
   3-4 DICAFFEOYL:

RIBOFLAVIN
RUTIN
SCOPOLETIN
UMBELLIFERONE

NUMBER OF CANCER-PREVENTIVE COMPOUNDS IN
ROSEMARY..13

CARNOSOL
CIRSIMARITIN
GERANIOL
LIMONENE
LIMONENE, (+):

LINALOOL
NEPITRIN
PINENE,ALPHA:
ROSMANOL

ROSMARIDIPHENOL
ROSMARINIC ACID
ROSMARIQUINONE
URSOLIC

NUMBER OF CANCER-PREVENTIVE COMPOUNDS IN
SAGE...38

ALANINE
APIGENIN
CAFFEIC ACID
CARNOSOL
CAROTENE, BETA:
CEDRENE, ALPHA:
CHLOROGENIC ACID
CHRYSOERIOL
CIRSILINEOL
CIRSIMARITIN
CITRAL
COUMARIC ACID, PARA:
DIOSMETIN

FERULIC ACID
GALLIC ACID
GERANIOL
GLYCINE
HISPIDULIN
LIMONENE
LIMONENE,(+)
LINALOOL
LINOLENIC ACID
LUTEOLIN
LUTEOLIN-7-0-BETA-
    D-GLUCOSIDE
OLEANOLIC ACID

OLEIC ACID
PANTOTHENIC ACID
PECTOLINARIGENIN
PINENE, ALPHA:
ROSMANOL
ROSMARINIC ACID
SALICYLIC ACID
SERINE
SITOSTEROL, BETA:
STIGMASTEROL
TYROSINE
URSOLIC ACID
VANILLIC ACID

NUMBER OF CANCER-PREVENTIVE COMPOUNDS IN
SOYBEANS...41

ALANINE
BENZOIC ACID, PARA-
    HYDROXY:
CAFFEIC ACID
CAROTENE, BETA:
CHLOROGENIC ACID
CHLOROPHYLL
COUMARIC ACID, PARA:
CYCLOARTANOL,24-
    METHYLENE:
DAIDZEIN
DAIDZIN
EDI-PRO-A
FERULIC ACID

FORMONONETIN
GALLIC ACID
GENISTEIN
GLYCITEIN
INDOL-3-ACETIC ACID
KAEMPFEROL
LINOLENIC ACID
LIQUIRITIGENIN, ISO:
METHIONINE
OLEIC ACID
PHYTIC ACID
QUERCETIN
QUERCITRIN
QUERCITRIN, ISO:

RUTIN
SALICYLIC ACID
SERINE
SINAPIC ACID
SITOSTEROL, BETA:
SQUALENE
STIGMASTEROL
TOCOPHEROL, ALPHA:
TOCOPHEROL, BETA:
TOCOPHEROL, GAMMA:
TYROSINE
VANILLIC ACID
VITAMIN A
VITEXIN
VITEXIN- 2 "-0-RHAMNOSIDE

NUMBER OF CANCER-PREVENTIVE COMPOUNDS IN
SUNFLOWER..*30*

ACETIC ACID ETHYL ESTER
CAFFEIC ACID
CAROTENE, BETA:
CHLOROGENIC ACID
CHLOROGENIC ACID, ISO:
COUMARIC ACID, PARA:
CYCLOARTANOL,24-
   METHYLENE:
EUGENOL
FERULIC ACID
HISPIDULIN

HYMENOXIN
LIMONENE
LINOLENIC ACID
LIQUIRITIGENIN, ISO:
OLEIC ACID
PECTOLINARIGENIN
PHYTIC ACID
PINENE, ALPHA:
QUERCETIN
QUERCETIN-3-0-BETA-D-
   GLUCOSIDE

SCOPOLETIN
SITOSTEROL,BETA:
SQUALENE
STIGMASTEROL
SUCCINIC ACID
TOCOPHEROL, ALPHA:
TOCOPHEROL, BETA:
TOCOPHEROL, GAMMA:
VANILLIN
VITAMIN C

NUMBER OF CANCER-PREVENTIVE COMPOUNDS IN
TARRAGON..*72*

AESCULETIN
ALANINE
ANETHOLE
APIGENIN
AXILLARIN
BENZOIC ACID,
   PARA-HYDROXY
CAFFEIC ACID
CAMPHOR, (DL):
CAROTENE, BETA
CARVONE
CEDRENE,ALPHA:
CHLOROGENIC ACID
CHRYSOERIOL
CINNAMIC ACID
   ETHYL ESTER
CIRSILINEOL
CIRSILINEOL
CIRSIMARITIN
CITRAL
COSTUNOLIDE
COUMARIC ACID,PARA:
COUMARIN
COUMARIN, DIHYDRO:
CRESOL, ORTHO:

CRESOL,PARA:
ESTRAGOLE
EUGENOL
EUGENOL METHYL ETHER
EUGENOL,ISO:
FERULIC ACID
FRAXIDIN,ISO:
GALLIC ACID
GERANIOL
GLYCINE
HISPIDULIN
HYPEROSIDE
KAEMPFEROL
LIMONENE
LIMONENE,(+):
LINALOOL
LINOLENIC ACID
LUTEOLIN
LUTEOLIN-7-0-BETA-
   D-GLUCOSIDE
MENTHONE
MYRCENE,BETA:
NARINGENIN
OLEIC ACID
PECTOLINARIGENIN
PHENOL

PHLOROGLUCINOL
PINEN,ALPHA:
PROSTAGLANDIN F-2-ALPHA
QUERCETIN
QUERCETIN-3-METHYL
   ETHER
QUERCETIN-3-0-BETA-D-
   GLUCOSIDE
QUINIC ACID,DI-0-
   CAFFEOYL:
RHAMNETIN
RHAMNETIN,ISO:
ROSMARINIC ACID
RUTIN
SCOPOLETIN
SERINE
SINAPIC ACID
SITOSTEROLL,BETA:
SQUALENE
STIGMASTEROL
TYROSINE
UMBELLIFERONE
VANILLIC A
VITAMIN C
VITEXIN, ISO:C

NUMBER OF CANCER-PREVENTIVE COMPOUNDS IN
THYME..36

ALANINE,
ANETHOLE,
APIGENIN,
BENZOIC ACID,PARA -
   HYDROXT,
CAFFEIC ACID,
CARVONE,
CHLOROGENIC ACID
CHLOROGENIC ACID,ISO:,
CHRYSOERIOL,
CINNAMIC ACID,
CIRSILINEOL,

CIRSIMARITIN
CITRAL,
COUMARIC ACID,PARA:,
DIOSMETIN
ERIODICTYOL,
EUGENOL,
EUGENOL,ISO:
FERULIC ACID,
GALLIC ACID,
GERANIOL,
GLYCINE,
KAEMPFEROL,
LIMONENE,

LIMONENE, (+),
LINALOOL,
LUTEOLIN,
LUTEOLIN-7-0-
   BETA-D-GLUCOSIDE,
MENTHONE,
NARINGENIN,
OLEANOLIC ACID,
PINENE,ALPHA:,
ROSMARINIC ACID,
TYROSINE,
URSOLIC ACID,
VANILLIC ACID

NUMBER OF CANCER-PREVENTIVE COMPOUNDS IN
TOMATOES..18

BENZALDEHYDE,
   PARA-HYDROXY:
CAFFEIC ACID
CAROTENE,BETA:
CHLOROGENIC ACID
CHLOROPHYLL A
CHLOROPHYLL B

COUMARIC ACID,PARA:
CYCLOARTANOL,
   24-METHYLENE:
EUGENOL
KAEMPFEROL
LYCOPENE

LANOSTEROL
NARINGENIN
QUERCETIN
RUTIN
SYRINGALDEHYDE
VANILLIN
VITAMIN C

NUMBER OF CANCER-PREVENTIVE COMPOUNDS IN
WHEAT..15

CAFFEIC ACID
CAROTENE,BETA:
CHLOROGENIC ACID
CHLOROPHYLL A
CHLOROPHYLL B

CITRININ
COUMARIC ACID,PARA:
FERULIC ACID
IONONE,BETA:
LINOLENIC ACID

OLEIC ACID
PHYTIC ACID
QUERCETIN
SINAPIC ACID
TYROSINE

4

FRIENDS AND ENEMIES

Now that you've had a chance to inventory the cancer-preventive compounds present in, **or missing from**, your diet, it's time to look at a few of these compounds in greater detail. Hopefully you'll come away with an understanding of the basic and fundamental role these, and other compounds just like them, play in the functioning of a healthy body.

After that you'll be exposed to some of the enemies of good health lurking in the typical American diet. Unlike the cancer-preventive compounds, these culprits have very short and simple names, such as sugar, fat and meat. If your diet is similar to that of 98% of the people in America, undoubtedly you're already very familiar with them. What you may be less familiar with is what they're doing to your body.

MOP

Found in carrots and parsnips, methoxypsoralen (MOP) serves as one of your body's natural seamstresses by helping to repair damaged DNA genes. As reported in *Scientific American* in August, 1988, MOP fits between the base pairs of DNA molecules and repairs any damages. Researchers found they could remove damaged white blood cells from humans, treat them with MOP, and return the repaired cells to the body in fully-restored condition. This is why carrots and parsnips should be a regular part of your diet.

PROTEASE INHIBITORS

Most Americans are meat-eaters, which is one reason they consume more protein than is really good for them. What you might not have guessed is that even vegetarians may consume too much protein for good health. Vegetarian protein, however, is far less detrimental than animal proteins, an excess of which has been positively linked to the development of cancer.

The "protein problem" is complicated somewhat by the fact that the Recommended Dietary Allowance (or RDA) for protein is set at 50 grams per day, which is much higher than the 28 grams really necessary for good health. When you consider that the average American consumes 120 grams per day, you can see why this may pose a real cancer threat (especially for weight lifters, who often consume 200 grams or more per day). Because of this excess protein intake, many of us are walking cancer time bombs just waiting to be detonated.

There is a way to defuse the bomb, however. You can make sure that you have an abundance of protease inhibitors, or protein stoppers, in your diet. These are compounds which actually prevent protein from being digested in your system.

Research has shown that kidney beans, chick peas, and tofu contain large amounts of protease inhibitors which can survive the cooking and human digestive processes. This means they can block natural carcinogens from forming tumors and even arrest the growth of tumors that have already formed. As the body produces tiny tumors on a daily basis, the role of protease inhibitors is a very important one.

Whole grains, such as flax and oats, also contain protease inhibitors, for those of you who are good about getting whole grains into your diet. A word of caution: an excess of protease inhibitors can cause kwashiorkor, or protein starvation. This happens when the proportion of protease inhibitors is too great for the amount of protein entering your system. In a sense, proteins go undigested and "wash" right through your body without providing important nutrients. It is unlikely you will develop kwashiorkor if you approach all aspects of your diet with moderation, but it bears mentioning nonetheless.

One thing to always keep in mind when planning your nutritional regimen is that protein in the diet is a mixed blessing. Too much can be just as harmful as too little.

ELLAGIC ACID

Ellagic acid is an organic compound that is a powerful cancer preventative. What makes it particularly unique is that it has the ability to counteract a number of the naturally occurring and manmade chemicals which are known carcinogens, a fact verified by research done by the American Health Foundation. Since it is impossible to avoid getting a certain amount of cancer-causing "chemicals" in your food, ellagic acid can be a real lifesaver.

Where can you get it? Try eating cherries and strawberries for starters.

GERANIOL

Geraniol is a dietary gem whose potency is very high at low concentrations. Dr. Charles Ellson of the University of Wisconsin Nutrition Science Department found that only 0.1% of geraniol increased the survival rate by 50% among rats with laboratory induced malignant tumors. In addition, Ellson found that geraniol adds an extra boost when combined with other anti-cancer compounds.

For those of you hooked on oriental cooking, you'll be happy to know that geraniol is abundant in ginger. It also occurs at high concentrations in rosemary and at lower concentrations in corn and peas.

ESCULETIN

When you eat too much animal fat and polyunsaturated fat, as most of us do on a daily basis, excess arachidonic acid is formed in the body. Now, if that was all that happened, you wouldn't be in such bad shape. Unfortunately, excess arachidonic acid produces certain bad types of prostaglandins that cause platelets in the blood to congeal, leading to a clogging of the arteries and eventually to strokes. It increases dramatically the production of certain cellular hormones. This accelerates the rate of normal cell reproduction, which leads to tumors. Tumors are simply areas where cells are reproducing out of control. If you don't hear an undercurrent of cancer here, then you are missing the point.

The good news is, esculetin helps prevent this from happening. Essentially, it helps stop arachidonic acid from creating the deleterious types of prostaglandins that wreak havoc on the body's blood and cellular systems. A nice secondary benefit is that esculetin promotes thinness. So, if you want to lose the weight that leads to strokes, degenerative heart disease and cancer, you may want to increase your consumption of fruits and vegetables, the majority of which contain esculetin. And remember, eating a lot does not lead to excess weight. Only eating a lot of the wrong thing does.

FIBER

The relationship between fiber and cancer prevention has been the object of research for some time. Over ten years ago, health science researchers established conclusively that fiber plays a strong role in the prevention of colon cancer. Now we also know that fiber can prevent colon cancer among people whose diets are high in fat. As fat is among the greatest contributors to this type of degenerative disease, the power of fiber is one to be taken very seriously.

As the role of dietary fiber receives more and more media attention, people are responding with increased interest. In the long term, this should result in a significant decrease in the number of colon cancer cases in the U.S., which makes fiber one of the few bright spots in the war on cancer.

Of course, there are a variety of fibers, from whole grain fibers to vegetable fibers. Most have the ability to "bind up" naturally occurring and manmade carcinogens and to prevent them from being absorbed into the human digestive system. They can also "dilute" these cancer-causing agents by means of their sheer bulk.

Not all fibers work alike, however. Even the size of the fiber makes a difference. Long fibers, like those found in fresh fruits, vegetables and coarse ground whole grains are much more beneficial than the fiber found in most fiber supplements and breakfast cereals. When fibers are finely ground, they lose their tendency to swell as they absorb water. The more finely ground the fiber, the more likely it will compact in the intestine and cause more problems than it can prevent. However, coarse fiber can irritate the bowel when consumed alone. Therefore, coarse fiber foods should be eaten with foods that contain soluble fiber or mucillage, such as those found in apples, bananas, flax, etc. Combining coarse fiber and mucillage is an unbeatable combination.

PUBLIC ENEMY # 1

To this point we have been reviewing a few of the friendly compounds that play a strong role in disease prevention. Now, let's look at some of your body's dietary enemies.

Public Enemy #1 is **SUGAR** — that's right, sweet little ol' sugar. Soft drinks, candy, alcohol, sugar-coated cereal, cake, cookies, brownies, syrup, canned fruit, chewing gum, jam, jelly, ice cream . . . . It's everywhere. And for a good reason. America is addicted to it. It's the mainstay of our junk food diet.

Oh, if your body could only talk! Here is a short look at what it must go through for you to have your "sugar fix:"

First, your blood registers an excess of glucose, the simplest form of sugar, which means it gets right into the system. Your blood sugar takes a quick jump, and you feel an instant rush of energy. Then a long, soft gland called the pancreas, located just behind the stomach, secretes pancreatic juice into the duodenum, where, in the islands of Langerhans, insulin is produced. This insulin takes the glucose and quickly moves it into the body's storage system in the form of saturated fat.

Because glucose is not a complex sugar and needs very little digestion, the body deals with it very quickly. No sooner do you feel a sugar high than you begin to feel a sugar low. Your blood sugar plummets, and you become listless and tired. Of course, the only remedy is to grab for more sugar, and this is the precise point where the "roller coaster addiction" to sugar begins.

69

But that's not all. The worst is yet to come. Due to the surge of insulin needed to quickly process the sugar, excess insulin continues to float around in your system. As long as that occurs, your body can't burn fat. In other words, you can't burn any excess sugar that has been placed in storage as saturated fat. This stored fat produces more cholesterol, and eventually cholesterol leads to degenerative heart disease.

Not such a simple sugar after all! By the way, your body can safely handle only sugar found naturally in fresh fruit and other high fibered foods, which slows the absorption. It's healthier to cut refined and artificial sugars out of your diet.

THERE'S BAD FAT!

A three member gang of fats is high on the list of dietary public enemies. Heading the gang is **saturated fat**.

In its most pure state, saturated fat resembles plastic. It is pliable, nonsoluble, and extremely difficult to digest. Eating a spoonful of it is the closest thing to swallowing a plastic bag, which is why it does nothing in the body but slump down in particularly vulnerable areas and refuse to move — say, around the middle or on the hips.

Another member is **hydrogenated fat**, made from polyunsaturated fats. Because it is not natural, but manmade, hydrogenated fat comes in eccentric shapes which have adverse effects on human cells. Defects in cell walls caused by this type of hydrogenated fat comes in eccentric shapes which have adverse effects on human cells. Defects in cell walls caused by this type of fat can actually create cellular leakage, as well as stimulate the production of adverse cellular hormones. It also forms cellulite on your hips.

Last but not least is **polyunsaturated fat**. Generally the problem associated with this fat is not due to the fat itself but rather to how much of it is consumed. Excesses of one polyunsaturate in particular, linoleic acid (an Omega-6 compound) has been linked to cancer. The effect of linoleic acid on the metabolism relates to the production of arachidonic acid. As you will remember from our discussion of esculetin earlier in this chapter, one of the things arachidonic acid does is accelerate normal cell reproduction, which leads to the formation of cancerous tumors. This is where excessive polyunsaturated fat intake and cancer are directly connected.

In effect, it can't be said that polyunsaturated fat starts cancer. It simply contributes to the acceleration of cancerous growth. Once again, the term "excess" is important. To maintain normal human growth, a 1% level of polyunsaturated fat is needed in the diet. At a mere 4% level, however, this fat has been proven repeatedly in cancer research to cause increased growth rate of tumors in humans and animals.

The balancing act between beneficial and detrimental intakes is a very fine one indeed. That is why it is so important for you to be particularly aware of the polyunsaturated fats you eat. Or, for that matter, all fats!

AND THERE'S GOOD FAT!

Now that you've learned about **bad fats,** let's take a look at **good fats**. And there are some! Many of us have become so accustomed to thinking that all fat is bad for us, we forget that the body's power plant actually runs on fat. It's one of our most concentrated sources of energy. That is why it is so important to understand which fats contribute to good health and which ones pose health threats.

There are only two safe, or "good," fats: mono-unsaturated fats and Omega-3 fats. Mono-unsaturated fats are obtained primarily from olive oil and canola oil. Unlike simple and complex sugars (glucose, fructose, and lactose), mono-unsaturated fats don't need to be converted into saturated fats before the body can begin using them. They supply *quick* and *long-lasting* sources of energy in their original forms.

What is interesting is that Middle Eastern cultures which depend on mono-unsaturated fats almost exclusively for their cooking needs show very low incidences of heart disease. America, on the other hand, depends much more heavily on saturated and polyunsaturated fats and continually rates exceedingly high in the area of degenerative illness.

The other "good" fat is linolenic acid, or Omega-3. Aside from being non-toxic to the body, linolenic acid is beneficial for several reasons. First, it employs the same enzymatic pathway that converts linoleic acid, the other essential fatty acid, into arachidonic acid, upon which the body depends for everything

72

from proper nerve response to cellular reproduction. This means linolenic acid prevents the excesses of linoleic acid, and subsequently arachidonic acid, which are directly connected to heart disease and cancer.

As a second benefit, linolenic acid burns easily and efficiently. It supplies the body with a quick form of energy, almost as quick as simple sugars. The difference is that linolenic acid causes no overproduction of insulin which contributes to the "roller coaster sugar rides" already discussed.

Excellent sources of linolenic acid are walnuts (3%), dark leafy vegetables (0.5%), canola oil (6%), and fortified, stabilized flax (17%).

BIG MEAT EATERS!

Americans are "big meat eaters." Roasts, steaks, chops, patties, cold cuts, loafs! You name it. If it moos, oinks, or baahs, we'll find a way to eat it. In fact, those of us who generally prefer "down home cookin' " over the more adventuresome international cuisines (Chinese, Japanese, Thai, Mexican, Italian, etc.) commonly refer to ourselves with pride as "your basic meat and potatoes person."

Well, living the good life on meat and potatoes may not be all it's cracked up to be.

One of the many health problems faced by this country today is posed by excessively high animal protein diets. There are several reasons for this. First, excess proteins in the body cause an excess of amino acids, a condition that can be toxic to the body. Moreover, proteins place an enormous strain on the digestive process because they are so difficult to metabolize.   Useful energy from other nutritional sources is actually siphoned off to prepare protein for use in the system.

And then we wonder why we feel so sluggish and listless throughout the day. Lethargy is a natural by-product of digesting excess protein.

Also, because excess protein from meat and dairy products must be processed through the kidneys before being dumped into the urine, the kidneys can suffer from undue stress. Prolonged high consumption of animal protein can, in fact, result in permanent kidney damage.

The toxicity of protein is related to its three constituent basic amino acids — lysine, phenylalanine, and tyrosine. One of these amino acids in particular, phenylalanine, has received considerable attention as a health threat. In addition to being linked to mental retardation, excess phenylalanine is known to add to a general deterioration of the human immune system. Unfortunately most of us are unaware that one of the two primary ingredients of a widely used artificial sweetener is phenylalanine. True!

Because meat and dairy products, our normal sources of protein, are high in saturated fat, all of the problems associated with a high-fat intake are also present with protein. One very real concern is that fat from these protein sources ties up calcium and makes it unusable in the body.

The process is virtually identical to the formation of "bathtub rings." Animal fats used to make soap combine with calcium in the tub water to form a hard, calcified ring around the inside of the tub. As you probably know, this ring is impervious to

74

normal scrubbing and must be removed with elbow grease and a strong cleanser.

What you won't be happy to learn is that the same process occurs inside your stomach and even on cell walls throughout your entire body. In essence, high fat consumption over the long term results in a body-wide calcification which turns you brittle. Have you ever heard of osteoporosis and premature aging? The brittleness resulting from a high fat diet is just another way of putting it.

At this point, you may be getting the impression it's dangerous to eat any meat at all. You're not alone. Vegetarianism has in fact been a major point of debate among food scientists and dietitians for some time. To be perfectly candid, good arguments can be presented for both sides, though a very interesting study by T. Collins Campell may help you formulate a stronger opinion on the subject.

Campbell, along with colleagues at Cornell University and experts from England and China, investigated a unique culture where vegetarianism is the norm — rural China. Because the rural Chinese have subsisted for hundreds, perhaps thousands of years, on a vegetarian diet of rice, vegetables, seeds, nuts, and sprouts, they were an ideal subject for study.

Campbell found that while the Chinese diet does not meet U. S. recommended allowances for calcium and iron, the Chinese showed few signs of iron-deficiency anemia or osteoporosis, as one would normally expect. Apparently the Chinese get most of their calcium and iron from whole foods, whereas primary sources for these minerals in the American diet are meat and protein-rich dairy products. What we are gradually coming to understand is that protein from meat and dairy products actually causes an excretion of calcium obtained from more beneficial food sources.

Also contrary to what Campbell expected to find, the high fiber diet of the Chinese does not interfere with vitamin and mineral absorption. Though the Chinese consume as much as 77 grams of fiber per day, 10 times more than the average American, there was no evidence even of vitamin B-12 deficiency. This was a unique discovery given the fact that B-12 intake among the Chinese is very low. Apparently microbes in the intestinal tract of vegetarians make necessary compensations by manufacturing this particular vitamin naturally.

A significant outcome of vegetarianism among the rural Chinese is a general retarding of physical and sexual maturation. Chinese children grow considerably more slowly and reach sexual maturity much later than American children. The average age for puberty in China is seventeen, as opposed to twelve in the U. S.

Campbell once again attributed these basic variances to differences in animal protein intake. As other experiments have shown, higher protein levels lead to faster growth rates, with animal protein accounting for faster growth than any other protein. In addition to containing more growth-stimulating amino acids, animal protein contains steroids as natural contaminants. As you may know, steroids are made up of a number of hormones which accelerate growth rates in all mammals.

The slow growth rate of the Chinese on animal protein-free diets has two predictable results. First, the national averages for heart disease and osteoporosis in China are much lower that those in the U. S. And second, breast cancer occurs much less frequently among Chinese women than among American women.

A further note of interest on the subject of the "protein-calcium connection" and its relation to osteoporosis was provided by Dr. D. M. Hegested from Harvard Medical School.   In the *Journal of Nutrition* (Vol 116, 1986, pp. 2316-19), Dr. Hegested presented a comparison of the incidence of hip fractures and calcium consumed in various countries.   The results were the opposite of what you might expect.

Available calcium in the food supply compared with the incidence of hip fractures in females of several nations

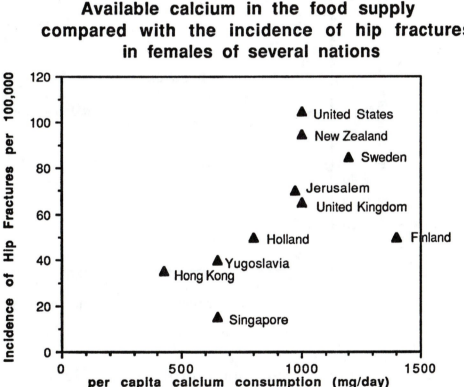

Next Dr. Hegested plotted hip fractures compared to protein consumed. Again, the results were different than expected. Higher consumption of protein above the minimal level appeared related to a greater frequency of hip fractures.

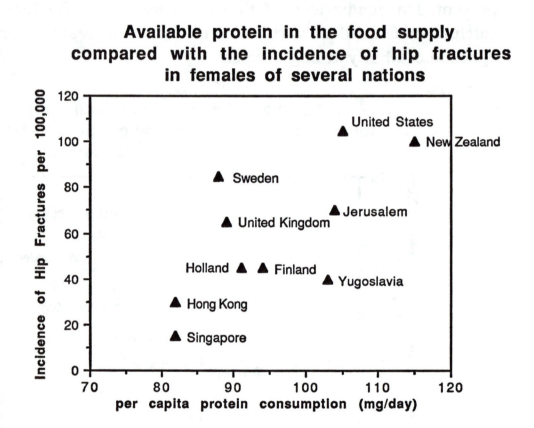

Available protein in the food supply compared with the incidence of hip fractures in females of several nations

These comparisons don't prove that calcium and protein cause hip fractures, but they do show an *association* between protein excesses and hip fractures. It looks as though we could learn a lot from how people of Singapore and Hong Kong eat.

HOW IT ALL ADDS UP

Hopefully it's apparent at this point that the typical American diet is suffering from an excess of sugar, protein and fat and a lack of fruits, vegetables, and whole grains. Not that we should be eating nuts and berries, and walking barefoot through the woods, but we might pause to consider the consequences of having fallen farther than ever from the perfect, natural diet provided us in the Garden of Eden or in the habitat of primitive man or woman.

Here are some disturbing facts. Our natural immune system is being steadily eroded by poor nutritional habits. We are faced with a number of truly frightening epidemics, including AIDS. The *New York Times* reported on August 24, 1990, that cancer rates for people over 55 are greatly increasing. Every region of the country is showing a climb in degenerative disease rates. In light of this, it's hard not to become discouraged.

Did you know that America ranks only 17th in the world for life expectancy behind such countries as Japan, Spain, Greece, and Italy? Yet we consume more energy than any other country in the world, have one of the highest per capita incomes, and spend more on health research and health care than any other nation. Doesn't it seem logical we should be somewhere at the top?

Most of us, I think, are under the impression that Americans are living longer, healthier lives than ever. The truth is, over the last century we have made only minor gains in life expectancy for adults. Since 1910, the life expectancy of a 40 year old male in this country has increased only 5 years.

Newborns live longer than they did in 1910 because of better infant care, but those of us who are middle age are not enjoying longer life.

This illusion of increased longevity is created in part by the complete faith we have come to place in modern medical technology. Exciting advancements in disease treatment and therapy make it seem as though our chances of living longer are greatly increased.

In reality, the progress we have made in longevity is miniscule compared to increased expenditures in health research. We are spending more and more for smaller and smaller gains. The best analogy that comes to mind is of a man swimming upstream against an ever-increasing current. Like the man, modern medicine is swimming harder and harder but doing little more than treading water.

Over the past 20 years, a ray of encouragement has come, though, in the area of heart disease. And not because of artificial heart progress, better transplant and bypass surgical procedures, or discoveries in blood pressure medication. Whatever major skirmishes have been won in the war on heart disease are the result of our own efforts.

How did we accomplish this?

Simple! We took direct action when the health hazards posed by a high sodium diet were revealed. We became "salt conscious." As a result, cookbooks were rewritten to reduce or eliminate salt as an ingredient, people began reading nutrition information on labels, and salt-crusaders preached the word of salt-free diets.

And it worked. In the span of a short twenty-year period, we engaged in a grass-roots dietary campaign against excessive use of salt. This resulted in dramatic decreases in arteriosclerosis and sodium-related degenerative heart disease.

Now, imagine for a moment what would happen if we waged a similar campaign to reduce the amount of saturated, hydrogenated, and polyunsaturated fats in our youngsters' diets, as well as our own diets. Essentially, we'd be eliminating still more of the major contributors to degenerative diseases. That, in itself, would be a tremendous additional step forward. It would also create a ripple effect leading to other health improvements. As we've pointed out, reductions in these fats significantly reduce the odds of developing various types of cancer.

Let's take this one step further. Imagine the effect of replacing these health threats in our diet with health benefits. We know that whole grains, vegetables, fruits and whole foods in general can prevent cancer, along with a number of other degenerative diseases. Isn't it logical, then, that the result of such dietary modification would be a staggeringly positive contribution to our national health?

The point is, good health and life expectancy gains are not products of high-tech medicine and its ability to preserve and prolong life. They are products of life style. Life style is a matter of choice, not a matter of genetic inheritance. Our "salt experiment" is proof of that.

If anything, the eating habits we learn from our parents, more than our genetic inheritance or our family medical history, determine longevity. Simply because a family has a record of cancer is no proof of susceptibility to this type of ailment.

However, when family members continue with the same high-salt, high-fat, low-whole-foods life style, they increase their chances of contracting cancer. That is why learning good nutrition habits at an early age is so important.

Somehow Americans aren't getting the message.

According the the National Cancer Institute, only 9% of the total population of the United States consumes four servings of fresh fruit and/or vegetables per day. Consequently, only 9% of Americans are actively fortifying their immune systems against cancer. The other 91% are leaving themselves wide open for health risk.

The National Cancer Institute has already declared that "cancer may not be a natural consequence of aging." Writing for the *Journal of the NCI*, Dr. Gio Gori and Dr. Ernest Wynder concluded that cancer prevention could be as simple as adopting the nutritional habits of the Japanese and other Far East cultures.

Here are the statistics upon which they based this claim:

American males vs. _Japanese males_ have:

- **2.8 times more lung cancer**

  (even though Japanese smoke more than Americans)
- **10.3 times more prostate cancer**
- **6.5 times more colon cancer**
- **4.2 times more bladder cancer**
- **3.4 times more rectum cancer**
- **3.6 times more mouth cancer**

American females vs. _Japanese females_ have:

- **5.6 times more breast cancer**
- **6.6 times more colon cancer**
- **11.7 times more uterine cancer**

- **5.9 times more ovarian cancer**
- **3.6 times more bladder cancer**
- **5.0 times more kidney cancer**

The Japanese keep cancer naturally in check through nutrition, something Americans did at one time but are not doing today. In a report issued in 1977, but generally ignored to date, the National Cancer Institute summed up its stance on cancer this way: "Present knowledge provides clues implicating dietary factors such as fat and meat intake and excess caloric intake." The report also indicated that a lack of whole grains and vegetables accentuated the cancer problem.

If you're beginning to sense something of a double-edged sword associated with nutritional deficiency, then you're approaching an understanding of what lies at the heart of our nation's crisis with degenerative diseases. Strictly in terms of our daily food supply, we are dumping into our bodies a regimen of "nutritional contaminants." These contaminants (including certain forms of fat and sugars) are proven to cause cancer. That in itself is dangerous.

But the sword's second edge is even sharper. Our bodies' natural immunities to cancer are being steadily depleted as a result of poor nutrition. In short, what we aren't eating is just as big a problem as what we are. In the end, the combined effect of these dietary sins astronomically increases our chances of getting cancer and other degenerative diseases. That, in a nutshell, is "how it all adds up."

5

IS CANCER A DISEASE?

Small pox. Pneumonia. Hepatitis. Syphilis. Strep throat. The "common cold." All of these maladies and numberless others that affect the human body are of viral or bacterial origin. They are neither the result of genetic mutation nor of an internally-generated physical change. Something outside the body has attacked its system and the result is a disease of a serious nature or, perhaps, a more innocent illness.

This is indeed not the case with cancer. Cancer is not the result of a bacterial or viral attack upon the body. You cannot "catch" cancer from another person. Unlike bacterial infections, cancer does not respond to antibiotics. Unlike viral infections, cancer does not respond to symptomatic treatment. If you are beginning to think that cancer sounds like something other than a disease, you're right on the money.

If not a disease, then what? Cancer is a molecular deviation of some organ, bone, blood or other cell in the body. Initially, although pinpointing the proof is difficult, one cell becomes molecularly changed. With staggering speed, additional cells become affected or, as we say, the cancer "spreads." Cancer is not unlike the wildest science fiction movie we're likely to ever see. An alien force has seized control of a part of us and there's not a whole lot we can do about it after the fact. Sure, surgical biopsies search for evidence of cancerous cells, as you know. The importance of screening through Pap tests, stool sampling, mammography, and periodic blood tests for those at high risk cannot be stressed enough. But once you've got it, you're in for a difficult time regardless of the treatments available.

To create perhaps a more easily understood frame of reference, let's assume that the body is an automobile. Let's make it a Mercedes. Usually, it simply "purrs" along, among the most reliable of cars, requiring minimum maintenance and, certainly, adequate fuel to keep it operating at peak efficiency.

But this Mercedes becomes the victim of a vandal. A cup of sand is dumped into the gas tank. Chances are you'll be quickly aware that something isn't right but, since you can't put your finger on the problem, you keep on driving. Now, I'm not a trained mechanic, but I've managed to get my hands under a hood often enough to know that you're going to have that Mercedes in for major surgery very soon. You can bet the fuel injectors are ruined, the pistons are ruined, the gas and oil filters must be replaced, and the valves and other vital parts will need attention. In all probability, the car can be rehabilitated, but it may never be quite the same as it was before. And, surely, your confidence will be eroded.

The vandal could have taken a different tack. Maybe a scant teaspoon of sugar was added to the gas tank every few days. The resulting problems are less obvious. In fact, you may be completely unaware that anything is wrong. But, little by little, week by week, that alien sugar is destroying the Mercedes until, one day, it stops dead in the road. After checking, the mechanic reports the car can't be fixed. Maybe he can do this-or-that to get it running again, but there's no guarantee, and he advises the car be junked.

That's very similar to the way cancer affects our body. In a true sense though, it is inaccurate to say that cancer can be cured, that the body can be fixed. Spare parts are not easy to come by for flesh-and-blood carburetors. And our "filters," our kidneys are far more complex than the Mercedes variety. Yes, today in some cases, cancer can be eliminated with apparent lasting success. But, as any victim can tell you, there remains the threat of a recurrence, and these victims are closely monitored throughout their lives.

Without the interference of the vandal but with proper care, maintenance, and gasoline of the right octane, that car we talked about is as indestructible as cars go. And if we treat our bodies with the same care we would a Mercedes, we can take advantage of many preventive-maintenance techniques for better health in general and to reduce the risk of cancer in particular.

To carry our automotive analogy one step further, consider that whatever we ingest — be it food, liquid, or air — enters the body unfiltered. The car's fuel, for example, goes through a filter at the pump and within the car before entering the carburetor. But our lungs, kidneys, liver, and intestines work to eliminate impurities after they've adulterated our system. In my opinion, we've been so brainwashed by television that most of us are addicted to foods, and the wrong foods at that; how many commercials can you recall that carry the message, "Just can't stop eating those—," or similar approaches? Without fundamental life style changes, we're on the road to "junking" our bodies with junk foods and other processed foods that are bad for us. There's little comfort in a doctor's diagnosis that we "suffer" from obesity, hypertension, diabetes, an "eating disorder" or other condition. Frankly, what we suffer from most is improper nutritional training or, if we know better, then let's eliminate the euphemism and call it stupidity.

While our nutritional plan is dependent upon a sensible selection of whole foods and their anti-carcinogenic values, we can't ignore another basic factor. Simply, we can't consume more calories in a day than we can use. An over-filled gas tank is a mess and risks fire. An over-filled body risks life itself. All excess calories with the exception of those consumed in the form of alcohol are converted to saturated fat and stored. Alcohol calories, incidentally, cannot be converted and are released only as energy, leading to an increase in the amount of food converted to saturated fats. Reversing the process is not easy because stored saturated fat is a compound not unlike plastic. Moreover, saturated fat tends to shut down the immune system, leaving us defenseless against a viral or bacterial attack.

Dr. William Lynne at the University of Texas Medical Branch in Galveston has documented the impact saturated fat has on "T" cells, the workhorses of the immune system. Dr. Lynne's research proves they simply stop functioning. Personnel managers might be amazed if they kept informal track of the absences due to illness experienced by their seriously overweight employees compared to the average for the company. Just as illuminating is a North Carolina State University study that reported saturated fat affects cell walls, and prevents the body from producing enough heat. In that study, mice on just a 30% saturated fat diet were literally in danger of freezing to death at normal laboratory temperatures. The rats could not burn the saturated fat fast enough to keep warm. Have you ever noticed how your slim friends appear comfortable while others are scurrying for sweaters or other cover-ups?

Let's get smart. Let's start doing what is best for our bodies at breakfast, lunch, and dinner. In fact, throughout the day. You will be amazed by the benefits. Somebody get the message to Dr. Ruth: good nutrition equates with a good sex life! Don't laugh. How good was your sex life when you were drunk or suffering a 7.7 hangover on the Richter scale? Good sex and good health go together and they disappear together.

In this book, we're talking a lot about cancer because the focus of new research information available today is primarily in that area. But what we are saying is profoundly significant to any "degenerative condition." Whether it's AIDS, Alzheimer, arthritis, diabetes, osteoporosis, kidney failure, or a respiratory difficulty, the best way to restore normal health is to control the molecules your body receives.

It's the time-honored "garbage in, garbage out" maxim of our computer-literate set. Symptomatic treatment of the condition with a drug may control the disease, but it won't change the underlying problem. Obviously, it is essential that you be under a qualified physician's care for treatment of your disease. This we recommend without qualification. But only you can take primary charge of your life; only you can "take out the garbage;" and only you can put "the right stuff," the right molecules, into your body. Working with your doctor, you can become the healthy and vibrant person you yearn to be. To be sure you're on the right track, though, throw your doctor a curve. You ask the questions. What does your doctor know about lignans? What does he or she know about linolenic acid and the differences between these compounds? If you get a blank stare or hems-and-haws as answers, you might find more sound nutritional advice elsewhere.

Most of us are probably aware that a healthy body carries out a daily task of fighting off all kinds of would-be intruders. That's one of the reasons why two people in a household may develop severe flu symptoms while a third remains unscathed. You can almost bet that the two ill persons never exercise; they dine on pizza and french fries; perhaps at least one of them smokes; and maybe they're even prone to hit the sauce a bit on the heavy side. The other healthy person takes brisk walks daily or jogs, is a steamed-broccoli freak, chomps on raw carrots, and has "flax for snacks."

Even if the above information is obvious to you, chances are you have never been told that *our bodies must line up defenses and fight off about a thousand cancer cells a day!* The body is not necessarily manufacturing these cancer cells, but they are a by-product of our acquired eating habits and partly caused by the environmental pollutants we encounter daily. That's why it is so vitally important that we pump in the right nutrients with their anti-carcinogenic compounds. These value-added "Preventive Compounds," arriving at the right time and in the right amounts, assist our bodies in killing the cancer cells before they start consuming our energy, destroying our protein, and plotting against us by building tumors, etc.

When we take advantage of this new information, we keep our batteries fully-charged. There is no energy wasted in fighting degenerative conditions. Athletes can perform at their peaks, or beyond expectations — and I assure you we've observed this through field work with hundreds of athletes. We all work better, think better, undoubtedly enjoy life more, and experience an absence of stress when we follow a nutritional life plan keyed to the principles espoused here.

6

GOOD NEWS FROM THE WAR ON CANCER

You and I can probably recall a dozen or more promising announcements in the last few years concerning cures or the isolation of chromosomes at the root of certain illnesses, birth defects, etc. Some of these promises have been cruel or premature at best. I particularly recall a Jerry Lewis telethon that truly seemed to include an announcement that a cure for muscular dystrophy had been found, that the years of research had paid off. Actually, we can understand their enthusiasm, but the more accurate condition was that progress was indeed finally being made.

So, our good news about cancer includes no suggestion that a cure has been found. The good news is that we *now* have ways of preventing cancer. With the generous help and continuing research of the National Cancer Institute, we have identified the five most potent cancer-preventing foods. As listed earlier, they are: flax, garlic, citrus, parsley, and licorice root. The hope is so significant that the NCI plans to spend $20 million over the next few years to study the effects of these foods in combinations and to collect other data. For example, one of the five may be more effective in preventing a particular form of cancer than another. And there's speculation that we may discover an ability to reverse the progress of some cancers with the addition of one or more of these foods to our diets.

My colleague, Dr. Herbert Pierson of the Dietary Prevention Branch of the NCI, and I are impressed with evidence that suggests flax is the one product that is the most effective cancer fighter of all. Flax has been shown to contain high levels of at least three compounds that have very high anti-cancer properties.

One of these compounds is **lignans** and its concentration in flax is a whopping 800 parts per million. That's 100 times higher than any other grain! This means that even a small amount of flax can go a long way in preventing breast cancer and cancer of the colon.

Dr. Lillian Thompson at the University of Toronto has reported a study in which rats were fed a cancer-causing chemical for one week. Then, they were fed a diet that contained just 5% flax for four weeks. Their tissues were then analyzed for pre-cancer cells, and urine tests were conducted to determine lignan concentration. Dr. Thompson found the lignan concentration had increased ten fold; pre-cancer cells had decreased by 40% to 60% (when compared to the control group that received no flax). Moreover, the growth rate of cancerous cells in the breasts and colons of the rats was decreased by 50%. To put this in perspective, we can deduce that a large number of the cancer cells were killed by the lignan concentration, in addition to the reduced growth rate of the surviving cells. This short term study should soon be followed by results from a longer study to find out if the lignans in flax can continue to kill cancer cells and, eventually, eliminate all of the cancer cells. With success, some day we may find ourselves monitoring our lignan level with a kit similar to those used by diabetics to test their sugar level. The results could provide an instantaneous answer to our personal concerns about developing cancer.

Lignans are reported to neutralize estrogen in the system which is known to stimulate tumor growth. Lignans also inhibit certain complicated chemical compounds, present in the body and called "free radicals," from acting on cells and starting them on the long road to becoming a tumor.

The second important compound flax contributes to our diet of whole foods is fiber. You've already read a lot about oat bran, but the fact is flax contains twice as much fiber as that highly-touted grain. Fiber acts as an anti-cancer compound by helping to remove those toxins produced in the gastro-intestinal tract before they can cause molecular changes in healthy cells and cause cancerous growths to begin forming.

Flax also contains alpha-linolenic acid (Alena), an essential fatty acid with Omega-3 activity. Certain fatty acids play healthy roles in digestion and growth, while others are quite harmful. ALENA, or alpha linolenic compound, inhibits the metabolism of the fatty acid, linoleic, which has been linked with helping cancer cells multiply more rapidly. Just a small amount of Alena can prevent a large amount of linoleic from causing trouble. And the Omega-3 activity of our new friend, Alena, has also been shown to help prevent heart trouble, arthritis, and other degenerative diseases.

If you're like so many of us who once thought flax was solely the source of linen, writing paper, and that wonderful oil that protected our baseball bats, think again. This all-purpose grain in your diet can mean a cancer-free life when coupled with other sensible whole food initiatives on your part.

Flax should be the center of any cancer prevention diet, but it shouldn't be left to stand alone. The diet should also be richly supplemented with garlic. Garlic has been used for thousands of years to cure and prevent hundreds of diseases. I find its the first thing I grab when any disease attacks. It's marvelous at knocking out flu symptoms, upset stomach, and food poisoning. I have seen miraculous overnight cures with garlic. In cultures that don't have doctors to patronize, it's the number one medicine. It seems to put the immune system into high gear. Thousands of scientific studies around the globe have attested to the power of garlic. It is unfortunate for our country that no one champions garlic here at home. There are thousands of reasons why garlic is a high priority compound to the "Designer Food Program" at the National Cancer Institute.

Citrus products are another high priority compound at the National Cancer Institute. Limonene from the oil in the rind of citrus was shown to reverse breast tumors in rats five years ago. Citrus oil is an FDA approved food. It's a shame that not very much has been done with citrus oil since them. I'm so glad that the NCI is picking up the research from where the University of Wisconsin dropped it five years ago.

Parsley is another important cancer-preventive food. Carrots and parsnips are also members of the group. Parsley has many compounds similar to broccoli at high concentrations that

94

have been shown to help prevent cancer. Parsley is often used as a condiment. It's a shame that the healthiest part of a meal is used for a decoration on the plate and sometimes the unhealthiest part is consumed as foods.

Listed here last among the "Big Five" is licorice root. Frankly, its compounds are highly effective in killing cancer cells. The problem is extracting them in a cost-effective manner so they can be added to our diets. Yes, it's the same food that flavors candy, certain liquors, etc., but those uses won't deliver enough of the compounds we need and certainly not within a whole foods regimen.

Can other things be done to add to the good news in the war on cancer? Yes, but simple as they are, implementing them won't be easy. Let's take the case of the hospitalized cancer patient. Radiation and chemotherapy are tightrope techniques of treatment. Too little and no positive results; too much and normal cells can be killed or become cancerous. That's why it is vital to know the track record of your doctor and treatment team with the particular type of cancer involved. Even with the utmost care, chances are the treatment will weaken the body's self-defense system, the immune system. A healthy immune system is needed to ward off bacterial and viral infections that lurk around even the best of hospitals.

The answer is to bring the whole food, cancer-preventive message of this book and the NCI "Designer Foods" into the dietary regimen for the cancer patient. Dietitians should create menus that provide patients with all the B vitamins, zinc, beta carotene, vitamin E, linolenic acid, lignans, limonene, quercetin, MOP's, Geraniol, and anti-oxidants their bodies can possibly absorb. Substances harmful to the immune system, such as saturated fats, sugars, milk proteins, and artificial-anythings, are an insult to the patient and to the practice of medicine. We're not implying that the right nutrients will cure the cancer patient, but they will make the success rate of all treatments climb, perhaps soar. And there's a very good chance those cancer-preventive compounds will prevent tumors from recurring and new ones from forming. That's worth a buck or two for the extra effort in the hospital kitchen, rather than depending upon the food service departments of Green Giant, Del Monte, or a chemical company.

While we're at it, let's appeal to the family and friends to forego the stop at Pizza Hut, or Burger King, or the candy counter to smuggle in goodies Aunt Betty is dying to eat. Aunt Betty is dying from cancer, people, and we can be allies in the fight for her recovery or cruel contributors toward her loss in the toughest war her body's likely to have ever fought.

Enough said for cancer.

7

WHO, WHAT, WHERE, WHEN

In 1971, the U.S. Department of Agriculture, in conjunction with universities in South Carolina and Nebraska, published "Evaluation of Research in the United States on Human Nutrition." Judging from the recognition this study received at the time of its release, its subject might as well have been something as obscure as the tensile strength of wet concrete in tropical climates. Neither the American Medical Association nor any public health agency gave proper attention to the findings of the study. No morning or afternoon talk show coverage. No press conferences by the Surgeon General. Nothing.

Yet "Evaluation of Research in the United States on Human Nutrition" made enough meaningful noise that it should have been heard from Miami to Pt. Barrow, Alaska. In essence, it said that nutrition is the key to a healthy population and a healthy country. Its implication was that an overwhelming majority of Americans need to replace poor eating habits with a new nutritional regimen based upon modern nutritional research.

In the course of its study, the USDA specifically itemized the impact of nutrition on heart disease, infectious diseases, mental health, infant mortality, aging, arthritis, dental health, diabetes, osteoporosis, obesity, anemia, alcoholism, allergies, digestive diseases, kidney disease, and muscle disorder. Unfortunately, all of this great information fell on deaf ears.

In 1971, 7% of this country's Gross National Product went for health care. Over the last twenty years this figure has nearly doubled. In 1990, our country will spend an astonishing 12% of its national pay check on medical care. Despite this enormous increase in medical care expenditures, our health problems remain essentially the same. The disease factor of the 90's is nearly identical to what it was in the 70's. There is only one difference. Today it costs us 3 to 5 times more for the same medical care we were getting 20 years ago.

The USDA task force could see this coming. That is why they presented such a radical departure from our normal way of dealing with health problems. Whereas the majority of research dollars today are spent on trying to find cures for diseases that already exist— a cure for cancer, a cure for AIDS, a cure for degenerative diseases of all sorts — the "Evaluation of Research in the United States on Human Nutrition" strongly implied the need for what might be called **disease prevention through diet.**

What's involved is making a wholesale change in our health- care priorities. Instead of putting energy into fighting disease once it has developed, focus on preventing it from ever happening in the first place. How do you do this? According to the USDA, a key factor is dietary control. It's already a proven fact that early dietary training can prevent cells from becoming nonfunctional and joints from becoming stiff and unusable in later life.

Actually there is nothing radically new about this approach. It's been around for centuries. Have you ever heard, "an ounce of prevention is worth a pound of cure?" "A stitch in time saves nine?" "Foresight is better than hindsight?" What's being said here is: **anticipate intelligently.** Prevent today what will only need curing tomorrow.

In this light it would appear that our present illness care philosophy, our obsession with "finding cures" for diseases, is the one which is really archaic. This is a sad condition when better diet can so easily improve the health of an entire population. According to the USDA report, every age, ethnic, economic and geographic segment of the country can be healthier with a more balanced nutrition conscious diet. Working people can be more productive, thus reducing the cost of labor in producing goods. The cost of health insurance can be lessened dramatically, as can the cost of Medicare. As we will see from the following excerpts of this report, better diet can touch every thread of the social and economic fabric of this country. This is one way President Bush can help our country save billions of dollars and make taxpayers richer so he can tax them more.

Here is what the USDA found:

Magnitude of Benefits from Nutrition Research

Part A.   Nutrition related health problems

Health problem	Magnitude of loss	Potential saving from improved diet in 1971 (in 1971 $$)
Heart and vasculatory	Over 1,000,000 deaths in 1967 Over 5 million people with definite or suspect heart disease in 1960-62 $31.6 billion in 1962	25% reduction 20% reduction
Respiratory and infections	82,000 deaths per year 246 million incidents in 19671 41 million work days lost in 1965-66 166 million school days lost $5 million in medical and hospital costs $1 billion in cold remedies and tissues	20% fewer incidents 15-20% fewer days lost 15-20% fewer days lost $ 1 million $ 20 million

----

Health problem	Magnitude of loss	Potential saving from improved diet in 1971 (in 1971 $$)
Mental health	2.5% of population of 5.2 million people are severely or totallyd isabled. 25million have manifest disability	10% fewer disabilities
Infant mortality and reproduction	Deaths in 1967—79,000 Death rate 22.4 per 1,000 Fetal death rate 15.6 per 1,000 Maternal death rate 28.0 per100,000 live births Child death rate (1-4 yrs.) 96.1 per 100,000 in 1964 15 million with congenital defects	50% fewer deaths 50% fewer deaths 50 % fewer deaths 50 % fewer deaths Reduce rate to 10 per 100,000 13 million fewer children with birth defects
Early aging and lifespan	49.1% of population, about 102 million people have one or more chronic impairments	10 million people without impairments
	Those surviving to age 65: White males 66% Black males 50% White females 81% Black females 64%	1% improvement per year to 90% surviving
	Life expectancy in years: White males 67.9 Black males 61.1 White females 75.1 Black females 68.2	Bring Black expectancy up to White

Health problem	Magnitude of loss	Potential saving fromimproved diet in 1971 (in 1971 $$)
Arthritis	16 million people afflicted 27 million work days lost 500,000 people unemployed Annual cost $3.6 billion	8 million people without afflictions 13.5 million work days 125,000 people employed $900 million per year
Dental health	44 million with gingivitis 23 million with advanced periodontal disease $6.5 billion public and private expenditures on dentists' services in 1967 22 million edentulous persons (1 in 8) in 1957 1/2 of all people over 55 have no teeth	50% reduction in incidence, severity and expenditures
Diabetes and carbohydrate disorders	3.9 million overt diabetic 35,000 deaths in 1967 79% of people over 55 with impaired glucose tolerance	50% of cases, avoided or improved
Osteoporosis	4 million severe cases 25% of women over 40	75% reduction
Obesity	3 million adolescents 30% to 40% of adults 60% to 70% over 40 years	80% reduction in incidence
Alcoholism	5 million alcoholics; 1/2 are addicted About 24,500 deaths in 1967 caused by alcohol Annual loss over $2 billion from absenteeism, lowered production and accidents	33% 33% 33%

Health problem	Magnitude of loss	Potential savings from improved diet in 1971 (in 1971 $$)
Eyesight	48.1%, or 86 million people over 3 years wore corrective lenses in 1966 81,000 become blind each year $103 million on welfare	20% fewer people with corrective lenses
Cosmetic	10% of women ages 9 or more with vitamin intakes below recommended daily allowances.	
Allergies	22 million people (9%) are allergic 16 million with hayfever, asthma 7-15 million people (3-6%) allergic to milk Over 693 thousand persons (1 in 3,000) allergic to gluten	20% people relieved 90% people relieved 90% people relieved
Anemia and other nutrient deficiencies	See Improved Work Efficiency, Growth and Development, and Learning Ability	
Digestive	8,495 work days lost 5,013 school days lost About 20 million incidents of acute condition annually $4.2 billion annual cost 14 million persons with duodenal ulcers $5 million annual cost 4,000 new cases each day	25% fewer acute conditions Over $1 billion in costs

Health problem	Magnitude of loss	Potential saving fromimproved diet in 1971 (in 1971 $$)
Kidney and urinary deaths	55,000 deaths from renal failure 200,000 with kidney stones acute conditions	20% reduction
Muscular disorders	200,000 cases	10% reduction in cases
Cancer	600,000 persons developed cancer in 1968 320,000 persons died of cancer in 1968	20% reduction in incidence and deaths

Part B. Individual satisfactions increased

Satisfactions	Magnitude of loss	Potential saving from improved diet in 1971 (in 1971 $$)
Improved work efficiency	0.5% increase -on the job productivity	
Improved growth and development	113,000 deaths byaccidents 324.5 million work days lost 51.8 million people needing medical attention and/or restricted activity	25% fewer deaths and work days lost
Improved learning ability	Over 6.5 million mentally retarded persons with I.Q. below 70 12% of school age children need special education	Raise I.Q. by 10 points for persons with I.Q. of 70-80

Despite the United States' ingenuity in nearly everything else, it can't seem to find a way of lowering the toll of **Heart and Vascular Disease.** The USDA offers insight into this ironic condition:

Heart and vasculatory diseases are the number one cause of deaths in the U.S., accounting for about 54% of all deaths; ranging from 10% of all deaths under the age of 35 years, and 33% between 35 and 45 years, to 71% at age 75 years and above. There were over one million deaths from heart and vasculatory disease in 1967. The way the incidence of heart disease is rising, more than 1.5 million Americans can be expected to suffer heart attacks and strokes in 1970. This projection was made in 1967 by a group of heart experts at an international conference on Thrombosis sponsored by the Academy of Sciences.

The most recent figures for incidence of heart and vasculatory diseases are from the Health Survey of 1960-62. At that time, definite heart disease had been diagnosed in 13.2% of the population and was suspected in an additional 11.7%. During 1960-62, there were 28 million adults between 18 and 79 years of age diagnosed or suspected of having heart disease. The condition is more frequently found in men than in women before the menopause and is much more prevalent in Blacks than Whites. The President's Commission on Heart Disease, Cancer, and Stroke estimated economic costs of deaths from heart disease at $31.9 billion in 1962.

Although the percent of all deaths due to the cardiovascular diseases has increased continuously since 1900, the death rate from

105

cardiovascular diseases has gone down. In 1900 cardiovascular diseases accounted for 20% of all deaths. Today, more than 50% of all deaths are from this cause. Meanwhile, in the age groups below 45 years, the death rates have gone down for both males and females. In the 45-64 age group, the death rate among females has gone down steadily since 1930. In men of the same age group, the trend was upward until 1940, reached a plateau for a period, and then started downward about 1950. Since then it has dropped about 7.5%. In the age group 65 and over, the rates have been relatively stable. However, if adjustment were made for the increasing proportion of older people in this age group, the trend would be somewhat downward.

Death rates from heart disease are much higher in the U.S. than in many other countries of comparable economic level. Among the developed countries, 26 have lower death rates from heart disease than the U.S. The rates of death range from 51.8 per 100,000 population in Japan, and 79.8 in France, to 312.9 in the United States, 344.5 in West Berlin, and 352.3 in Scotland.

Epidemiological data indicate a high variance in death rate from heart and vascular disease among geographic areas in the U.S. Highest rates for white males were in the Southeast, for white females in the Southeast and Upper Michigan. The effects of early environment, including diet, is apparent in the statistics. Persons born in areas where the cardiovascular mortality was high, were more likely to die from this cause even though they moved to low rate areas. However, their chances were better than if they remained in their state of birth. Persons from low rate areas fared best if they remained in their birth place. Those who moved to high rate areas were less likely to die of heart disease than those who were born and lived in the high rate area.

Any consideration of the reasons underlying geographic differences in death rate must include diet. What foods are eaten? Do the foods differ in nutrient content or value among the areas? What differences exist in the mineral content or the water supply? Areas with the highest death rate for men are those recognized as having depleted soils. Higher death rates from cardiovascular disease also are found in areas where the water is hard.

The cause of the high death rate from heart disease in the U.S. is not known. Several high risk factors have been identified including family history, sex, age, smoking, stress, blood pressure, diabetes, overweight, lack of exercise, blood cholesterol, blood triglycerides. The importance of diet compared to the other risk factors is not known. A great deal of attention has been given to the possible relationship between diet and heart disease because most of the conditions are associated with an alteration in fat metabolism, reflected in increased levels of blood cholesterol and/or blood triglycerides. Fat transport systems are not normal in many cardiovascular patients; five types of hyperlipoproteinemia have been identified and diets devised to control the conditions. The diets vary for each of the five types and involve control of calories, cholesterol, type, and amount of fat or carbohydrate.

Substantive data has not been obtained on the role of diet prior to or during the development of cardiovascular problems. Being overweight is a problem because of the frequent association with high blood pressure and diabetes. In addition, additional body mass puts added strain on the heart. The relationship between high blood sugar levels and stroke is clearly established although the reason is not. Depending on the individual, the blood cholesterol level may be reduced by one or more of these dietary changes: reduction in the amount of fat, increasing the proportion of fat occurring as polyunsaturated fatty acids, or changing the type of carbohydrate. Very likely other nutrients can and do exert an effect. For example, an increased intake of chromium may increase the glucose tolerance of many individuals and thus might reduce the risk of heart disease for some persons.

A number of studies have been made on the relationship of diet and diet adjustment to the incidence of cardiovascular disease in selected populations. None of these have been conclusive. While diet may alter the risk factors, there is no clear statistical proof that the development of coronary heart disease can be slowed up by changing diet. There is no proof that lowering the dietary cholesterol intake affects the coronary patient. Scientists do not agree on the value of diet adjustment in preventing death in coronary patients. A number of diet studies have been of men who had suffered heart attacks. Coronary relapses were usually 25-50% less among those men on diets adjusted to reduce the intake of fat and cholesterol and to increase the proportion of polyunsaturated fatty acids. However, there was no difference in the total number of deaths. Interpretation of the results is complicated by the fact that adherence to the diets was only 50%.

There is no proof, but considerable evidence shows that to be effective, any change in dietary patterns should begin at an early age in order to delay the onset of these diseases. The first changes in the vascular system may have occurred by the age of 3, although coronary heart disease may not be diagnosed until the fourth or fifth decade. Good nutrition, including control of weight and diabetes by those having a family history of heart disease, should be encouraged from birth.

Selected References

American Heart Association, 1968. The national diet. Heart Study Final Report. Amer.Heart Assoc.,Inc. New York,Monograph 18.

American Heart Association, 1970. Coronary heart disease in seven countries.Ed., A. Keys, Amer. Heart Assoc.,Inc. New York.Monograph 29.

Committee on Nutrition, 1965. Diet and heart disease. Amer. Heart Assoc., Inc., New York.

Hursh, L.M., 1970. Heart disease. What do we know about diet as a risk factor? National Dairy Council,Chicago.

Levy,R.I., 1970. Hyperlipoproteinemia. Speach given at the Second Graduate Institute of Nutrition, Alton Ochsner Medical Foundation, New Orleans.

Mann, G. V. 1970 Comments on feeding studies in man. Third International Congress on Food Science and Technology, Washington, D. C.

The following chart shows that for men over 35, the death rate from heart disease has been holding steady or going up ever since 1930 despite huge expenditures for heart disease research. Only younger people and women have experienced fewer deaths from heart disease, yet most research has been spent on preventing heart disease in older males. As a matter of fact, the Office of Science and Technology just released a study criticizing past scientific studies for being "male chauvinistic," since most studies in the past have nearly all concentrated on studying men's health problems, such as prostate problems.

DEATH RATES FOR CARDIOVASCULAR DISEASES

White Population, U.S., 1930–60

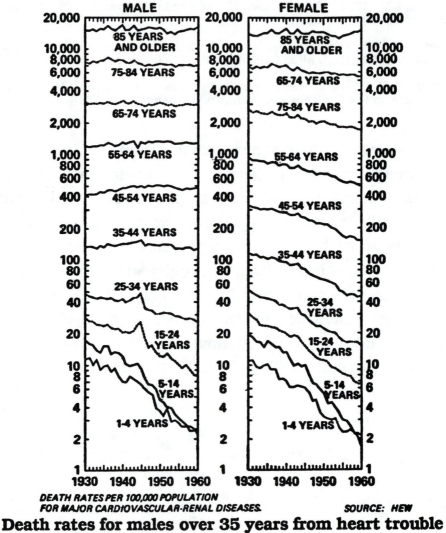

DEATH RATES PER 100,000 POPULATION
FOR MAJOR CARDIOVASCULAR-RENAL DISEASES.   SOURCE: HEW

Death rates for males over 35 years from heart trouble have not changed in the last 60 years, despite massive federal expenditures for such research.

From what we know today about **Respiratory and Infectious Diseases,** we are faring no better than we were twenty years ago. Here is what the USDA had to say about the subject in 1971:

Despite great advances in the control of infectious diseases in the past decades, acute respiratory infections remain the most frequent cause of illness and the most important cause of loss of time from work and school in the U.S. Pneumonia and influenza ranked fifth and other bronchopulmonic diseases tenth as causes of death in the U.S. in 1967; together they accounted for over 85,000 deaths. Acute respiratory infections are the most important single cause of illness. One-third to one-half of industrial absenteeism from sickness is caused by acute respiratory infections. In addition, mild infections may reduce efficiency without occasioning absenteeism. Young adults and children suffer the highest incidence of these infections, while the long lasting morbidity associated with chronic diseases is more frequent in older adults. The economic importance of morbidity from acute respiratory infections is impossible to determine precisely, but it has been estimated to be well over five million dollars per year. In addition, one billion dollars alone are spent for cold remedies and facial tissues.

Diet and the nutritional state of the individual involved are clearly associated with the incidence, duration, and severity of respiratory and infectious diseases. Nutrition is most likely to be a factor when the lower respiratory tract is involved, when bacteria are involved, or a chronic condition exists. Individuals in a good nutritional state are less likely to succumb to the disease and those with high levels of nutrient reserves are more likely to recover quickly. These reserves are of special importance when the disease state results in loss of appetite due to coughing and vomiting, and increased caloric expenditure due to added difficulty in breathing.

There are many reports that malnutrition lowers resistance to infection and that nutritional deficiencies may be precipitated by an acute infection in subjects with borderline nutrient inadequacies. Few statistics are available to show a direct relationship between nutrition and infection. One of the best studies was carried out in Guatemala at INCAP. Three matched villages were studied. In two, health measures were introduced, the third remaining as a control. The health measures in one village involved adding supplementary food to the diet of children during and after weaning; in the other village, preventive and curative medical care was offered. Overall death rates declined in all three villages beyond what was expected from trends prior to the study. Reductions in mortality were as follows: in the medical care village 31% (50% beyond that expected), in the feeding village 56%, and in the control village 38%. Fully half of the deaths occurred during the second year of life.

Further evidence of the relationship between nutrition and infection rate has been observed. Virus infections hit harder among the undernourished, and the severity of the infection is directly proportional to the degree of malnutrition — these data are from studies with mice. Acute diarrhea in young infants results from a synergism between poor nutritional state and infection.

In children, acute infections such as pneumonia, rheumatoid arthritis, acute tonsillitis, and rheumatic fever reduce the levels of Vitamin A in the blood as does vaccination against small pox and measles. Xerophthalmia, night blindness, frequently follows these infections indicating the depletion of body reserves of Vitamin A. Vitamins B-1, B-6, and C, and protein also are implicated.

Unfortunately, there are no satisfactory ways to determine the extent of body stores for most nutrients or to identify the level of nutrient intake needed to maintain adequate stores for resistance to infection.

Despite major advances in drug treatment prior to 1950, the incidence of respiratory and infectious disease remains high for the very young, 1 to 4 years, whose body reserves are low. The incidence increases with age where the cumulative effects of a lifetime of chronic marginal nutrient intake and reserves show up.

The manner by which good nutrition and diet combat infectious diseases is not well understood. Healthy cells and membranes may be more resistant to the entry of microorganisms. Protein, several vitamins, and minerals are needed to produce the antibodies to resist and recover from infectious diseases, although their role in the production of antibodies is not clear.

Recent studies with animals have shown a direct relation between specific nutrients and production of antibodies to specific stimuli such as disease organisms or organ transplants. The relationship exists when a specific nutrient, usually a vitamin, is lacking in the diet. Increased resistance to disease has not been demonstrated when individual vitamins are added to marginal or normal diets.

Lung irritants present in the atmosphere, such as ozone and nitrogen dioxide, are an increasingly important contributor to respiratory problems. Vitamins A and E may help protect the lungs from the adverse effects. Vitamin A is essential for production of healthy mucus-secreting tissue in the lung while Vitamin E may protect the Vitamin A from destruction by air pollutants.

Diet is additionally involved in the transmission of several infectious diseases including salmonellosis, typhoid fever, dysentery, hepatitis, and gastroenteritis. Most of these diseases are transmitted

113

through contamination of food and water supplies. Statistics on the incidence of illness from food poisoning are inadequate. Only those cases are recorded where the causative organism is isolated from both the food and the stricken individuals. Probably not more than 1% of all cases of food poisoning are reported. The causative organisms, primarily salmonella, clostridium perfringens, and staphylococci, are widely distributed in food. They become a health problem when the food is improperly handled and the microorganisms have the opportunity to grow, reproduce, and in some instances produce toxins. About 99 out of 100 cases of food poisoning are due to improper handling of food during preparation and storage by the consumer.

In 1966, it was estimated that two million Americans or 1% of the population suffered from attacks of salmonellosis often self-diagnosed as "24 hour flu" or stomach upset. If the average duration of each incidence is two days, then a total of 1.5 million work days were lost. The estimate of two days per incident is considered conservative.

Chronic and respiratory diseases other than tuberculosis are at the present time rapidly increasing in the U.S. For example, since 1949, the death rate for pulmonary emphysema with or without chronic bronchitis, has increased faster than that for any other leading cause of death. The rate of increase in death and incidence is of epidemic proportions. About 1% of deaths of males and 0.5% of deaths of females are caused by chronic non-tuberculous respiratory diseases. Atmospheric pollution, cigarette smoking, and constitutional factors are implicated as important causes of the chronic respiratory diseases. Some of them such as bronchial asthma may be allergic disorders.

Selected References

Anonymous, 1967. Salmonella. FDA Papers 1 (1): 13.

Anonymous, 1970. Vitamins A and E help maintain lung health.   Chem. Eng. News 48 (27): 38.

Axelrod, A., 1970. Nutrition and immune processes. Symposium   on Relationships between Nutrition and Infectious Disease. Tenth Annual Meeting, The American Society for Clinical Nutrition, Inc. Atlantic City.

Grayston, J.T., and E. R. Alexander, 1967. Acute respiratory infections. In: Preventive Medicine, eds., D. W. Clark and B. MacMahon. Little, Brown and Co. Boston, p. 439.

What is your response when you read a statement such as this: "A direct relationship can be drawn between nutrition and much of the mental illness resulting from organic brain disorders?" If you're appalled, you will be interested in what else the USDA had to say about the effect of nutrition on **Mental and Emotional Health.**

Mental illness is difficult to define and even specialists in the field are dissatisfied with present classifications. Thus, data on its incidence vary widely. Estimates of impaired disability due to disturbances of thought, mood, perception, and behavior vary from 1% to more than 20% of the population. The National Association for Mental Health estimates that 19 million people in the United States (about 1 in 10) are afflicted with some form of mental or emotional illness requiring mental care. Moreover, mental disorders are a significant factor in many physical illnesses. Estimates, based on a study by the Commission of Chronic Illness in Baltimore in 1952-55, and other data indicate that at any point in time 12% of the population are suffering from psychiatric disorder and that 2.5% (over 52 million persons) are severely or totally disabled by it. Only 19% were considered entirely free of psychiatric symptoms. Prevalence of mental illness increases with age and is higher in the lowest socio-economic groups.

A direct relationship can be drawn between nutrition and much of the mental illness resulting from organic brain disorders. Dietary improvement results in increased resistance to infection, better management of alcoholics, fewer circulatory disturbances and cardiovascular conditions, control of metabolic disturbances due to diabetes, hyperthyroidism, and nutrient deficiencies. The relationship of nutrition and mental disorders not associated with organic brain damage is less clear. There is no doubt that mental disorders can lead to poor eating habits and malnutrition. Also, it is clearly established that good nutrition is necessary for proper development and function of the central nervous system. Recovery from mental disability can be delayed if the condition is complicated by nutritional inadequacy.

Conceivably as much as 80% of the U.S. population could benefit from improved mental health with 12% having a major benefit. Benefits would be economic, through reduced hospital and psychiatric costs, improved ability and opportunities on the job, and fewer work days lost. Social benefits would be of even greater importance of the individual and their families.

Selected References

Norman, E.C., and J. R. K. Robson, 1969. Nutrition and mental health. Mental health considerations in public health.Public Health Service publ. 1898. U.S. Dept. of Health, Education, and Welfare, Wash., D.C.

Pasamanick, B., 1961. A survey of mental disease in an urban population. IV. An approach to total prevalence rates. Arch. Gen. Psychiat. 5: 151.

Srole, L., T. S. Langner, S. T. Michael, M.K. Opler, and T.A.C. Rennie, 1961. Mental health in the Metropolis. The Midtown Manhattan Study, vol. 1. McGraw-Hill Book Company, New York.

Though rates of infant mortality and reproductive problems are higher in the 90's as a result of increased drug abuse among pregnant mothers, the figures were still distressingly high in 1971. The USDA in that year pointed out the correlation between nutritional deficiencies and **Infant Mortality and Reproduction.**

In 1968, there were approximately 3.5 million children born in the U.S. Of these live births, 75,000 infants died within the first year of life. The infant mortality rate in the U.S. has shown a constant decline during this century, but it has not declined as rapidly, or to as low a level, as in several other countries. In 1950, the U.S. ranked 6th among a group of countries with characteristics which make comparison possible. In 1961-63, the U.S. had moved to 10th place and to 13th in 1968. Sweden had the lowest average annual infant mortality rate, about 13 per thousand in 1968. In 1968, the infant mortality rate in the U.S. was 21.7, a slight decrease from 22.4 in 1967. The mortality rate for white infants in 1967 was 19.7 per thousand as compared with 35.5 for nonwhite infants. A large part of these infant deaths were neonatal or occurred during the first month of life. Neonatal death rate was 16.5; with the rate for white infants being 15.0 as compared with 23.8 for nonwhite infants. The large proportion of the neonatal deaths occurred in infants who were small at birth, either because they were "prematurely" born, or because they were "small-for-date" infants. Since 1960, about 325,000 "premature" babies, "babies with birth weight of 5.5 pounds or less," have been born in the U.S. each year.

The infant mortality rate for nonwhite was 40.3 in 1965, nearly double the rate in the white population. The same causative factors apply that make for high rates among the poor: premature termination of pregnancy, lack of health and medical care services, inadequate diet and health practices, and inadequate living conditions. The impact of the level of living on infant survival is illustrated by the fact that the post-neonatal (age 1-11 months) death rate in the 17 states with the lowest per capita income was over a third above the national average in 1965.

The incidence of low birth weight in the U.S. is increasing. In 1950, 7.6% of live-born infants were "premature"; in 1960, 7.7%; and in 1964, 8.2%. Among the white infants, the incidence has hovered about 7.0%. The incidence among nonwhite infants increased from 10.4% in 1950 to 13.8% in 1964. To a large extent, these small babies are the result of poor fetal nutrition. Recently developed techniques for taking intra-uterine fluid samples will make it possible to identify and study nutritional problems during the fetal period. Until the development of this technique, very little was known about the direct interrelationship of nutrition and fetal development in humans.

A number of studies have been done with animals showing the severe effects upon the full-term animal fetus of nutritional deficiencies during pregnancy. Zinc deficiency will cause skeletal malformations as cleft palate, cleft lip, club feet, missing eyes, missing vertebra, and abnormalities of other body systems. A manganese deficiency during pregnancy produces abnormal body righting reflexes in the young.

The first evidence that a change in maternal nutrition could disrupt the normal development of mammals appeared in 1935. The relationship was established between diets deficient in Vitamin A and a variety of birth defects including missing eyes in pigs. Since that time, a number of abnormalities have been deliberately induced by nutritional deficiencies. Among the nutrients studied were riboflavin and folic acid. Significantly, folic acid and Vitamin A are two of the vitamins most likely to be deficient in the U.S. diet.

One of the earliest deficiencies to be recognized for its effects on prenatal development was a deficiency of iodine. This results in the birth of a somewhat overweight, but seemingly normal, infant. However, by the sixth month, the clinical picture of cretinism is clearly defined. This is of particular economic significance in the U.S. at the present time because of the increasing prevalence of goiter in several parts of the U.S. among girls of childbearing age. This increased incidence may be due to the increasing consumption of prepared foods made with salt which has no iodine added.

Since 1910 the percentage of infant deaths due to birth defects has steadily increased. Many millions of children have handicaps. In fact, the 1964 Vital Statistics Survey in the U.S. showed that congenital defects, including genetic metabolic disorders, was the leading cause of death in the first year. At least 62,000 deaths each year in all age groups in this country may be attributed to birth defects. Actually, as a cause of death, birth defects are outranked only by heart disease. The National Foundation has estimated that today in the U.S. there are 15 million persons with one or more congenital defects that affect their daily lives. There is considerable evidence relating to the relevance of birth defects to poor nutrition. The Health Insurance Program of New York and others have found that babies who weighed less than 5.5 pounds at birth are twice as likely to have birth defects. Some of these relationships have been discussed elsewhere. The incidence of blindness is from two to three times as high in infants of low birth weight.

Malnourishment in the mother usually results in the birth of a baby who is underweight. These babies are more likely to have birth defects. This has particular significance in the U.S. where there are probably more child pregnancies than in any other nation in the world. In 1965 in the U.S., there were more than 196,000 live births to girls 17 years or age or younger. Statistics are not available to show the relation of the age of the mother to the incidence or birth defects. However, young mothers are in the sex-age group most likely to have nutritional deficiencies as indicated by the National Nutrition Survey of 1968 in Louisiana, 40% of 7-17 year olds had unacceptable plasma Vitamin A values. This vitamin deficiency has been implicated in birth defects.

Complications during pregnancy resulting in maternal death may also be related to the nutritional state of the mother. In 1967, the maternal death rate was 28.0 per 100,000 live births. The rate for white mothers was 19.5 and for nonwhite mothers was 69.5. While hygiene and other factors are also causative agents, the role of nutrition may be very important particularly with the nonwhite mothers, many of whom are from low economic groups. There are a number of ways in which nutrition influences maternal death. The frequency of misshapen pelvic bones, a cause of difficult labor and frequency of adverse effects on the infant, has been much reduced by the prevention of childhood rickets. Because the principal cause of rickets is an inadequate intake of Vitamins A and D and is more often present among economically deprived populations, we have an example of the influence of economic status and malnutrition in early life on the outcome of pregnancies many years later.

Nutrition has been recognized as a possible major cause of the toxemias of pregnancy for several years. The specific nutrient involvement is not well understood. The relative importance of nutrition in the cause and course of toxemia in pregnancy has been the subject of controversy for many years. Greatest interest has centered on the intake of calories, protein, and salt. It appears likely that the problem is the result of a very complex metabolic disturbance involving abnormal hormone activity and an unbalanced dietary intake. Vitamin B-6 also has been implicated. The clinical pattern and geographic distribution of pre-eclampsia is reminiscent of primarily nutritional disorders, particularly pellagra.

The increased nutritional needs of women during pregnancy has been recognized for many years. Yet information from human metabolic studies on the nutritional requirements of this important group is only fragmentary, and few new studies have been made in the past 15 years.

INFANT MORTALITY RATE
SELECTED COUNTRIES

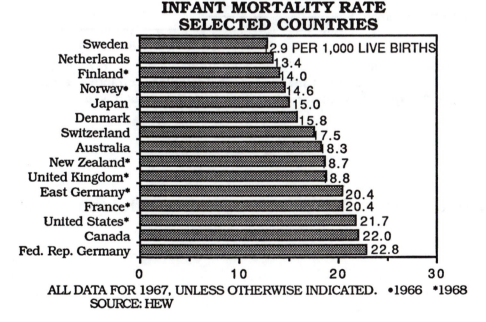

Country	Rate
Sweden	12.9 PER 1,000 LIVE BIRTHS
Netherlands	13.4
Finland*	14.0
Norway•	14.6
Japan	15.0
Denmark	15.8
Switzerland	17.5
Australia	18.3
New Zealand*	18.7
United Kingdom*	18.8
East Germany*	20.4
France*	20.4
United States*	21.7
Canada	22.0
Fed. Rep. Germany	22.8

ALL DATA FOR 1967, UNLESS OTHERWISE INDICATED. •1966 *1968
SOURCE: HEW

In 1968, the United States ranked 13th in Infant Mortality Rate. In 1990, it ranked 17th.

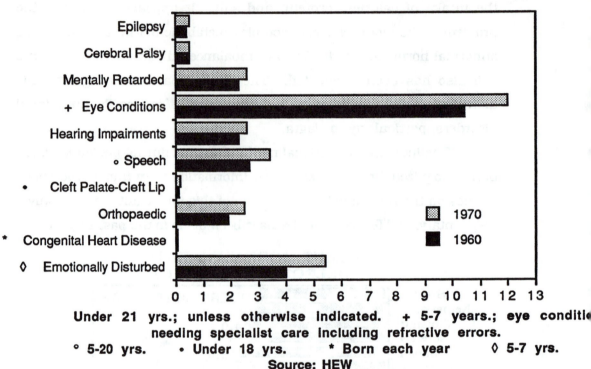

MILLIONS OF CHILDREN HAVE HANDICAPS

Under 21 yrs.; unless otherwise indicated.   + 5-7 years.; eye conditi◄
needing specialist care including refractive errors.
° 5-20 yrs.   • Under 18 yrs.   * Born each year   ◊ 5-7 yrs.
Source: HEW

More children each year are being born with birth defects.

Selected References

Bergner, L., and M.Wl Susser, 1970. Low birth weight and prenatal nutrition: An interpretative review. Pediatrics 46: 946.

Buck, C.W., 1967. Prenatal and perinatal causes of early death and defect. In: Preventive Medicine, eds., D.W. Clark and B. MacMahon. Little, Brown and Company, Boston, p.143.

Drillien, C.M., 1970. The small-for-date infant: Etiology and prognosis. Symposium on the Small-for-Date Infant. Pediat. Clin. North Amer. 17:1.

Hunt, E., 1970. Infant mortality trends and maternal and infant care. Children 17:88.

Hurley, L.S., 1968. The consequences of fetal impoverishment. Nutr. Today 3(4): 3.

Kark, R.M., 1968. Some aspects of nutrition and the kidney. In: Modern Nutrition in Health and Diseases, ed. 4, eds., N.G. Wohl and R.S. Goodhart. Lea and Febiger, Philadelphia, p. 819.

National Academy of Sciences, 1970. Maternal nutrition and the course of pregnancy: Summary Report. Committee on Maternal Nutrition, Food and Nutrition Board, National Research Council.

National Academy of Sciences, 1970. Maternal Nutrition and the Course of Pregnancy Committee on Maternal Nutrition,Food and Nutrition Board, National Research Council.

U.S. Bureau of the Census, 1969. Statistical Abstract of the United States: 1969. 90th ed., U.S. Dept. of Commerce, Washington, D.C.

U.S. Children's Bureau, 1967. Some facts and figures about children and youth. U.S. Dept. of Health, Education, and Welfare, Washington, D.C.

Usher,R.H., 1970. Clinical and therapeutic aspects of fetal malnutrition. Symposium on the Small-for-Date Infant.Pediat. Clin. North Amer. 17:169

Here is what was reported by the USDA about **Arthritis** in 1971. According to present research, the situation has worsened in the past twenty years.

Arthritis represents a number of musculoskeletal conditions which cause a greater loss of time from work than any other set of health problems with the exception of nervous and mental disorders and respiratory diseases. This loss was recently estimated at 27 million days annually. About 16 million people in the U.S. are afflicted. About one of four victims of arthritis is restricted from carrying on any major activities and one of ten is confined to home. Present estimates are conservative because there is little precise information regarding the true prevalence of the chronic rheumatic disorders in the general population. Recent estimates are that arthritic conditions cause unemployment each year to the equivalent of nearly one-half million people, cost the Government nearly 200 million dollars annually in lost income taxes, and account for about 12% of welfare expenditures. The total cost to the individuals involved and to the Government from arthritis and related disorders is estimated at 3.6 billion dollars annually. No price tags, however, can be placed on the untold suffering, pain, invalidism, and mental anguish which these disorders impose on individuals and their families.

Selected References

Arthritis Foundation, 1966. Today's facts about arthritis. The Arthritis Foundation, New York

Bick, E.M. 1967 Musculoskeletal system. In: Preventive Medicine, eds.

D.W. Clark and B. MacMahon. Little, Brown, and Company, Boston, p.403

National Institute of Arthritis and Metabolic Diseases, 1967. Special report: Arthritis. Prepared for 1970 appropriation hearings. U.S. Public Health Service, U.S. Dept. of Health, Education, and Welfare, Wash., D.C.

Number and Percentage With One or More
Chronic Arthritic Conditions
By Sex and Age: United States, July 1965 - June 1966

Sex and age	Total population in thousands	Persons with one or more chronic conditions	
		Number in thousands	% of population
Both sexes			
All ages	190,710	93,668	49.1
Under 17 years	66,840	14,950	22.4
17-24 years	22,393	9,671	43.2
25-44 years	45,185	26,756	59.2
45-64 years	38,713	27,316	70.5
65 & over	17,578	14,976	85.2

Data based on household interviews of the civilian, non-institutional population.

Source: National Center for Health Statistics, 1967. PHS publ. 1000, series 10, no. 37, table 9. U.S. Dept of Health, Education and Welfare.

While most of us consider dental hygiene a matter of how often we brush and floss and what brand of toothpaste we use, for the sake of our teeth and gums we should probably be paying more attention to the food we eat. The USDA affirms this view in its assessment of the impact of nutrition on **Dental Health and Cost of Dental Care.**

Diet serves three major roles in the maintenance of good dental health. Adequate nutrition is essential for the proper development of tooth structure before eruption and later for the maintenance of a firm, healthy tooth surface and resistance to the carcinogenic organisms in the mouth. These micro-organisms in the mouth are generally accepted as responsible for conversion of sugars to acids in the mouth, the latter dissolving the calcium in the tooth to form the hold. Some sugars (and starches) have very low carcinogenicity. The presence of sucrose, especially the sticky sweets eaten between meals, encourages the increase in numbers of carcinogenic organisms. A change in food habits is necessary to make this means of control effective.

The third critical area for diet in dental health is in the maintenance of healthy gums and teeth in adults to prevent or modify the onset of periodontal disease. The Health Examination Survey, conducted during 1960-62 by the U.S. Department of Health, Education, and Welfare, estimated that about 44 million adults, age 18 to 78 years had gingivitis, and about 23 million had chronic destructive disease indicative of advanced periodontal disease. Both dental caries and periodontal disease also are influenced by a number of non-nutritional factors, particularly oral hygiene.

An examination of the economics of health services in the U.S. indicates that the consumer spends 1/7 th to 1/9th of his health dollar for dental health services, a total of about 3 billion dollars in 1966. This cost represents the 20% of the population estimated to receive adequate dental care during the calendar year. At that rate, care for the total population of the country would have approached 15 billion dollars or 2% of the country's gross national product. The size of the dental health problem is reflected in the fact that in 1957 there were 22 million persons in the U.S. who had no natural teeth. This is equivalent to one out of every eight persons past the age of 55 years having no natural teeth. Over 98% of the U.S. population is afflicted with dental decay, and he proportion is rising. Dental caries without proper dental services and hygiene are the main cause of the problems. The preventive role of proper diet is not clearly established.

The influence of nutrition in dental health begins before birth. Many changes in oral structures of experimental animals have been reported in relation to prenatal nutrition. These include basic changes in the dento-facial pattern ranging from minor abnormalities to cleft palate and harelip; changes in size and shape of both molars and incisor teeth, delay in eruption of molars; and an association with increased dental caries. A deficiency or an excess of a nutritional factor normally required, or an antagonist which can disrupt the normal metabolic process may interfere with embryonic development. Some of the nutritional factors which have been associated with these changes include riboflavin, folic acid, and their anti-metabolites; Vitamin A; and diets high in sugar or phosphate. Each factor tends to be involved in a characteristic pattern of effects which are not necessarily limited to the oral structures. Changes in the maternal diet can affect the fetus without being detrimental to the mother. The mechanism of this nutritional influence appears to result in the death of the cell or in alteration in the rate of cell growth.

Clear-cut cause and effect relationships between nutrition and periodontal disease have not been established. Gingival inflammation can be induced by nutritionally inadequate diets. Healing of existing lesions has been delayed by protein-deficient diets. Also, the morphology of the dental plaque closely associated with the presence of periodontal disease can be varied by alterations in the composition of the diet.

Selected References

Carlsson, J., and J. Egelberg, 1965. Effect of diet on early plague formation in man. Odont. Revy 16: 112.

Fisher, M.A., 1970. New Directions for dentistry. Amer. J. Publ. Health 60: 848.

Knutson, J.W., 1967. Prevention of dental disease. In: Preventive Medicine, eds., D.W. Clark and B. MacMahon. Little, Brown and Company, Boston, p. 229.

Larson, R.H., 1964. The effect of prenatal nutrition on oral structures. J. Amer. Dietet. Assoc. 44: 368.

National Center for Health Statistics, 1969. Selected examination findings related to periodontal disease among adults, United States, 1960-1962. Public Health Service publ. 100, series 11, no. 33. U.S. Dept. of Health, Education, and Welfare, Washington, D.C.

Unfortunately because the USDA's findings on **Diabetes and Carbohydrate Disorders** were so under-publicized, the incidence of these disorders has increased significantly in the last twenty years.

Problems of carbohydrate metabolism, including reduced glucose tolerance and intolerance to certain disaccharides affect a large proportion of the adult population. Severely reduced glucose tolerance, resulting from the inability of the body to efficiently utilize glucose is commonly referred to as **diabetes mellitus**. Less severe reduction in glucose tolerance does exist unrecognized in large numbers of persons. The diabetic population is increasing. Diabetes stood 7th among the causes of death in the U.S. in 1969 accounting for over 35,000 deaths. Over 4 million diabetics were estimated in the U.S. in 1967. There are an additional 5,600,000 potentially diabetic persons. Thus, 1 in 20 has diabetes or is potentially diabetic. Nearly 7 out of 10 known persons with diabetes had their diabetes discovered at age 45 years or older.

In diabetes, the body is unable to metabolize carbohydrates normally, being unable to convert carbohydrates into the stored form, glycogen, or to utilize them for the energy required for normal body functions. Glucose disappears from the bloodstream at a slower than normal rate following carbohydrate intake. The condition is associated with deficiency or inadequate utilization of insulin. As the disease progresses, abnormal carbohydrate metabolism becomes associated with a derangement in the metabolism of fats and proteins. Health conditions associated with diabetes are extreme tiredness, leg pain, eye trouble, sudden weakness, frequent urination, thirst, itching, loss of weight, changes in appetite, and degenerative vascular disease.

Diabetes has been known for some time to be a hereditary disorder which can be controlled by insulin therapy and diet management. During the past decade, the trace mineral chromium has been shown to improve the body's ability to use carbohydrate, particularly when the reduction in glucose tolerance is associated with aging. It has been postulated that the decreasing ability to handle glucose with age may reflect chronic marginal intake of chromium throughout life. It is known that the original content of chromium or its biologically available form, as of other trace elements, is markedly reduced by refining and processing of foods. U.S. Public Health Service studies have suggested that as many as 14% of the U.S. population may have reduced glucose tolerance. A recent study in 1965 found that 77% of "normal" subjects over 70 years of age have abnormal glucose tolerance. The reduced glucose tolerance, a characteristic of the aging process, has been associated with increased incidence of coronary heart disease and stroke.

Blood sugar levels increase with age. Evidence of reduced glucose tolerance is apparent before age 30. This reduction in glucose tolerance may result from aging, a high prevalence of diabetes-related genes or, as recently suggested, a reduction in body chromium stores resulting from a chronic marginal intake during the lifetime. Women tend to have a slightly higher blood sugar level than men. The tendency increases with succeeding pregnancies and may be due to decreased body stores of trace elements such as chromium.

Considerable attention is now being given to the significance of lactose intolerance in nutritional problems in the U.S. Lactose is the principal sugar naturally occurring in milk. Normally, it is changed during digestion to glucose and galactose which are absorbed. In the adult, and occasionally in the infant, not enough lactase is produced to break down the lactose. In these "lactose intolerant" individuals, the sugar passes into the intestine where it is acted on by microorganisms with the production of gas and accompanying discomfort from diarrhea and intestinal distension. The incidence of lactose intolerance in healthy adults is shown in table on page 18. As many as 19% of adult Caucasians, 74% of Blacks, and 95% of Orientals in the U.S. may be affected.

Persons who are unable to metabolize lactose find it necessary to exclude milk and many milk products from their diet. This is particularly important in evaluating and improving the diets of low income families. About 75% of the black adults in this group probably cannot consume milk without distress. About 45% of black school children in Baltimore, MD, had a reduced ability to metabolize milk sugar. Milk given with the school lunch was more likely to be rejected by these children even though small amounts of milk could be consumed without major discomfort.

Monosaccharides also may present a metabolic problem. An inborn error in the metabolism of galactose results in abnormally large amounts of this sugar in the blood. The condition is characterized by nutritional defects, mental and physical retardation, enlargement of liver and spleen, osteoporosis, and cataracts. Eyesight is frequently affected.

Selected References

Levine, R., 1968. Nutritional aspects of diabetes mellitus. Borden's Rev. Nutr. Res. 29: 15.

Lutwak,L., 1970. The significance of lactose intolerance in nutritional problems. Eastern Experiment Station Collaborators' Conference on Human Nutrition, October 28, 1969. Agricultural Research Service, ARS 73-67. U.S. Dept. of Agriculture, Washington, D.C.

McDonald, G.W., and G.F.Fisher, 1967. Diabetes prevalence in the United States. Public Health Rep. 82: 334.

Paige,D.M., T.M. Bayless, G.D. Ferry, and G.S.Graham, 1971. Lactose malabsorption and milk rejection in Negro school children. Unpublished.

Sharkey,T.P., 1971. Diabetes mellitus-present problems and new research. J.Amer. Dietet. Assoc. 58: 201.

National Center for Health Statistics, 1966. Blood glucose levels in adults, United States, 1960-1962. Public Health Service publ. 100, series 11, no. 18 U.S. Dept. of Health, Education and Welfare, Washington, D.C.

National Institute of Arthritis and Metabolic Diseases, 1969. Special Report: Diabetes. Prepared for 1970 appropriation hearings. U.S. Public Health Service, U.S. Dept. of Health, Education, and Welfare, Wash., D.C.

WHO Expert Committee 1965 Diabetes mellitus. World Health Organization Technical Report series no. 310. World Health Organization, Geneva.

Lactose Intolerance in "Healthy" Adults

Group	Lactose intolerance By blood sugar
Caucasians: (U.S., Great Britain, Australia) (several studies combined)	19 %
Black, U.S.A. (several studies combined)	74 %
Black, Central Africa, various countries	88 %
Black, Bantu, various tribes	59 %
Oriental, U.S.A.	95 %
Oriental, Australia	85 %
Oriental, India	22 %
Oriental, Thailand	97 %
Australian Aborigine	79 %
North American Indian	67 %
South American Indian (Columbia)	100 %
Greek Cypriot	88 %
North African Arab	100 %

Source: Lutwak, L. 1970 The significance of lactose intolerance in nutritional problems. Eastern Experiment Station Collaborators' Conference on Human Nutrition, Oct. 28, 1969. ARS 73-67. U.S. Dept. of Agriculture.

As the USDA pointed out, **Osteoporosis** was (and continues to be) a major health problem among American adults.

Osteoporosis is a disease of the bone characterized by increased porosity and softness in which the amount and strength of the tissues has been decreased. The bones are susceptible to fracture, and osteoporosis is one of the most common and yet least understood afflictions of bone. It occurs during middle or old age and is observed more frequently in women than in men. Osteoporosis is one of the major causes of disability in age. The spine is affected first. Thinned by disease, the bones of the spine are compressed by body weight resulting in low back pain, back deformity, loss of weight and the capacity of physical activity.

The significance of the disease as a basis of vulnerability to fracture and disablement is of real or potential importance to millions of persons over 40 throughout the world. Recent surveys indicate that osteoporosis is more widespread than arthritis and about 3 times as common as diabetes. Using the severe criterion of vertebral compression, these surveys suggest that approximately 25% to 30% of women and 15% to 20% of men over the age of 50 have osteoporosis of this high degree. An extensive study of osteoporosis in 2,000 women of Puerto Rico and Michigan indicated that nearly 50% of women over 45 years and 80% of women over 65 have "significant vertebral atrophy."

Selected References

Krook, L., Lutwak, P. Henrikson, F. Kallfelz, C. Hirsch, B. Romanus, L.F. Belanger, J.R. Marier, and B.E. Sheffy 1971. Reversibility of nutritional osteoporosis: Physiochemical data on bones from an experimental study in dogs. J. Nutr. 101: 233.

Lutwak, L. 1964 Osteoporosis-a mineral deficiency disease? J. Amer. Dietetic Association 44: 173

Lutwak, L. 1970 Survey of osteoporosis and pre-osteoporosis in a general population. Grad. Sch. Nutr. News, Cornell Univ. 7: 4.

Whedon, G.D. 1967. Battling the bone-thinner. Today's Health 45: 66.

If you're "in the pipeline," "on your way up the corporate ladder," but overweight, you may want to consider a different diet for reasons other than just looking good. This and many more conclusions can be drawn from the USDA's evaluation of the problem of **Obesity.**

Obesity is a prevalent health problem, at every age, in both sexes, and at every economic level in the U.S. today. Precisely how prevalent is difficult to assess, and there are no exact statistics. Almost 3 million adolescents (10%) in the U.S. are estimated to be seriously ill with overweight. In adults, the percentage of persons above their best weight is considerably higher. A person is generally considered to be obese if he weighs more than 20% above the average for his age and height. Obesity is more prevalent in women than in men and is more likely to occur as age increases. The greatest increase in weight occurs in the 20 to 30 age group. About 60% to 70% of men and women over 40 years are above their ideal weight.

Obesity and overweight are not considered to be a cause of death; however, they are closely associated with increased mortality from other conditions. Insurance statistics reveal that overweight people are more likely to develop certain diseases and to die at a younger age than people of normal weight. Diseases such as diabetes mellitus, gall bladder disease, gout, kidney and digestive disease, hypertension, and possibly coronary heart disease are significantly associated with obesity. Obesity increases surgical risk; is a hazard in pregnancy; prevents ambulation and self care in arthritis and fractures of the lower extremities in the aged; places a greater load on the heart and circulatory system; and increases the work in breathing. Reduction in weight to normal levels increases the likelihood of success in treating these health conditions. Weight reduction alone is not a cure, but it may modify the condition so that it is no longer critical. In addition to health problems, there are a number of social and psychological consequences arising from obesity. Good nutrition and maintenance of normal weight may prevent many health conditions from becoming debilitating.

There has been considerable research on various aspects of the causes of obesity, the nature of the disorder, and its treatment. Obesity is not a disease entity as such but a symptom of some underlying difficulty which may have many causes. A number of diverse factors are indicated: genetic, physiologic, psychologic, and social economic influences contribute to the development and perpetuation of the condition. Culture, activity, food habits, and way of life, all are involved.

Obese children and adolescents are more likely to remain obese as adults and to have difficulty in losing fat and maintaining fat loss. A longitudinal study of obese children showed that 86% of the men and 80% of the women who were over weight as children were overweight as adults. This has been shown to occur in developing countries where the incidence and severity of undernutrition is high. It probably is a factor in the high incidence of obesity in low income families in the U.S.

Malnutrition during pregnancy and early life may be reflected in obesity in adulthood. The total number of cells in the body are determined during the prenatal period, infancy, and early childhood. Later periods of growth in adulthood influence the size of the cells rather than the total number. Poor nutrition and undernutrition during the period of cell formation means that the adult will have fewer cells to carry on body processes and store fat. Malnourished children are likely to be obese adults, because fewer cells are available to the body for fat storage. Even though their height-weight ratio is close to average, these

135

individuals have a lower proportional protein and higher fat content in their body mass than do well nourished people. Overfeeding early in life may establish metabolic pathways which predispose the adult to obesity.

A very important factor in the development of obesity is the amount of exercise. The periods of rapid growth and high activity during adolescence are accompanied by high caloric requirements. When calorie needs are less, excess calories are retained as fat unless diet is adjusted. This should be a normal process regulated by appetite. When this does not occur, body fat increases over a period of time leading to obesity.

The wide variation in the efficiency with which people use calories suggests that heredity is also a factor in obesity. Studies of obese and normal adolescents and young adults show that the non-obese individual tends to burn up rather than store excess calories in short-term dietary excesses while the obese individual stores them as fat. Obese persons also are less likely to mobilize body fat to meet short-term calorie deficits than the non-obese. In addition, some persons convert carbohydrate to fat at an increased rate.

Food habits are important in both the development and control of obesity. Traditional and family eating and cultural patterns are often conducive to overeating and obesity and contribute to the high incidence of obesity in some families. Food preferences may be established as early as three years of age. Because food provides so many satisfactions besides nutritional needs, bad habits are not easy to change.

There are many economic costs arising from obesity and overweight, including the greater likelihood of early death and lost productivity. In addition, there are direct costs to the individual such as increased insurance premiums. Costs due to increased likelihood of developing certain diseases have been included elsewhere in the cost of these health conditions. Obese persons tend to be inactive and lethargic which may result in a reduced work efficiency.

The social costs of obesity are less easy to identify and gratify. Obese individuals are less attractive and are less readily accepted in the community. They are at a disadvantage in employment because of lesser agility, and they create a poor image in their relationships with other persons. Because of these factors and the greater likelihood of developing debilitating health conditions, obesity is frequently a handicap to career advancement.

Selected References

Anonymous, 1967. The obese patient: problem in management. Dairy Council Dig. 38 (1): 1.

National Center for Chronic Disease Control, Heart Disease Control Program, 1966. Obesity and health. Public Health Service publ. 1485. U.S. Dept of Health, Education, and Welfare, Washington, D.C.

Shipman, W.G. 1968 Predicting results for obese dieters. Nutr. News 31 (2): 5

Shipman, W.G., and M.R. Plesset 1963 Predicting the outcome for obese dieters J. Amer Dietetic Assoc. 42: 383

Percentage of Persons Deviating From Best Weight

Age (years)	MALES		FEMALES	
	10-19% above best bestweight	20% or more more above best weight	10-19% above best weight	20% or more more above weight
20-29	19	12	11	12
30-39	28	25	16	25
40-49	28	32	19	40
50-59	29	34	21	46
60-69	28	29	23	45

Adapted from Metropolitan Life Insurance Co. New York. Frequency of overweight and underweight, Statistical Bulletin 41 (4); January 1960.

Source: National Center for Chronic Disease Control 1966 Public Health Service publ. 1485. U.S. Dept. of Health, Education and Welfare.

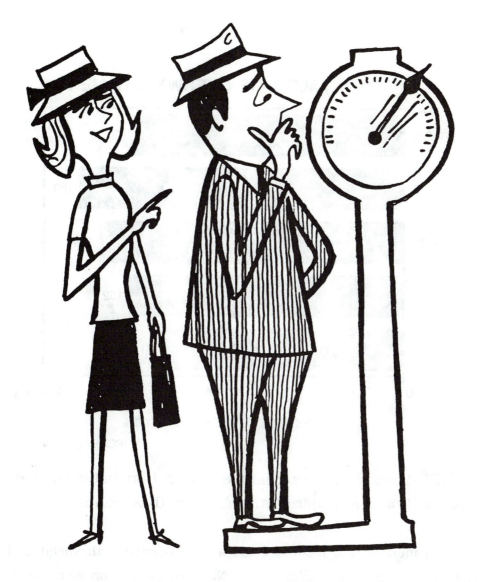

" You've gained 10 pounds
in 6 months!!...In 30 years
you'll weigh 770 pounds ."

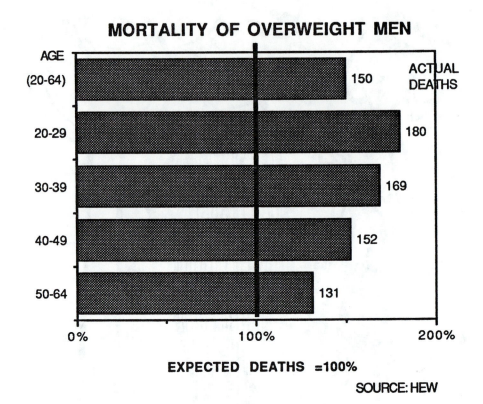

MORTALITY OF OVERWEIGHT MEN

AGE			ACTUAL DEATHS
(20-64)			150
20-29			180
30-39			169
40-49			152
50-64			131

0%   100%   200%

EXPECTED DEATHS =100%

SOURCE: HEW

The USDA found a very positive connection between poor diet or malnutrition and America's problem with **Alcohol**.

Alcoholism is a metabolic disease associated with social and physiological stress. According to the National Council on Alcoholism, 5 million alcoholics live in the U.S. This estimate is for 1970. Firm figures for incidence are not available because many alcoholics, particularly women, are not identified. Alcoholism is occurring much more frequently among very young people. The incidence is high among the lower social and economic classes. Persons with a history of

140

alcoholism have a death rate 2 1/2 to 3 times higher than standard risks. The National Council on Alcoholism estimates an annual loss to industry of over 2 billion dollars, resulting from absenteeism, lowered productivity, and accidents associated with alcoholism.

Good diet is an important factor in maintaining the productivity and health of alcoholics. It has generally been supposed that it is alcoholism, which is usually accompanied by a lack of interest in food, that leads to malnutrition. Not until recent months has poor diet been implicated as a cause. There is now some evidence with rats that a craving for alcohol can result from a chemical imbalance created by inadequate diet. Switching to a well-balanced diet was accompanied by a reduction in alcohol consumption.

Alcohol is a food contributing seven calories per gram of alcohol. It has been estimated that alcohol contributes 15-20 % of the total caloric intake in U.S. diets. The alcoholic individual substitutes alcohol for much of the normal food intake and as a consequence the intake of proteins, minerals and vitamins may be grossly deficient. About 50% of alcoholics have anemia due to hemorrhage, ulcers, or malnutrition. Many of the symptoms characteristic of alcoholics may be attributed to nutritional deficiencies rather than to toxicity of alcohol *per se.* Weakness, numbness, fatigue, and lack of interest typical of alcoholism also are characteristic is thiamine deficiency. When Vitamin B-1 is supplied, many of the symptoms disappear. Skin conditions characteristic of pellagra are sometimes seen in alcoholics and may be reversed by increasing niacin intake. Lack of Vitamin B-6 and pantothenic acid also may be responsible for neurological changes. A reduction in serum magnesium levels is occasionally seen in delirium tremors. Diets containing good quality protein and vitamins may help prevent many adverse changes in alcoholics and permit them to be gainfully employed.

Chronic intake of large amounts of alcohol is associated with the development of fatty liver and ultimately cirrhosis. In 1967, cirrhosis of the liver ranked 11th as the leading cause of death accounting for almost 28,000 deaths. There has been a marked increase in the death rate from cirrhosis of the liver during the past decade. Alcohol was the major factor in 88.5% of the deaths from cirrhosis in Baltimore in the years 1957-58 and 1965-66. The increase in the death rate from cirrhosis was thought to reflect the improved control of tuberculosis since 1961. Prior to that date, many alcoholics died from tuberculosis before cirrhosis had progressed far enough to be fatal.

Nutrition has contributed significantly in alleviating the results of alcoholism. There are still many people who could benefit from existing knowledge who have not been reached. These are the people whose condition has not reached the clinical stage. More help could be given if we understood better the factors responsible for fat deposition and mobilization in the liver. This knowledge is also fundamental to understanding the problems of obesity and of the undesirable changes in fat metabolism associated with heart and vasculatory disease. More complete knowledge of the mechanism of fat metabolism is required before sound recommendations can be made for altering diets.

Selected References

Davies, Karl M., 1965. The influence of alcohol on mortality. Proc. of the Home Office Life Underwriters Ass. XLVI: 159.

Kuller, L.H., K. Kramer, and R. Fisher, 1969. Changing trends in cirrhosis and fatty liver mortality. Amer J. Publ Health 59: 1124

Register, U.D., M. Johnson, C.I. Thurston, and A. Sanchez, 1970. The role of dietary factors in free-choice consumption of ethanol in rats. Federation Proc. 29: 632 (abstract)

Ever wonder why so many people wear glasses in the U.S.? The USDA Task Force found a definite correlation between nutrition and **Eyesight**, especially with relation to our nations' children.

The eye is particularly sensitive to nutritional inadequacy. Vision is one of man's most precious faculties. Good nutrition and intact vision are inextricably linked together throughout all phases of life. The eye as well as the brain has its most rapid rate of growth while the fetus is taking form and growing in the uterus. The eye continues to grow rapidly during most of the prenatal period and after birth commencing to slow in the third year of life. The eye increases in size hardly at all after age five. The brain-eye system is most vulnerable to the effects of deprivation of food during the early months and years of life. Some of the results of nutritional inadequacy during this early period do not become apparent until later in life when the eye is more susceptible to infection. Degenerative changes occur at an earlier age and progress to greater severity.

The social and economic costs of poor eyesight and blindness are great. 48% of the U.S. population over three years of age wore corrective lenses in 1966. Included were over 8 million children, 15% between the ages of 3 and 16 years and about 78 million or 88% of the population 45 years of age or over. In 1968, almost 81,000 blind persons received public assistance at an estimated cost in public assistance of over 103 million dollars. Statistics are not available on the number of persons who are partially or severely handicapped in their employment because of poor

143

vision nor are the number of accidents which occur from this cause. About 81,000 persons become blind every year.

Lack of Vitamin A is responsible for the most widespread form of blindness of nutritional origin in the world today. Insufficient Vitamin A results in damage to the cornea. In its early stages, it is reversible if treatment is instituted in time. The disability changes in the eye take place only after a long period of deprivation of vitamins. The incidence of adverse eye changes due to Vitamin A deficiency in the U.S. is not well documented. Recent developments indicate that Vitamin A deficiency is much more common than predicted. A nationwide survey of household food consumption in 1965 indicated that 27% of all households consumed diets below the recommended daily allowance for Vitamin A. More recent, preliminary results form the National Nutrition Survey begun in 1968 are showing that about 33% of children under five years of age and 29% of those aged six to nine years have blood Vitamin A levels below that considered adequate. In some areas about 40% of children up to 17 years of age had unacceptable plasma Vitamin A levels. About twice as many children in low income brackets had unacceptable Vitamin A levels as in more affluent families. Of even greater concern are clinical observations made in Iowa where adverse changes in the eye indicative of Vitamin A deficiency are being found in individuals having plasma Vitamin A values twice as high as the level generally accepted as being satisfactory.

There are indications, not well documented, that myopia in children is probably due to malnutrition. The normal, well-developed young child is long sighted. If all goes well, the refractive state of the eye gradually arrives at adult status before school age. About half of U.S. children have less than 20/20 vision. There is evidence that severe nutritional stress during the period of active growth may throw the delicate compensating mechanisms off balance and lead to myopia. Additional evidence comes from the observation that premature infants are much more myopic than full-term infants. Also, a recent study of 553 blind children born in New York State over a 12 year period revealed that many were of low birth weight indicative of poor nutrition during fetal development.

Deficiencies of the B-complex vitamins, thiamine, niacin, riboflavin, and vitamin B-12 are associated with impaired vision. In some instances, adverse changes in vision thought to be due to Vitamin A have responded to Vitamin B therapy but not to additional Vitamin A. The B vitamin deficiencies are more likely to be associated with deterioration of vision resulting from optic nerve degeneration. This condition is more often found in the adolescent school child or in young adults eating a monotonous poorly balanced diet. B vitamin deficiency also is likely after periods of calorie restriction, whether deliberate or involuntary. Dimness of vision from B vitamin deficiency may be recognized with greater frequency in the future as greater demands are placed on acuteness of vision by wider education and the need for more skilled labor.

Problems of eyesight also are associated with other diet based problems. It is not uncommon to find cataracts in diabetics and in galactosemia. The latter condition occurs as a result of the inability to metabolize galactose from milk sugar.

Selected References

McLaren, D.S., 1963. Malnutrition and the eye. Academic Pres, New York.

McLaren, D.S., 1968. To eat to see. Nutr. Today 3(1):2.

National Cancer for Health Statistics, 1967. Current estimates from the Health Interview Survey, United States, July 1965-June 1966. Public Health Service publ. 1000, series 10, no. 37. U.S. Dept. of Health, Education, and Welfare, Wash.,D.C.

National Center for Health Statistics, 1968. Current estimates from the Health Interview Survey, United States, July 1966-June 1967. Public Health Service publ. 1000,   series 10, no. 43. U.S. Dept of Health, Education, and Welfare, Wash., D.C.

Stern,J.J., 1968. Nutrition in ophthalmology. In: Modern Nutrition in Health and Disease,ed,4,eds M.G. Wohl and R.S. Goodhard. Lea and Febiger, Philadelphia, p.1025

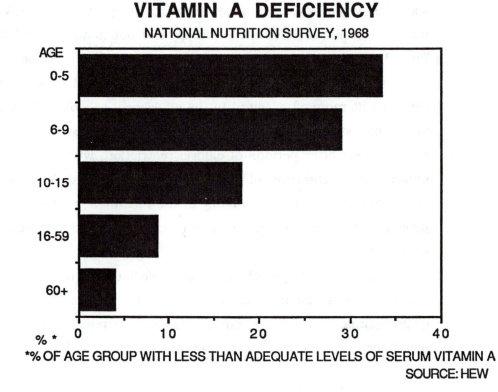

VITAMIN A DEFICIENCY
NATIONAL NUTRITION SURVEY, 1968

*% OF AGE GROUP WITH LESS THAN ADEQUATE LEVELS OF SERUM VITAMIN A

SOURCE: HEW

Proportion of Children Reaching Visual
Acuity Levels of 20/20 or Better

Age(years)	United States 1963-65	Private patients Houston, TX 1950	School children Toronto, Canada 1952

Percentages

6	51	44	-
7	46	52	72
8	51	56	84
9	58	61	83
10	58	69	80
11	56	75	78

1.) U.S. Health Examination Survey 1963-65.
2.) Stataper, F.J. 1950 Age norms of refarction and vision. A.M.A. Arch. Ophth. 43 (3); 466-481, March.
3.) Morgan, A.L., J.S. Crawford, T.J. Pashley, and J.R. Gatey 1952 A survey of methods used to reveal eye defect in school children. Canadian M.A.J.A. 67; 29-34.
Source: National Center for Health Statistics 1970 PHS publ. 1000, series 11, no. 101. U.S. Dept. of Health, Education, and Welfare.
COMMENT: Differences in rates among the three studies is due in part to differences in the procedures used to evaluate acuity. Procedures are not standardized.

Though **Kidney Disease** is a very gray area in medical science, the USDA sheds considerable light on the connection between renal failure and nutrition.

Very little is known concerning the mechanism of prevention and control of kidney disorders. Very few major illnesses fail to involve the kidneys. By selective excretion of certain substances and reabsorption of others, the kidneys play an important role in regulating the composition of blood and other body fluids. They continually process blood to eliminate harmful waste products of metabolism. When kidney function is impaired, diet regulation is critical to maintain life. The alternative is kidney dialysis or transplantation. Because the kidney is so closely related to nutrient metabolism in its function in disposing of metabolic waste, it would be reasonable to consider the role of diet and nutrition in preventing the development or in modifying the severity of kidney disease. Almost no attention has been given to this aspect of kidney disease, although it would benefit many more people at much less expense and inconvenience than the more drastic methods of transplant and dialysis.

A disturbance in mineral metabolism particularly calcium, is the first nutrition-related function to appear in chronic renal failure. One of the problems arising is the production of kidney stones. The incidence of kidney stones may be as high as 9.47 persons per 10,000 population. Vitamin D, excessive dietary alkali, excessive dietary calcium, and Vitamin A deficiency have all been implicated. Diets high in carbohydrates also may be conducive to stone formation. The incidence of calculi is greater when sucrose is the source of carbohydrate than when starch or dextrose are eaten. Starch produces fewer calculi than dextrose or sucrose. This has great significance in U.S. diets where there is a trend towards a decreasing consumption of starchy foods and an increase in the production of carbohydrate calories from sugars. This shift in recent years in U.S. diets may be conducive to an increased incidence of kidney stones.

Many researchers consider that the occurrence of urinary calculi falls into the general class of deficiency disease. The relation of diet to urinary calculi formation is unknown. Many of the same dietary factors may be involved as in the formation of kidney stones. Vitamin A deficiency has been suggested as a cause in animal studies but has not been demonstrated in human patients. Animal studies also suggest that pyridoxine deficiency may be a factor, particularly in relation to the magnesium and calcium content of the diet.

Selected References

Kass, C.H., 1967. Renal and urinary disorders. In: Preventive Medicine, eds., D.W. Clark and B. MacMahon. Little, Brown and Company, Boston, p. 539.

National Institute of Arthritis and Metabolic Diseases, 1969 Special Report: Kidney disease and the artificial kidney. Prepared for 1970 appropriation hearings. U.S. Public Health Service, U.S. Dept. of Health, Education, and Welfare, Washington, D.C.

Review, 1963. Nutritional aspects of urinary calculi. Dairy Council Dig. 34(5): 1.

Do you ever wonder why your child has such a short attention span? A large part of this inattentiveness is likely due to poor nutrition. Have you also wondered why enormous brain power, money, and energy continue to be spent on solving a raft of problems with **Learning Ability** and the educational system of this country? Findings of the USDA in 1971 provide interesting answers to these questions. There may be a simpler solution than overhauling our educational curriculum. It might be as simple as overhauling our diet.

Improved diet may improve learning ability in a number of ways, some of which have already been discussed. Some specific nutritional deficiencies limit ability to learn, for example, by causing blindness and by causing apathy and tiredness. Improper diet may also affect learning directly through its effect on brain and central nervous system development during the fetal period, infancy, and early childhood. Malnutrition in school age children and adults may handicap learning ability by shortening attention-span and decreasing the ability to work at the same task for any sustained period.

The President's Committee on Mental Retardation is studying the relationship between mental retardation and nutrition and plans to submit a report by June 1, 1970. The Committee has not been able to establish a causal relationship between nutrition and mental retardation because of the complexity of the problem and lack of basic data. They note, however, that among the poor, severe mental retardation is two or three times the average. They suggest that this greater incidence of mental retardation may be due to poor nutrition, prematurity, poor hygiene, or a combination of the three.

The incidence of mental retardation is high. Over a quarter of a million people were institutionalized in the U.S in 1967. In addition, there are many thousands in jails and correctional institutions. About 3% to 4% of the total number of the persons classified as retarded are accounted for by the institutional figures. Over 6.5 million persons may be involved. Improved diet, based on research yet to be done, during the critical years of pregnancy, infancy, and childhood, has a good possibility of increasing the mental performance of about half the potential retardates. Benefits would be realized from the savings on institutional costs, improved possibilities for employment and reduced likelihood of civil offenses.

The consequences of malnutrition in terms of impairment of learning ability depends on the time in life when the deprivation occurs as well as its extent and duration. For the brain, the most critical period is the five months prior to birth and about ten months after birth. By the end of the second year, the brain has practically completed its growth. Studies on rats have shown that the brain grows both by increase in the number of cells and by increase in the size of each cell. Severe malnutrition during the period of cell division permanently reduces the total number of cells and cannot be repaired by subsequent proper diet. Malnutrition during the cell growth phase is reparable by improved diet. Direct application to humans is not possible, because similar studies are not possible with human infants. However, the brains of infants who died of marasmus were found to have fewer brain cells than those infants who died from accidents.

Interest in the role of nutrition in mental development and learning ability has been stimulated by problems in developing countries where lack of food and undernutrition have great economic significance. The implications for children from low income families in the U.S. are now being studied. The National Nutrition Survey found evidence of retarded physical growth in about 3.5% of children from low income families. It is possible that these children also may have lasting damage to mental capacity. Severe deficiency of individual nutrients and undernutrition in general have been shown to adversely affect development of the brain and central nervous system in animals. Studies in developing countries have suggested that findings with animals may be extended to severely undernourished children. There is little or no information concerning the effects of chronic low level nutrient deficiencies found in the U.S. upon permanent mental damage.

A number of studies are in progress on the effects of feeding programs for preschool and school age children upon their mental ability as indicated by I.Q., grades and learning ability. Preliminary results in a New Orleans, Louisiana, study using nonverbal performance tests have shown no difference between normal and anemic children of a very young age (4 years, 5 months to 4 years, 9 months).

However, anemic children about a year older had slightly lower I.Q.'s than comparable normal children. Follow-up after a year of kindergarten showed that the anemic children receiving a multiple mineral and vitamin supplement had gained as much as ten I.Q. points more than the anemic children who didn't get the supplement. While there were no differences between the normal and anemic children on short-term attention tests, the performance in the anemic children deteriorated rapidly when the reaction time was longer, and they made more errors on rapid tests. Similar results were found in Philadelphia, Pennsylvania, where the I.Q.'s of anemic children, 4 and 5 years of age, were similar to those of nonanemic children, but their attentiveness was significantly less. Because attentiveness is essential to learning, the potential for learning could be expected to increase when the diet was improved. This is an example of what might be accomplished for children by improving their diet. Conceivably, improved diets from prenatal to school age might increase the learning ability of 50% of children sufficiently to increase their I.Q. by ten points.

Selected References

Correa,H., 1969. Working capacity, productivity and economic II, August 26, 29, 1968, San Juan.

Correa, H., and G. Cummins, 1970. Contribution of nutrition to economic growth. Amer. J. Clin. Nutr. 23:560.

Correa,H., and G.Cummins, 1970. Some economics of malnutrition in the United States. To be published.

Howell, D.H., 1970. Clinical problems of iron deficiency in early life. Iron nutrition in infancy. Report of 62nd Ross Conference on Pediatric Research,October

After examining the relation between nutrition and learning ability, the USDA concluded its study with a look at **Reducing Losses of Nutrition During Food Preparation.** Because of the growth of microwave cooking and improvements in cooking utensils, much of what is covered by the USDA has now become current cooking practice for many Americans.

Improved food preparation techniques would reduce the loss of some nutrients and increase the availablity of others. As a result, the nutritional value of diets could be improved without modification of feeding patterns. The nutrients most likely to benefit are the water soluble vitamins, minerals, and amino acids. Water soluble vitamins and minerals leached into cooking water may be reclaimed. Up to 50% of the water soluble vitamins, thiamine and ascorbic acid may be lost if the cooking water is not used. Even greater losses, up to 90%, occur when cooked foods are held for long periods of time or are reheated. One of these procedures and sometimes both are necessary in food service operations and at home when prepared foods are used.

Processors' attention is centered on palatability, not nutritive value, when prepared food products are designed and methods for reheating are recommended. New processing techniques coupled with improved methods of handling and preparing processed foods could ensure vitamin losses no greater than 25%. This would mean fewer persons with diets inadequate in Vitamin C. Based on findings of the National Nutrition Survey 1968-69, 27% to 41% of households now on the poverty level and 20% to 40% of those above the poverty level have diets less than adequate in Vitamin C. The number of households with inadequate diets may be reduced by 1/4 through use of improved food preparation and handling procedures.

Cooking food has been shown to reduce the availability of amino acids. In meats, as much as 60% of methionine and lysine may be made unavailable; in some cereal products, the amount may be higher. The decreased availability of amino acids is often associated with development of desirable flavor. The reduction in available amino acid content of food as a result of cooking is probably insignificant nutritionally in U.S. diets which are generally high in protein. Methionine and lysine are the amino acids likely to be affected and are also those most likely to be deficient in cereal based diets. Preparation procedures designed to minimize the binding of these amino acids would benefit population groups whose protein intake may be marginal for economic or ethical reasons, or individual preferences.

Selected References

Ten-State Nutrition Survey in the United States, 1968-70. Preliminary Report to the Congress, April 1971. HEW, Center for Disease Control, PHS.

Because of the flak received from the meat and dairy councils and lobbies, as well as the food giants, the USDA has not updated its report on the beneficial effect of good nutrition since 1971. Obviously the controversial findings of the original report rankled many groups and professions who stood to lose by it, including the medical profession. We would like to offer our gracious thanks to the USDA for making this material available. Such vital information should not be censored or repressed.

8

FINDING
THE CHAMPION WITHIN

Each New Year's Eve, as the confetti falls, thousands of resolutions are made. "I'll quit smoking, lose ten pounds, lower my cholesterol, start an exercise program." The intention is good. But then the new year wanes and resolutions fall by the wayside. Wouldn't it be nice, just once, to celebrate last year's success on New Year's Eve, rather than using the occasion to start all over again?

The key to lasting success is replacing empty resolutions with permanent solutions. At one time or another most of us have resolved to change our lives by going on a diet. In many respects this is exactly the right approach. A change of diet can improve everything from looks to energy level. The right diet can even help us live longer. But most of us make the mistake of losing sight of the big picture. Dieting for a change in appearance won't release our true potential. Concentrating only on problem areas, such as pudgy stomachs and fatty thighs, leaves the champion within each of us trapped inside.

Finding the champion within and reaching a personal peak performance level depends upon building a solid foundation of healthy habits, a good "dietary life style." The core of that foundation is the network of biochemical molecules which makes up each of the body's cells. If the foundation crumbles, the building soon crumbles. Each molecule we consume in our food either makes our body stronger or weaker. There is no such thing as a neutral "filler molecule."

A strong body gives us a positive mental attitude, a strong desire to do what's best, not necessarily what's convenient, for ourselves and for others. Without a strong foundation, the effort to put the right molecules in the right place at the right time is wasted energy.

Each of us has a natural potential based on our genetic makeup. If we have built well by always eating what is healthy for the body, we are likely operating close to that potential. If we have eaten poorly, we undoubtedly have great room for improvement. Because the brain and body cells are in a constant state of renewal, we can replace bad cells with good ones and actually rebuild a better self, provided we eat right.

Increasing our potential involves change, and it's not easy to change habits formed over a lifetime. What makes it even more difficult is our constant exposure to influences, such as advertising, which turn many of us into our own worst enemies. We get hooked into eating sugary, greasy, preservative-laden foods, believing them to be more convenient and tastier. In the long run, neither is true. The time we save now by eating quick meals may be the time we spend later in the hospital, for as sure as death and taxes, a poor diet eventually will catch up with us.

To make positive changes, it's helpful to become familiar with current research and learn the facts about nutrition. This chapter, "Finding The Champion Within," will help you do both. It combines the latest nutritional information with testimonials from real life and provides practical knowledge which can help you realize your true mental and physical potential. Armed with a little information about how your body works, you'll be able to make changes in your life you never thought possible.

THE SCIENCE BEHIND THE SUCCESS

The guiding principle beind the science of food and human physiology is simple: the human body is in the process of contantly renewing itself through cellular repair and replacement. It is this condition which creates an ongoing opportunity for mental and physical improvement. Your skin, for example, is not the same skin that covered you seven years ago. It is made of entirely new cells. The fat beneath your skin is not the same fat that was there a year ago. Your oldest living blood cell is only 120 days old, and your entire digestive tract is renewed every three days.

Although this continual change may seem chaotic, it takes place according to molecular rules called biochemical pathways. With the correct pathways, a body can improve itself, enhance performance during adult life, and ultimately prolong health in old age. It's important to know that these correct pathways depend directly on what you eat and consist of combinations of essential nutrients which work for, rather than against, releasing the champion within. The best diet, like the best body, is a constantly changing mixture of nutrients. Alchemists have not yet found a way to turn stones into gold nuggets, and people have not, and will not, find a single food to eat repeatedly that will build a strong body. The magical transformation of nutrients into energy in healthy body cells occurs only when a mixture of the most nutritious foods are included in the diet, foods that can provide the body with *all* of the basic nutrients.

The following sections on basic nutrient groups explain the roles, required amounts and exceptional sources of each nutrient. Where necessary, explanations of the food industry are included to help you avoid advertising and marketing traps set by companies concerned with an ever rising sales curve, not your health. Hopefully, after finishing the last chapter, both you and your body will be able to make the changes, and the choices, of champions.

THE SEVEN ESSENTIAL NUTRIENT GROUPS

A chemical analysis of a healthy, 150-pound human body would show that it contains about 90 pounds of water and 30 pounds of fat. Another 30 pounds are mostly carbohydrates, protein, and the bone materials of calcium, magnesium, boron and phosphorus. Vitamins, minerals, and protective compounds account for only a fraction of a pound.

Based on what your body is made of, it is easy to determine what your body needs. If your body were a book, its table of contents would have seven main chapters, based on the seven groups of essential nutrients: water, fats, carbohydrates, protein, vitamins, minerals and oxygen. Each of these chapters, or nutrient groups, is necessary for a complete story. To build a healthy body, your diet must include all seven "chapters" of nutrients in their proper place and ratio.

Your body can also be compared to a garden. Fats, carbohydrates, and protein provide energy for growth. Water, oxygen, vitamins and minerals provide the environments of soil, rain, and sunlight in which that growth happens. Truly you are more like a tree or a flower than you may think. Like a flower, you need natural, whole foods to flourish. You can't live on Twinkies any better than an orchid can grow in the dark.

Whole foods, sometimes referred to as natural or organic foods, are composed of hundreds of different kinds of materials. Because most of them were once alive themselves, as plants or animals, they are made up of the essential nutrients needed for life. Each grain of wheat is made of some of the same molecules needed by your body.

With every bite of food you take, an intricate system of chemical reactions breaks this food down and rearranges the molecules into groups of nutrients to be used by your body. During this process, referred to as metabolism, each nutrient taken in is broken down into a molecular structure and put back together in a different form. The repeating cycles of this process are the metabolic pathways.

An inherited genetic code, recorded in your DNA molecules, gives instructions for the raw materials of food to be assembled into the cells, tissues and organs of your body. You can't change your genetic code, but you can affect your metabolic pathways by controlling the raw materials you take in. Any food you eat is composed of dozens or even hundreds of different kinds of materials in the form of atoms and molecules.

As I've said, body fuel can come in the form of fat, carbohydrates and protein. The amount of energy these nutrients release is measured in calories. Although calories are often thought of as a part of food, they are not; they are only a measure of the potential energy of a food. This includes the energy the body spends during metabolism, exercise and repair and even during the process of storing energy itself in the form of deposit fat. A gram of simple carbohydrate contains 4 calories; a gram of complex carbohydrates contains 3 calories; a gram of protein contains 2 to 4 calories; and a gram of fat contains 8 to 11 calories, depending on how much energy the body uses to release this caloric energy. Cultures such as China that live on mostly carbohydrates can consume as much as 25% more calories that Americans, yet obesity is almost non-existent in China. Even registered dietitians can't explain this finding.

When all of the calories in your food are not used immediately after eating, they are stored in the form of fat. As unappealing as this may sound, stored fat is a vital necessity. It is what keeps you alive through the night and allows you not to have to eat constantly. Stored fat is your energy reserve. Whenever you eat more calories than you use, the excess becomes fuel for future use. This is true for everything you eat. An excess of meat (a protein-rich food) gets stored in exactly the same way as an excess of potatoes (a carbohydrate-rich food). Although not a nutrient, alcohol is metabolized by the body and yields 7 calories per gram. It, too, is converted to fat when not used immediately. Without fat and the process of fat storage and fat burning, you'd spend your time doing nothing else but feeding yourself.

THE ENERGY SOURCE

Nearly all foods contain mixtures of the three energy sources—fat, carbohydrates and protein—but they are sometimes classified by the predominant nutrient. Though we usually think of beef purely as protein, modern beef actually contains more fat than protein. Likewise, though considered mainly a source of carbohydrates, many grains actually contain both essential fatty acids and protein. The only exceptions to the "multiple nutrients rule" are sugar, which is pure carbohydrate, and refined oil, which is pure fat. Consequently they are some of our least beneficial foods.

Armed with a knowledge of your needs, you can more easily choose nutritional food and provide yourself with the best source of energy. As long as the nutrients you need are in the food you eat, you can maintain and repair the complex machinery that keeps you going. The best way to maintain your body and maximize your amount of energy is to get a wide variety of whole foods—foods that are not laced with preservatives and have not undergone drastic reductions in nutritional value as a result of refining and processing for purposes of convenience.

Problems nearly always arise when foods are nutrient poor. This deficiency often occurs among people on high-fat, high-sugar diets made up mainly of junk food; and even among health conscious people who eat organic food but are unaware of how to balance the essential nutrients. It is important to be aware of the amount of each nutrient the body needs and how the food industry changes our foods, for better or for worse.

WHAT IS THE RDA ANYWAY?

Before we examine each of the seven classes of nutrients and their effects, a few pointers about "recommended dietary allowances" (RDA) will be helpful. It's important to distinguish between the literal meaning of the words and the legal meaning adopted by the U.S. Government and various food manufacturers.

In most cases, the Recommended Dietary Allowances may be only vaguely related to the amount of each nutrient you need every day. When manufacturers print RDA charts on product packages, they are referring to research done by the National Academy of Sciences. The tenth and most recent edition of Recommended Dietary Allowances was published in 1989.

Though results are published by the government, committees selected to set the allowances for each nutrient are composed of independent scientists. After analyzing relevant research, they arrive at a recommendation, not a requirement, based on an average for infants, children, males, females, pregnant women and nursing mothers. Further divisions by age in the first four groups account for 17 different sets of recommendations.

Though certain human variables are factored into the RDA, each allowance, in essence, is only a suggested amount based on generalized opinions of scientists, rather than on personal need. The RDA does not pretend to specify for each individual how much of any given nutrient is needed to reach a level of peak performance. What it does specify is how much it takes to prevent illness.

The U.S. RDA, often confused with RDA, is simply a broader estimate covering a wider range of individuals. Instead of encompassing the seventeen sets of children and adults covered by the RDA, the U.S. RDA makes only one average recommendation based on the highest requirement for a nutrient set by the RDA. For instance, the U.S. RDA for iron is 18 milligrams. This is the same amount set by the RDA for an adult female. The RDA for an adult male, however, is 10 milligrams of iron, 8 milligrams less than that quoted by the U.S. RDA. It is this more generalized average, the U.S. RDA for adults, which must, by law, be included on any product offering nutritional information. Therefore, when you buy a box of cereal that says it provides 10% of the U.S. RDA for protein, that recommendation is not necessarily geared to your particular situation. Perhaps you are a pregnant mother, a long distance runner or someone else with higher protein needs. If so, the cereal you are eating may not be supplying you with 10% of your particular daily requirement for protein. And that is where the nutritional information of food products, based on the U.S. RDA, may be misleading.

Now, let's take a look at what keeps us living.

ESSENTIAL NUTRIENTS

When carbohydrates are mentioned, what do you think of? Sugars and starches, of course. But most fibers are also carbohydrates.

Carbohydrates are often thought of as fattening, but, as explained earlier, fat is only created when excess nutrients are eaten. For energy, the body prefers carbohydrates over all other sources. They are clean burning and produce no toxic by-products, as protein does. Present in all plant food, carbohydrates are composed of sugars which come in three main sizes: sugars with a single ring of carbohydrates, sugars made from pairs of single ring carbohydrates, and large molecules that are actually long chains of single ring carbohydrates. The chemist's term for these three types of carbohydrates are monosaccharides, disaccharides, and polysaccharides.

Simple Sugars (monosaccharides and disaccharides)

Like fats, sugars are defined by the complexity of their structure. Also like fats, different types of sugars vary greatly in the harmful and beneficial effects they can have on the body. While known as simple sugars, monosaccharides and disaccharides are also known as simple carbohydrates. Because of the simplicity of their structure, both can be quickly converted to energy by the body.

The six common sugars found in foods are: glucose, fructose, galactose, sucrose, lactose and maltose. Most common among these is sucrose, which is purified and granulated from sugar cane and sugar beets to provide the brown, white and powdered varieties available in the supermarket. Since our ancestors did not have a source of pure, refined sucrose, the human body has not evolved to cope with large quantities of it. While the body needs sugar, it is true that complex carbohydrates, which convert to sugar, are a better source of energy than sucrose.

Simple carbohydrates are well known for increasing serum cholesterol levels. Sucrose and lactose (milk sugar) have been found to increase levels the most.

Though not poisonous, as some might claim, sugar can be harmful, as it invariably displaces other more valuable nutrients while offering little or no nutritional value in itself. For example, 200 calories worth of sugar are essentially empty calories. The same number of calories consumed by eating three pieces of whole wheat bread, on the other hand, provide 14 percent of the protein, 18 percent of the thiamine and 12 percent of the niacin needed to keep you functioning on a healthy level. Even more beneficial, whole grain bread contains valuable fiber and supplies energy as needed, not all at once, as sugar does.

Complex Sugars (Polysaccharides)

As with fats, the more complex structures offered by complex sugars and carbohydrates are best for maximum performance. These polysaccharides come in three forms: starch, glycogen and cellulose.

Under a microscope, starch appears as a long, straight or branched chain of hundreds of glucose units. A single starch molecule may contain 3,000 or more glucose units linked together, often as many as a million in a cubic inch of food. In a plant, starch serves as energy storage needed for growth and stamina, somewhat like glucose. Grains are the richest source of starch. In many societies, at least half, in some cases two-thirds of a person's energy is derived from grain. Legumes (beans and peas) and tubers (potatoes and yams) are also rich in starch.

Glycogen, the second polysaccharide, is absent from plants and found in animal meats only to a limited extent. Unimportant as a dietary element, glycogen is the body's storage form of glucose. Just as lipids are stored as body fat, glucose is stored by the liver as glycogen. Though only 100 to 200 grams of glycogen can be stored in the body, this storage process is vital to life. Not only does every cell depend on glucose to a greater or lesser extent, but the brain and nervous system depend solely on glucose for energy.

The third important polysaccharide is cellulose. Like starch, cellulose is found abundantly in plants and is composed of glucose units connected in a way different from how polysaccharides are joined. However, unlike starch, which is digested by enzymes in the mouth and stomach, cellulose is not digestible by human enzymes. As such, cellulose provides no energy but has an entirely different function in the body, which will be discussed later when we examine fiber.

Understanding how the various beneficial sugars interact with the other nutrient groups and how they differ among themselves is important to achieving maximum performance and realizing the champion within.

Effects of Sugar Levels

Regardless of which carbohydrates are eaten, the body invariably converts them to its own energy source of blood sugar, more properly called blood glucose. A certain amount of glucose in your blood is indispensable to feeling well. If your blood glucose concentration falls below normal, you may become tired, hungry, and shaky; if it rises above normal, you may become sleepy. If either extreme is pushed far enough, you can enter a coma. Optimal functioning is only possible when blood glucose remains within a certain range of concentration.

As we've pointed out, every body cell depends on glucose to a greater or lesser extent. Ordinarily the cells of your brain and nervous system depend solely on this sugar for their energy. Brain cells are continually active, even while sleeping, so they continually draw on the supply of glucose contained in the fluid surrounding them. To maintain this supply, blood replenishes the glucose as cells use it up.

Maintaining proper glucose levels is critical to homeostasis, a condition of balance the body is constantly striving for. Homeostasis is a big part of maintaining peak performance. When you wake up in the morning, your blood contains between 80 and 120 milligrams of glucose for each 100 milliliters of blood. This range, known as the fasting level of concentration, is normal and is accompanied by a feeling of alertness. If you don't eat, the blood glucose level gradually falls as cells all over your body keep drawing on the diminishing supply. At 60 or 65 milligrams per 100 millileters, the low end of the normal range is reached and you may feel hungry, irritable or tired. The normal response is to eat and raise the blood glucose level.

Because it is important that the blood glucose level not rise too high, the body works to prevent this. The first organ to respond to raised blood glucose is the pancreas, which detects the excess and puts out a hormonal message to correct it. Then the liver and muscle cells receive the message, remove the glucose from the blood and store it as glycogen.

Special cells of the pancreas, called beta cells, are sensitive to the concentration of blood glucose. When the concentration increases, beta cells respond by secreting more of the hormone insulin into the blood. As the circulating insulin bathes the body's other cells, many respond by taking up glucose from the blood. Most of the cells can only use the glucose for immediate energy, but the liver and muscle cells have the ability to store it for later use: they assemble the small glucose units into long branching chains called glycogen. The liver cells can also take the glucose apart and convert it to a saturated fat for export to other body cells. The fat cells can pick up this ready-made fat the liver cells have sent to them, or they themselves can make saturated fat from glucose.

After you eat, your blood glucose concentration returns to normal, and any excess glucose is put into storage as glycogen and saturated fat. During the hours that follow, before you eat again, the hormone glycogen opposes the action of insulin and works to bring glucose back out of storage as needed. Thus, the stored liver glycogen can keep replenishing the blood glucose as brain cells and other body cells keep drawing on it to meet their energy needs. Also muscle glycogen can be dismantled to make glucose, but this glucose is used primarily within the muscle cells themselves where it serves as an important fuel for muscle action.

The maintenance of a normal blood glucose level thus depends on two processes. When the level gets too low, it can be replenished quickly either from liver glycogen stores or from food. When the level gets too high, insulin is secreted to siphon the excess into storage. How you eat determines whether or not you can stay between these two extremes. There are three main guidelines to follow. First, when you are hungry, you should eat without waiting until you are famished. Second, when you do eat, you should eat a balanced meal including all the essential nutrients. Third, you should consume the number of calories that your body will need until the next meal. In other words, **breakfast** and **lunch** should anticipate active periods and be the largest meals, and supper should be the smallest (dreams don't use many calories). "Dinner" should be reserved for feast days, a few times a year.

For one reason or another, some people's blood glucose regulation fails and problems occur. The two most common problems are hypoglycemia and diabetes.

The term hypoglycemia simply means low blood glucose and refers to a symptom, not a disease. Signs such as weakness, rapid heartbeat, sweating, anxiety, hunger, shakiness, mental fatigue, confusion and amnesia can indicate problems. In many cases they indicate the body has bottomed out and may be dangerously low in blood glucose.

For example, poor circulation has the same feel as glucose deprivation, a cutting off of the brain's energy supply. Also poor circulation—perhaps due to heart disease, poor lung function, and dehydration—can actually cause glucose deprivation by lowering blood volume. Eating a large meal can even cause symptoms of hypoglycemia as the brain synthesizes compounds that favor sleep and as the blood is temporarily rerouted to the digestive tract to pick up nutrients, thus reducing blood flow to the brain. The same condition is caused by the rebound effect of eating a large dose of sugar. In fact, over-consumption of sugar is one of the most common ways of preventing peak performance.

A second condition that results from problems in glucose regulation is diabetes. This is a disease characterized by a deficiency of insulin in the blood or by a surplus of ineffective insulin. Either the pancreas fails to synthesize insulin (Type I Diabetes) or cells fail to respond to the insulin that is present (Type II Diabetes). In either case, the problem results in an excess of blood sugar due to blood glucose rising too high and insulin failing to bring it back down to normal.

Because insulin is so important in maintaining the necessary blood glucose level, it is easy to see that a steady level must be kept. A person whose glucose levels are a series of peaks and valleys is unable to function at their best simply because their body is constantly fighting to recover from one extreme or the other. This constitutes a definite health risk. Recent studies have also indicated that frequent snacking on nutritious foods during the day may be more beneficial than our usual pattern of eating generally a small breakfast, modest or large lunch, and large meal in the evening.

FIBER

A great deal of research has been done lately on fiber, extolling the virtues of its many different forms. Researchers in Africa formed a "fiber-hypothesis" which suggests that consumption of unrefined, high-fiber carbohydrate foods protects against many western maladies, such as constipation, hernia, hemorrhoids, gallstones, diabetes, coronary heart disease, obesity, bowel cancer, breast cancer and high blood pressure. Their hypothesis grew from the fact that rural Africans naturally have a diet high in fiber and show a low incidence of many of these chronic conditions.

The science of nutrition, however, is too complex to pin a problem on a single cause. Many researchers believe that higher intakes of salt, sugar, and animal fat, and not low intakes of fibrous foods, account for the higher incidence of the above problems. In truth, high incidence of degenerative disease is a combination of these factors. The ideal diet therefore should be low in saturated fats, refined sugar and sodium and include several sources of fiber.

Types of Fiber

Not all sources of fiber are equal. As with fats and sugars, fibers come in a wide variety of forms, some of which are beneficial and some of which are useless, even harmful to your health. As a general definition, fiber is any substance in plant food (specifically that part which makes up the cell walls) that is not digested by human enzymes. Crude fiber and dietary fiber simply are more precise terms. Crude fiber is fiber that remains in food after a harsh, acidic chemical procedure in the laboratory. Dietary fiber is the fiber that remains in food after digestion in the body. Because the body must work harder to digest foods containing dietary fibers, the net yield of calories is lower. High fiber foods also exercise the intestinal muscles more vigorously to give them better tone and health.

Another difference among fibers is their ability to dissolve in water. Soluble fibers, such as pectin, mucilage and guar, form gels when mixed with other liquids. This slows the absorption of sugar. Insoluble fibers, such as cellulose, help to speed the passage of digested food. Each type has its own unique advantages.

Nearly every form of fiber can do a body a lot of good. By helping to regulate and exercise the digestive system, fiber is responsible for preventing many diseases and reducing the effects of aging.

The only danger involved with eating fiber comes from not drinking enough water. Fiber without adequate water can either cause gas or cause the food mass in the stomach to become hard and dehydrated. With sufficient water, high-fiber foods are very soft and gentle to the digestive tract.

Many weight loss drink mixes contain high levels of sugar and low levels of fiber and thus can cause constipation. Energy drinks high in fiber can be useful and have been proven successful, but only when backed by sound nutrition. When buying any energy drink, look for one made from whole grains and high in essential fatty acids and vitamins and devoid of sucrose and lactose.

Carbohydrates (the body's main energy source) and fibers are a necessary part of a healthy diet. Understanding how they work with the other nutrient groups and how they differ among themselves will allow you to make the choices necessary for a long and healthy life.

FATS

Fats play one of the most important roles in helping you obtain peak performance every day. Compared to protein and carbohydrates, fat provides the most energy and constitutes the form in which excess energy is stored. Unfortunately, many people are convinced that the less fat you have on your body, and the less fat you eat, the better off you are. This is simply not true. Like all nutrients, fat is beneficial in the right quantities. It is as harmful to eat too little as it is too much.

Fats have two distinct uses in the human body, structure and energy. Fats used for structure are called essential fatty acids (EFA) because they are indispensable. EFA are used for building cell walls, parts of all organs (especially the retina of the eye), ovaries and testes, brain cells, and semi-permeable membranes throughout the body. Semi-permeable membranes control the entrance of all nutrients into the cell and the exiting of all waste products, many of which are toxic. Membranes are made of layers of proteins for strength and layers of fat which control the migration of water in and out of cells. Having both layers made perfectly is very important. Without proper structure, cells cannot function normally, nor can minds and bodies.

The best fats have one thing in common: they burn cleanly. This means they don't contain an abundance of unwanted substances, such as excess cholesterol, unwanted animal steroid hormones, oxidized fats, or oxidized cholesterol (found in dried milk and other dried animal products.)

When we refer to "fat," we are actually referring to what doctors, nutritionists and scientist call lipids. Lipids help maintain the structure and health of all cells. They are a part of every cell in the body, their function being to send and receive fat-soluble substances, such as vitamins and hormones, in and out of cells. Special cells also contain large stores of lipids, specifically to meet the body's moment-to-moment needs for energy. These cells provide two-thirds of the body's energy. Moreover, they are an integral part of the body's insulation system. A layer of body fat beneath the skin protects each and everyone of us from the cold. Also a pad of hard fat beneath each kidney protects it from being jarred and damaged during movement.

The importance of fat to the body makes it an essential dietary component. That's why it's important to understand the difference between useful or necessary lipids, called essential fatty acids, and lipids which can do irreversible harm to our bodies.

Triglycerides

Like nutrients, lipids are divided into different groups. The largest group, triglycerides, make up 95 percent of our body fat and include the most important lipids of all, the essential fatty acids.

To understand fats and how they can either help you reach peak performance or keep you from it, it helps to understand their molecular structure. Like people, triglycerides come in many sizes and varieties, but they all share a common structure; all have a backbone of glycerol to which three fatty acids are attached. All glycerol molecules are alike, but the fatty acids vary in three ways: length of the carbon chain, the position of any double bonds, and the number of double bonds, which indicates the degree of saturation.

Fatty Acids

A fatty acid is an organic acid consisting of a string of six or more carbon atoms with hydrogen attached and an acid group at one end. The simplest organic acid is acetic acid with a chain only two carbons long. Natural fatty acids mostly occur with even numbered carbon chains.

Besides the length of their carbon chain, the other difference in fatty acids is their level of saturation, hence the term saturated fat. Saturated fat is composed of saturated fatty acids. A fatty acid is considered saturated when all of its carbon atoms are loaded with hydrogen atoms. Saturated fats are the ones to be avoided, though adding linolenic acid to the diet will speed up the rate at which the body can burn them. Studies by Storlien in Australia showed that it took nearly 50 hours to burn saturated fats as compared to 15 hours for oleic or linolenic acid. Oleic acid is a monounsaturated, 18-carbon fatty acid which burns rapidly in the body. This makes oleic acid (from olive and canola oil) an ideal energy yielding fat in the diet.

Linoleic acid is an essential fatty acid which, according to recent research, is not an ideal energy source. The body requires 40 hours to burn it, about the same amount of time it takes to burn saturated fat. Because of this, consumption should be held to 2% by weight of the total diet. Oleic and linolenic fatty acids provide better sources of concentrated energy.

Essential Fatty Acids

Essential fatty acids are important to the production of prostaglandins, whose function in the body is similar to that of hormones. They send messages from one cell to another and each one has its own important function. One dilates and constricts blood vessels. Another alters transmission of nerve impulses. Still another modulates body tissues' responses to hormones. Others act on the kidney, affecting its water secretion, or in breast milk, protecting the infant's digestive tract. About 100 different prostaglandins have been discovered in the body so far. The half life of most of them amazingly is about 30 seconds, and they are effective at concentrations of one part per billion.

Instrumental in the production of prostaglandins are the two essential fatty acids: linoleic acid, an 18-carbon fatty acid with two double bonds; and linolenic acid, an 18-carbon fatty acid with three double bonds starting at the third carbon atom. A balance between these two in the diet is important to maintaining a properly functioning body. In most Americans' diets, this balance is upset by consumption of far too much linoleic acid and far too little linolenic acid.

Phospholipids and Sterols

While triglycerides are the largest class of lipids (fat), the smallest classes are phospholipids and sterols. Together these two classes make up only 5 percent of dietary lipids. Among the phospholipids, lecithin is the best known. Appearing in many different forms, it is used in the body to make cell membranes and to keep cells functioning.

Many different sterols are used by the body in stomach acids, adrenal hormones and sex hormones, but the one that has been receiving the most attention lately is cholesterol. Like lecithin, cholesterol is needed metabolically, but is not an essential nutrient. The liver manufactures 50 trillion molecules (50,000,000,000,000,000) of cholesterol per second to supply the body with electrical insulation and to keep cell walls flexible. Without some cholesterol, we would all have premature wrinkles.

The misconception about cholesterol is that any amount in the diet is bad. Actually, only excess cholesterol is bad. Because it has been associated with heart disease, manufacturers have made a big issue of their products being cholesterol free. It is important to remember, however, that the raw materials used by the liver to make cholesterol can all be made from glucose, amino acids, or fatty acids—which means cholesterol can be made from carbohydrates, protein or fat. In other words, the body manufactures it.

CVD: What does it mean?

More than half the adults who die in the United States each year die of cardiovascular disease (CVD), a disease of the heart and circulatory system. The underlying condition of these deaths is artery disease, which is so widespread it has been called epidemic.

Artery disease often begins with hardening of the arteries, or atherosclerosis. With atherosclerosis, soft mounds of lipid accumulate and form plaque along the inner walls of the arteries. This layer of plaque gradually enlarges, which makes artery walls lose their elasticity and restricts the flow of blood.

As blood normally surges through the arteries with each beat of the heart, the arteries expand with each pulse to accommodate the flow. Arteries, hardened and narrowed by plaque, cannot expand, resulting in a rise in blood pressure. This increased pressure puts a strain on the heart and damages the artery walls further.

As pressure builds up in an artery, the arterial wall may become weakened and balloon out, forming an aneurysm. If and when an aneurysm bursts in a major artery, massive bleeding and possible death can result.

In addition to being elastic, the inner walls of the arteries must be smooth for blood to move over the surface with as little friction as possible. Clotting is an intricate series of events triggered when the blood moves over a rough surface, such as the edge of a cut. As long as the inner wall of an artery remains smooth, clots will not form. As plaques encroach on the inside of the artery, however, their roughness can cause clotting to begin.

Once formed, a clot may linger and gradually grow until it shuts off the blood supply to that portion of the tissue supplied by the artery. The tissue then may die slowly and be replaced by scar tissue. Or the clot may break loose and travel along the system until reaching an artery too small to allow passage. In this case the tissues fed by this artery will be robbed of oxygen and nutrients and will die suddenly. When a clot lodges in an artery of the brain, killing brain tissue, a stroke has occurred. When a clot lodges in an artery of the heart, causing sudden death of part of the heart muscle, a heart attack has occurred.

Though national advertisers might lead us to believe that only those in high risk groups (men over 45 and women after menopause) need to reduce their risk of cardiovascular disease, the truth is that atherosclerosis begins early. Fatty streaks have been observed in the aortas of infants less than a year old, and plaques are well developed in most individuals by the time they are 30. No one is free of the condition. The question is not whether you have it, but to what extent.

Atherosclerosis takes a heavy toll among people in their productive years, long before retirement. Many health agencies have devoted millions of research dollars and hours to the battle against atherosclersis, but so far all that can be said for sure is that no single cause has been found. There are many "risk factors" including smoking, gender, heredity, high blood pressure, lack of exercise, obesity, stress, high blood cholesterol, calorie excesses and nutrient deficiencies, and personality characteristics. So far, the relationships among these factors remain only conjecture.

There are things you can be doing, however, to lessen the risk of cardiovascular disease. Substituting polyunsaturated fats for saturated fats may help, but it leads to other degenerative diseases. A smarter approach is to eliminate saturated fats as best you can, use **monounsaturated** fats (olive oil and canola oil) whenever fats are needed, and eat vegetables and whole grain breads and cereals as much as possible as sources of energy and fiber. Also add as much linolenic acid as possible to the diet to help burn the saturated fats, balance the polyunsaturated fats, and produce rejuvenating hormones.

PROTEIN

The importance of protein is evident from the meaning of the word in Greek—first things. Three quarters of all the solid matter of your body is protein. All enzymes and most hormones, every cell and muscle, every piece of tissue in your body is made of protein. The human body in fact contains an estimated 10,000 to 50,000 different kinds of protein with a tremendous range of possible surface structures, each empowered to perform a distinct, individual and specialized function. Each of these proteins must be custom-built to specifications of your body. In other words, it is this wide array of proteins, together with their catalysts and enzynes, that makes you different from any other person on earth.

Aware of the importance of protein, most people associate it with strength and success more than any other nutrient. In fact, it has received so much emphasis that many people consume too much protein at the expense of other nutrients. An understanding of the quantity and quality of protein needed for a proper diet will help put it in perspective. As only one of many essential nutrients, it is needed in correct proportions (about 45 grams per day) to achieve maximum performance.

Amino Acids

Like carbohydrates and lipids, protein is a chemical compound composed of carbon, hydrogen and oxygen atoms. What makes it different is the presence of nitrogen atoms. All atoms in a protein are arranged into amino acids, which are its building blocks. When your body needs a particular protein, the proper amino acids are linked together in a chain. The amino branch of one molecule joins with the acid branch of the next, and the link is bonded by enzymes called peptides.

Amino acid chains are therefore sometimes called polypeptides rather than proteins. No matter how many amino acids join together, there are always branches free to make further bonds. Protein molecules have been found to contain chains of as many as five hundred amino acids. Many of these are the same type but bonded in specifically different sequences.

The ability to create either highly active chemicals or hard, fibrous structures shows the versatility of amino-based proteins. But for all their variety, they are still only chains or minute molecular strands. By cross-linking and interweaving with other molecule chains of the same protein, they form multi-layered latticeworks. Then, folding back on themselves, forming loops and superimposing themselves on other latticeworks, they gradually grow into the highly complicated

182

and specialized three-dimensional structures that make up everything in your body. Carbohydrates and fats can't do this, which is why protein, the product of an almost limitless number of amino acid combinations, is so vital in the right proportion.

The side chains on amino acids are what make proteins so different by comparison to carbohydrates and lipids. A polysaccharide, for example, is composed of glucose units, one after the other. It may be several thousand units long, but every unit in the chain is a glucose molecule identical to all the others. In the case of a protein, 22 unique amino acids may appear, each differing from the others according to the groups of molecules attached to them. One amino acid may have an acid group attached to it, another may have a basic amino group attached to it, and still another may have neutral side chains, including complicated ring structures. These acidic, basic and neutral groups confer different characteristics on the amino acids.

Amino acids are divided into two basic groups, fibrous protein and globular protein. Fibrous protein creates solid, straight tissue, such as muscle. Globular protein is somewhat different. Unlike the fibrous protein structures laid down in interwoven chains, globular molecules are often composed of single chains which fold and curl back on themselves. Globular proteins create enzymes and hormones, which are soluble, highly reactive chemicals.

While the true number of amino acids is unknown, the number of essential amino acids is nine. They are "essential" once again because they cannot be manufactured by the body. Essential amino acids are very important to the brain where they determine not only emotional and mental states but also the energy levels, growth, and general health and functioning of the body as well. Many of our most mysterious diseases are related to malfunctions of the brain and may be amino acid-related: Alzheimer's, senility and schizophrenia.

The Purpose of Protein

One of the many functions of protein is to maintain the body's fluid balance. Fluid is present in several body compartments, chief among them being the spaces within the cells. As fluids flow back and forth between these compartments, proteins, together with minerals in the fluids, help maintain an even distribution of nutrients.

Also, major proteins in the blood stream are antibodies that help fight disease. When a body is invaded by a virus, the virus enters the cell and multiplies there. One virus may produce 100 replicas of itself in an hour. The antibodies, large protein molecules circulating in the blood, present a defense against viruses, bacteria and other foreign agents. The body creates a unique antibody for each virus that enters. Even more amazing, it never forgets how to reproduce these antibodies when needed. It is this memory for antibodies which constitutes our immune system.

Another group of proteins in the bloodstream are referred to as transport proteins. These serve to carry nutrients and other molecules to various cells in the body. Calcium and iron enter the body with the help of a protein through the membrane of the intestines. Specialized lipoproteins transport the lipid molecules to and from storage. Also, many vitamins are moved from one place to another with the help of proteins.

Perhaps protein is best known for its role in growth and body formation. It is responsible for the construction of scars, bones, teeth and even pigment in the retina.

Protein Deficiency

Protein is involved in nearly every function of the body, as are all the other nutrients. This illustrates the most important rule of nutrition: no nutrient functions alone.

Because malnutrition of any kind causes the body to use protein, protein deficiency can be found in any person who suffers from a general lack of food. When children are deprived of food, any food, they suffer a calorie deficit and begin using the protein of their own body to create energy. Unlike other deficiencies, protein deficiency is rarely caused by a lack of that specific nutrient.

The Dangers of Excess Protein

Most people in the Western world eat too much protein. The recommended dietary allowance is about .35 grams per pound of ideal body weight, assuming the quality of protein is high and calorie intake is adequate. The per capita level of protein has averaged about 1.6 times the RDA since 1900. That is exactly double what it should be.

The form in which you get your protein is important. Diets containing animal proteins tend to produce a hypercholesterolemia (cholesterol overload), whereas those containing plant proteins produce low plasma cholesterol levels.

Fake Amino Acids

Aspartame, a sugar substitute sold commercially as Nutra Sweet, is advertised as the more pleasant replacement for saccharin. It tastes like sugar and is made of two apparently harmless amino acids, the building blocks of protein. Discovered in 1965, it was approved for limited use in 1981. In 1983, the FDA approved its use in soft drinks. Within 3 years, its use increased to 10% of the overall sugar intake and continues to rise. While food manufacturers readily add it to presweetened cereals and drink mixes, it is not suitable for use in foods that are heated for any length of time, as it breaks down into chemicals that are no longer sweet.

As often as it was applauded by the industry, aspartame was assailed in other quarters. The first problem it created was phenylketonuria (PKU). Today one out of 20,000 babies is born without the ability to metabolize phenylalanine, one of the two amino acids that make up aspartame. Toxic levels of aspartame

186

can result in mental retardation for infants unable to metabolize it. As a result, the FDA requires all packaged goods containing aspartame to bear a warning notice for the benefit of people with PKU. Unfortunately, foods served at restaurants or cafeterias are not covered by this regulation, and the food industry continues to add 5 million pounds per day to our food supply.

Scientists also believe that high doses of aspartame pose risks to the unborn babies of pregnant women who do not have the disease themselves but may carry the trait for the disease. Just a few artificially sweetened foods per day may cause their babies to be born mentally retarded. Other scientists are concerned that aspartame might alter brain activity, cause brain tumors, and bring about behavior changes in consumers. In fact, many people complain of headaches, dizziness or menstrual problems after consuming the product.

VITAMINS

A relatively recent addition to the list of seven essential nutrients, vitamins are needed for peak performance. Unlike fats, carbohydrates and protein, they are not energy nutrients, they are energy releasers. Essential to many chemical reactions in the body that affect your performance throughout the day, vitamins take part in metabolism and help deliver energy to individual cells.

Like all other nutrients, vitamins are divided into different groups based on their chemical make-up. The body must metabolize or break down every food put into it in order to use the nutrients or store them for later use.

187

Water-Soluble Vitamins

The body uses vitamins in two ways. Water-soluble vitamins are distributed to the water-filled compartments of the body to be circulated in the bloodstream before elimination. Fat-soluble vitamins are immediately stored for later use in lipids. Because of this difference, water-soluble vitamins are depleted more easily, but are less likely to reach toxic levels. Both types of vitamins, however, are necessary for balanced nutrition.

The two water-soluble vitamins, B and C, were named after the test tube designations used for experimental collection. Researchers discovered that the test tube containing vitamin B actually contained a number of different vitamins. These were eventually numbered and given names of their own.

B Vitamins

Each B vitamin has its own unique role in nutrition. For example, when food is taken into the body, it is immediately put on the "disassembly line." During metabolism, the body mechanically takes apart the molecules and reassembles them to form needed cell structures. The machinery used for this disassembly is built of enzymes, and the switch that turns each enzyme on is a co-enzyme, a B vitamin. Without coenzymes, enzymes cannot function, and without enzymes, the body's entire food factory comes to a screeching halt.

The eight B vitamins that function as coenzymes are: thiamine (B-1), riboflavin (B-2), niacin (B-3), pyridoxal (B-6), folacin (also known as folic acid), cobalmin (B-12), biotin, and pantothenic acid. If the body lacks any one of these B vitamins—niacin for example — the enzymes involved in every step of the glucose-to-energy pathway fail to function. As energy for the body's activities is made available by means of these steps, everything slows to a stop. Signs of niacin deficiency begin with dermatitis, a flaking of the skin. Eventually diarrhea may result. Because glucose is the brain's only source of energy, insanity can occur in severe cases of niacin deficiency. These are only the most obvious signs. Any lack of niacin affects the body in many more subtle ways.

Another B vitamin, folacin can have a similar effect on health, but without clearly noticeable symptoms. Folacin creates a coenzyme to assist in the replication of intestinal cells. Because cells that make up the lining of the intestinal wall change constantly, a deficiency in folacin can have serious effects on digestion.

Oddly enough, though we know a great deal about their individual molecular functions, we are unable to say precisely why a deficiency of any one B vitamin produces a particular disease. This is partly due to the fact that deficiencies of single B vitamins seldom show up in isolation. All in all, the benefits of B vitamins are much better known.

Niacin, or vitamin B-3, has been credited with lowering cholestrol levels, and even with reversing the process of atherosclerosis. B-6, pyridoxine, is known for its beneficial influence on neurotransmitters of the brain and for relieving seizures and convulsions in infants. Studies are currently being done relating B-6 to relief of stress and strengthening of the immune system. Vitamin B-6 is used in hundreds of reactions in the body and works with zinc to properly metabolize essential fatty acids.

Vitamin C

Nearly 200 years after citrus fruit was first found to cure scurvy, its beneficial active compound was isolated and named ascorbic acid, or vitamin C. The main role of vitamin C is the formation of collagen, the single most important protein in connective tissue. Collagen holds together everything from scars to cells, and helps artery walls withstand the constant expansion and contraction of heart beats. Vitamin C is also involved in the metabolism of several amino acids and is released by the adrenal glands during times of stress. As an anti-oxidant, it has been shown to block some of the cancer-causing substances found in food, such as nitrosoamines.

Though vitamin C comes in tablet form, the best sources, as with other vitamins, are whole foods rich in a multitude of nutrients. Citrus fruits are well-known for their vitamin C content, but C can also be found in broccoli, brussel sprouts, greens, cabbage, cantaloupe, strawberries, and others.

Fat-Soluble Vitamins

Like water-soluble vitamins, fat-soluble vitamins—A, D, E, and K—are essential for maintaining peak performance. Their method of storage makes them less vulnerable, however, than water-soluble vitamins. Found in the fat and oily parts of foods, they tend to move into the liver and adipose tissue and remain there, rather than be regularly excreted. This method of storage makes it possible to go for long periods of time without them, but they are no less important.

Vitamin A

Vitamin A, also known as beta carotene, has long been known for its role in vision. When the eyes are functioning properly, they receive light and transform it into signals that travel to the brain, where a mental picture is displayed. For this to happen, they must transform light energy into nerve impulses. These transformers are the molecules of pigment in the cells of the retina. Retinal, which is part of this pigment, is a compound the body can synthesize only when vitamin A is present.

As important as sight may seem, only one-thousandth of the vitamin A in the body is in the retina. Much more is in the body's skin and linings of internal organs. Vitamin A even plays a role in maintaining the integrity of the mucous membranes. When vitamin A is not present, tissues are dry and unable to protect themselves against infection. Vitamin A is also important in building bones. With the help of vitamin A, certain enzymes are activated to remove parts of a bone no longer needed as the bone grows. Interestingly, an unborn baby has a tail but loses it before birth due to processes involving vitamin A.

The most common signs of vitamin A deficiency are related to the eye: nightblindness, drying eyes, spots on the cornea and, in extreme circumstances, blindness. Other signs of deficiency can be seen in the skin, body linings, bones and teeth. White spots often appear on the nails. The lungs are more susceptible to infection, diarrhea may occur, joints may be painful and teeth may crack.

On the other side of the coin, excess of vitamin A can cause toxic reactions. Red blood cells may lose some of their oxygen. Loss of appetite, fatigue, headaches, nausea, vomiting and weight loss may occur.

The best way to avoid both deficiencies and excesses of vitamin A, as with all vitamins, is to eat an abundance of whole food. The safest form of vitamin A, beta carotene, is in fact found only in plants.

Vitamin D

While vitamin A helps to reconstruct bones, vitamin D helps to mineralize them. By raising the concentration of calcium in blood, vitamin D helps to create a sturdy skeleton.

One of the amazing facts about vitamin D is its unusual origin. Using the much maligned substance cholesterol, the body creates vitamin D with the help of the sun. When ultraviolet rays hit the compound sent by the liver to the skin, this compound (7-dehydrocholesterol) is converted to vitamin D. Fortunately the sun is not the only source of vitamin D. It can be obtained from eggs, liver and fish.

The consequence of vitamin D deficiency is a disease known as rickets, whose symptoms are similar to those of calcium deficiency. Bones fail to calcify and form abnormally. An overdose of vitamin D can be equally serious. Toxicity can be produced by high levels of fortification in many western foods, notably milk. When toxicity occurs, more calcium is drawn into the blood, causing soft tissues to calcify.

The most preferred way to reach peak performance is to obtain vitamin D through natural sources such as sunlight. Though we have undoubtedly been exposed to the cancer scare about getting too much sun, it has recently been documented that polyunsaturated fats (corn oil, soy oil, safflower oil, etc.) have a negative reaction when exposed to sunlight, a reaction which promotes the development of skin cancer. Oils taken in naturally by eating seeds and beans do not seem to cause a problem. However, when oil is *extracted* from corn, soybeans, safflowers and vegetables, the density and high concentration of fat can be harmful. While peanut oil is a monounsaturated oil, aflatoxins found in some peanut oils make it less than the oil of choice. Thus, it is important to use virgin olive oil or canola oil (monounsaturated oils.)

Vitamin K

Closely allied with vitamin D is vitamin K. Its primary function is in the formation of blood clots, though it also participates with vitamin D in regulating calcium levels in blood. Because vitamin K is manufactured by the body, deficiency and toxicity are rarely problems. Vitamin K is found in vegetables.

Vitamin E

Last of the fat-soluble vitamins is vitamin E. Its function in the maintenance of healthy body cells is very similar to that of vitamin C. In the lungs, vitamin E protects cells from continuous exposure to oxygen, other gases and air pollutants. Vitamin E also protects polyunsaturated fatty acids, such as the linoleic and linolenic acid, from oxidation. A deficiency of vitamin E suppresses the immune system and supplementation stimulates it in several species of animals.

Many claims have been made about the benefits of vitamin E. Two in particular relate to its proven corrective role in neurological dysfunction and cysts or soreness in breasts.

A curious aspect of vitamin E is its extreme vulnerability to fish oils. Fish oils are highly oxidizing and cause a lowering of vitamin E levels in blood, even when 1000 IU are taken per day with fish oil capsules. It's a mystery where all the vitamin E goes, but until the problem is solved, it is recommended that people avoid consuming high levels of fish oil. Eat the whole fish instead, and cut off the fat. Vitamin E is found in the germ of whole grains.

Both water-soluble and fat-soluble vitamins are closely related to the body's energy system and also to the last group of essential nutrients, trace minerals. Knowing how each of them works contributes to an understanding of the importance of a varied diet. There is no magical vitamin pill that can cure any illness, just as there is no constellation made up of only one star. To find the champion within requires the entire array of vitamins and minerals working hand in hand with the energy nutrients.

MINERALS

Water

Though water is not a mineral, its close association with minerals makes it a logical place to begin a discussion of our last group of essential nutrients.

One of the most important roles of the body's water is maintenance of blood pressure. This pressure against the capillary walls ensures that nutrients, oxygen and waste can move in and out of cells. When blood reaches the capillaries, whose thin walls permit fluid passage, much of its fluid and small dissolved molecules exit. Fluid from the tissue cells then seeps back into the capillaries, which then carry carbon dioxide and other waste away. When blood pressure falls, this process is threatened, at which point the kidneys set in motion a mechanism to raise the blood pressure and hopefully to restore the normal process.

Sodium and Potassium

While many dietary factors affect blood pressure, sodium and potassium produce the most noticeable changes. When sodium is retained by the body, the vital mineral potassium is traded for it. This exchange disrupts what is known as the electrolyte balance. For normal electrolyte balance, sodium and potassium levels need to remain about equal. For several reasons in recent history, this balance has been disrupted, the result being increased high blood pressure in many populations.

One way to upset the balance is by consuming foods high in sodium and low in potassium. Foods that naturally contain sodium such as vegetables, normally contain potassium as well, because most other forms of life have a similar electrolyte balance to maintain. However, when we add salt to food, a compound high in sodium, the balance is disrupted. While the body can deal with minor disruptions, major disruptions, such as those caused by processed foods, have more serious consequences. When foods are processed, their cells are damaged. This causes them to spill their sodium and potassium contents. In most cases the sodium is put back in as salt for flavor and preservation, but potassium is not replaced. Thus, the more whole and unprocessed a food is, the more ideal its sodium-potassium ratio. The more processed a food is, the poorer its ratio. That is why one is well advised to stay away from processed foods.

Calcium, Magnesium, Boron

The reason for examining these three minerals together is their close interconnectedness in the human metabolism. None can work independently of the others. What is also unusual is that an excess of any one of them can cause symptoms of deficiency in the others.

Along with protein, **calcium** is one of the most overrated nutrients in the American diet (see Appendix D, "Calcium the Killer"). Though the worldwide average RDA for calcium is 400 milligrams per day, in the U.S. the RDA is set at 800 milligrams, exactly double. The reason for this increase has absolutely no foundation in scientific research, which leads to a number of

196

questions. It has been postulated that special interest groups, such as the meat and dairy lobbies, are at the root of the problem. Because protein consumption is so high in the U.S., the RDA for calcium has been adjusted accordingly so as not to upset the "economics" of meat consumption. If protein consumption were reduced to a reasonable and healthy level, 400 milligrams of dietary calcium would be more than sufficient, provided magnesium and boron intakes remained at a healthy level.

This is not to imply that calcium is not important, because it definitely is. For one thing, it is linked to blood pressure. There is abundant documentation that people who drink hard water, high in calcium and magnesium, have lower blood pressure, on the average. Generally speaking, the higher the calcium intake the lower the blood pressure in the United States.

Another role of calcium involves the transportation of molecules in and out of cells. It is essential for muscle and nerve action and must be present for blood to clot.

The role we all are most familiar with is the one calcium plays in bone formation. Without it, bones deteriorate and eventually become porous, a condition known as osteoporosis, which literally means "porous bone." What is less known is that calcium cannot and does not work alone. Without adequate supplies of magnesium, boron and vitamin D, all of the calcium in the world is for naught. Each is an essential bone tissue component.

In the case of **magnesium,** hundreds of enzymatic reactions, such as converting calories, facilitating proper muscle action and maintaining regular heartbeat, can't happen without it. Unfortunately the magnesium level in the American diet is horribly inadequate due to low consumption of vegetables and whole grains. Moreover, most supplements do not provide magnesium in a usable form, as magnesium in and of itself is insoluble, and therefore useless in the human body.

Recently discovered as a nutrient important to good health, **boron** also serves several functions. In a recent study conducted by Dr. Forrest Nielsen of the U.S. Department of Agriculture Human Nutrition Research Laboratory, it was found that within eight days of supplementing 3 milligrams of boron, a test group of post-menopausal women lost 40% less calcium and 33% less magnesium in the urine. The same women retained the equivalent of 1000 milligrams more calcium than the control group in a twenty day period, which translates into a 5% yearly increase in calcium bone content.

Dr. Nielsen's study further revealed that beneficial hormonal levels were also affected. Among women, the most active form of estrogen increased significantly. In men, testosterone levels rose upon boron supplementation. The conclusion was that boron works with the body's own hormones to produce beneficial effects without exposure to the dangers associated with traditional hormonal therapy. Most post-menopausal women lose 1 to 5% yearly.

Boron is also essential to the process of locking calcium and magnesium into bone matter. Its negative ion combines with positive ions of these two other minerals and cements them in place. Beyond that, it is indispensable to the conversion of vitamin D from food and from sunlight on the skin into active vitamin D.

While good sources of boron include apples, pears, and leafy vegetables, the USDA found that stabilized flax is the best source of all. Only two tablespoons per day meet the recommended dietary allowance of 2 milligrams.

Phosphorus

The only mineral more plentiful than phosphorus in the body is calcium. About 85% of this phosphorus occurs in combination with calcium in bones and teeth. It is this bond which gives bones their rigid structure. Also found in DNA cells, which contain the code for all growth, phosphorus is so abundant in natural foods, and especially processsed foods, that deficiencies of it are virtually unknown. High consumption of soft drinks can overload the body with phosphorous, defeating its purpose.

Iron

Iron is vital to cell respiration, the process of generating energy. Every human cell— in fact, every living cell of every kind— contains iron. Iron is also found in many of the enzymes that break down nutrients into their usable parts and is involved in carrying oxygen throughout the body. Because iron is used to create every blood cell in the body, deficiencies can have serious effects, most notably fatigue, lowered immunity and reduced learning ability. Iron deficiency, otherwise known as anemia, is especially a problem for women, who lose blood regularly through menstruation, and for children who are growing and constantly increasing their blood volume.

When attempting to increase your iron supply, it is not enough to eat high-iron food. You must also increase your body's capacity for iron absorption. To do this means knowing what contributes to, and what detracts from, the absorption process. The main contributor is vitamin C, found in all citrus fruit; the main detractors, oddly enough, are coffee and tea. Thus, when any good source of iron such as meat is eaten, the presence of coffee dramatically reduces absorption. For those who eat little or no meat, an excellent supplement of this mineral is carbonyl iron. Also because vitamin C increases absorption, a combination of orange juice and an iron source such as wheat bran is ideal.

Zinc

Another mineral whose deficiency causes very serious consequences is zinc. As noted in the discussion of protein, wherever zinc is found, protein will also be found helping zinc to do its job. Zinc is so tightly connected with the health of human tissues that in times of deficiency the body will break down its own tissue to get at it.

Other important functions of zinc relate to the development of healthy teeth, the building of the immune system to protect against infection, and the metabolism of protein and fatty acids. Zinc deficiency can alter growth in children, cause diarrhea, disturb the metabolism, alter the sense of taste and slow the healing process. Its symptoms are so diverse that deficiency is incorrectly diagnosed as malnutrition. Fortunately, zinc does not pose the same absorption problems as iron. Dietary sources are whole wheat, fresh greens, seafood and animal protein.

Iodine

The last of our essential minerals is iodine. Best known for its role in the thyroid, it is involved with regulating body temperature, metabolic rate, reproduction, growth, and proper muscle function. Its most common sources are seawater and soil, through which it enters indirectly into the diet by means of the food production chain. In many locations, such as the central areas of the United States, Canada and Africa, the soil is iodine poor and seawater is not available. To compensate, iodine is added to salt. Because of iodized salt, nearly all maladies associated with iodine deficiency, such as goiters and other diseases of the thyroid, have been eliminated.

A FINAL NOTE: WHO IS HUNGRY?

Many theories have been put forth to explain appetite. The glucostatic theory of hunger proposes that the blood glucose level determines whether or not we feel the need to eat; the lipostatic theory maintains that hunger depends on the size of our fat stores; and the purinergic theory says that circulating levels of purines, molecules found in DNA and RNA, rule our hunger pangs. Any and all of these theories may be correct, though in the final analysis, hunger is a signal from the brain that it's time to replenish the body's nutrients.

201

Unfortunately the way we respond to this signal is influenced or determined by the food industry, which has a vested interest in how often and what food we eat. Often the food we reach for is not the best food for us.

As James Hightower puts it in his book, *Eat Your Heart Out*, "It is not that food firms are trying to produce bad food. Rather, what they are trying to produce is profits, and they have learned that in order to expand their markets, in order to keep growing and commanding a bigger share of the market, they feel they must process and sweeten, process and add salt, process and add color dyes and flavor chemicals."

Researchers at the Monell Chemical Senses Center found that low-calorie sweeteners such as Aspartame can actually lead to obesity. Apparently the taste of sweeteners triggers the bodys' conversion of blood glucose into saturated fat. This causes low blood sugar, which in turn sends out the signal to eat. The end result is a self-perpetuating cycle between low-cal sweeteners and higher food consumption, ultimately leading to weight gain. Is this happening to you?

Like artificial sweeteners, processed foods in general are more profitable for a variety of reasons. With much of the food value removed and dozens of preservatives added, processed foods last practically forever. When flavors, colors, texture, and even the food itself is synthesized, food manufacturers are freed from dealing with the cost and bother of preserving real foods such as fresh vegetables and fruit. More importantly, foods can be designed to push "consumer hot buttons," industry lingo for the real or imagined needs of the public.

Shelf-life is clearly one of the industry's most vital priorities. It is not at all unusual for freshness codes on food packages to indicate a product will still be at optimum freshness almost a year after it arrives in the store. An article in *Progressive* by Daniel Zwerdling ("The Food Monsters," 1980, p.22) reported that food engineers at the Campbell Soup Company are working on a process to keep their foods fresh for two to three years.

Prolonged shelf-life, heralded by the food giants, would be a shining scientific accomplishment indeed if it were not for the fact that organic microbes are after the same nutrients your body is. Many of these microbes resemble those in your digestive tract. That food won't spoil is simply an indication that microbes responsible for spoilage can't survive on it. If they can't survive, this should be a definite sign your body can't either. Rarely does this enter the minds of company executives obsessed with prolonging the shelf-life of their products. What matters to them is: (1) they will be able to stock pile when commodity prices are low and have their stock last long enough to get them through periods of high commodity prices; (2) they can centralize their location and ship processed foods from one spot to all parts of the nation and every corner of the world; and (3) grocers will snap up a product that lasts a year and turn down foods that may spoil in a couple of days or weeks.

It is particularly ironic that food giants love to brag about product "freshness" in their advertising. Bread manufacturers assume they can proclaim everlasting freshness if their product stays soft and white for several days on the shelf. When canning companies put out firm and brightly-colored canned corn, they may venture to name a brand line "Fresh." Orange juice producers may invent an overly tart, substandard fruit juice and say that it has been "fresh frozen."

The way things are going in the food industry, there may come a time in the near future when food companies will bypass Mother Nature altogether. According to the United States General Accounting Office, almost 80% of the additives in food are cosmetic. Instead of real lemonade, what you drink consists of sodium caseinate and artificial flavoring. Instead of real food, the processed food you eat is a conglomerate of high-priced chemistry experiments designed to simulate food. In the words of Albert Clausi, vice-president of General Foods, "In my business, commodity is sort of a bad word." When did fresh, real food to which the term commodity refers become a "bad word"?

I hope I'm not suggesting that the food industry is intentionally trying to sabotage the American diet or that memos float around offices saying, "Make the stuff less nutritional." In reality, few people in the food industry probably realize what is happening. Food manufacturers undoubtedly believe they have the consumer's interest at heart. They make what we want to eat. When consumers buy processed products for the sake of convenience, manufacturers respond with the message: "We're giving them what they want." Likewise, researchers are praised and promoted when they make "differentiations" which improve product sales, and with alarming frequency these changes amount to adding sugar, fat and salt and processing out nutrients, all of which are catastrophic to our health.

9

FAT AT 32 ... FIT AT 42

At age 32, Roy Pirrung of Sheboygan, Wisconsin, was 45 pounds overweight, smoked 2 packs of cigarettes a day, and puffed and wheezed just to walk up stairs.

At age 42, Roy is a fit, trim, 5'7" ultra-marathoner who is one of the best long distance runners in the world! He exudes good health, and this is his story.

There must be an epiphany, a sudden moment of recognition, for a person to completely turn his or her life and health around. Roy had his epiphany while on a ladder painting his house. From that vantage he could see a woman, bordering on criminal obesity, chugging along in her jogging clothes. As he watched her, he couldn't help but think about his own battle with losing weight. Roy had always had a weight problem. He'd diet religiously, take off a few pounds, only to slide back into his careless eating habits.   The lost pounds were always replaced with a few extra, which meant Roy was "dieting" to become progressively heavier.

In 1981, the fat was climbing again as Roy stood on his ladder and arrived at a conclusion about himself. If this very fat woman, jogging slower than a walk, could discipline herself to exercise and be concerned about herself, so could he. At that moment, as a birthday gift to himself, he vowed that he would change his life style, clean up his diet, quit smoking, and start running his way to good health.

He began by buying magazines such as *Runner's World* and became particularly fascinated with marathons. One of the many articles read at that time dealt with the importance of nutrition and diet. Stressing the connection between eating properly and maintaining peak performance, the article emphasized eating whole grain products, vegetables, and fruit, and avoiding sugar, soft drinks, tobacco and junk food in general.

Roy took the article to heart and consulted with his wife. The two of them resolved to revamp their diet and make an earnest effort to improve their life style. Only one year later, Roy completed his first full-length marathon, a distance of over 26 miles, and has never stopped to look back.

By the end of 1982, Roy had long given up smoking, his weight was down to 140 pounds and he was feeling stronger than ever. One day, not long after his first marathon, he was out for a run, when a woman stopped to offer him a ride. It was the same woman he had seen jogging by his house. During the course of their brief conversation, Roy learned that his entire fate and "new life" depended on a misperception. The woman was not out jogging for the health of it. This was simply her way of getting down to McDonald's for her morning coffee and sweet roll. For Roy it was a good chuckle, knowing that his life would never be the same because of that coffee and sweet roll.

In October on 1983, Roy ran once again in the Milwaukee Lakefront Marathon. As he remembers, "My training and nutrition programs were getting me places I never dreamed possible. With ease I completed the marathon in 2:38:47. I was ecstatic and could not wait to take on the hills of the famous Boston Marathon.

"April of 1984 found the family flying to Boston. I remember the flight as being totally non-smoking because there had been so many requests by runners for the non-smoking section that they just made the entire flight free of smoke.

"I completed the Boston Marathon in the low 2:40 range with some severely blistered feet. My thrill at having run so well displaced any pain I may have felt, because for the first time I knew I was a real athlete.

"The Ice Age Trail 50-Mile Run was my first ultra-race and it earned me a fifth place finish in 7 hours and 12 minutes. Another runner challenged me to enter a 24-hour run at Fruth Field in Fond du Lac, Wisconsin. I accepted, as by now challenging myself had become a part of me.

"The gun went off at 8 a.m. that Labor Day Weekend and I steadily clicked off the miles. The state record stood at 119 miles and I went through 100 miles in a little over 15 hours and still felt pretty good. (My challenger was taking a nap!) The following day at 8 a.m. I had completed 137.99 miles, 18 miles over the record.

"With this exhilarating experience, a whole new world of running opened up to me. I began researching and reading up on this unique aspect of ultra running. The 24-hour event led me to be a guest speaker at the All Nations Running Events alongside two of my heroes, Patti Cattalano-Lyons and 10,000-meter Olympic champion Billy Mills."

As Roy's full time job with the Kohler Co. in Sheboygan, Wisconsin, is very physically demanding, he had to condition himself and plan his time off for racing very carefully. He began setting a personal goal to run the granddaddy of all ultra-marathons, the Spartathlon, a grueling 155 miles from Athens to Sparta, Greece.

To get to Greece he needed to prove he was now a world-class runner. In September, 1988, he ran the TAC/USA 24-Hour National Championships in Atlanta, Georgia.

This is Roy's description of how the race went: "We were on the outer edge of Hurricane Gilbert's path. The weather in Atlanta was cooler than normal, with rain ranging from mist to drizzle to heavy downpour. The rain let up after about 6 hours. I had held back during the early miles to see what the weather would do to everyone. I was feeling great and ready for more.

"By 100 kilometers, I assumed the lead more or less by attrition. Those who had gone out hard were paying for their decision. I began to gain on the rest of the field. I had wanted to reach the 100 mile mark in 15 hours, but was ahead of schedule with a 14:37 split time. Not only was I ahead of my schedule, but I was also ahead of the competition by quite some distance.

"I felt strong throughout the entire race. I had eaten properly as I had brought a supply of Natural Ovens breads, fruits, and bottled water and had kept well-hydrated not only on the inside but on the outside as well. At the end of 24 hours, I had won the open division as well as the Masters to secure my second and third National Championship titles. The runner-up had 133 miles, 795 yards, compared to my new road-course American Record of 145 miles, 1464 yards.

"To start 1989 off on the right foot, I accepted an offer of sponsorship from Paul and Barbara Stitt, owners of Natural Ovens of Manitowoc, Wisconsin, and Essential Nutrient Research Corporation (ENRECO). It was Paul who introduced me to a new product called ALENA Energy Drink.

"The Energy Drink is a combination of stabilized, fortified flax, oats, malted barley and a number of other ingredients which has truly become a source of energy for me. My training took on an entirely different meaning. Workouts seemed easier, I recovered quickly, and was ready for another hard workout the following day. I was amazed and let the Stitts know of my discovery.

"Paul had no idea his food, developed primarily for arthritics and cardiac rehabilitation patients, could have such a positive effect on a healthy person. His research immediately took on new meaning for me. To have a product help those with some physical problem as well as those without any ailments was extraordinary.

"I began setting new personal records (PR's). This was done without any additional training or changes in my regular program. The only change was the inclusion of the Energy Drink everyday for breakfast.

"I did a 50-mile road race into a strong 35 mph headwind and set a new PR by over 2 minutes. The 50 had seemed so easy, and I could only credit the Energy Drink.

"One month later I did a one-mile road race to see how the Energy Drink had influenced my speed. I had done no specific training for a one mile event, as everything had been geared to the ultra distance.

"Much to my surprise, at age 41, I completed this one mile dash in 4:51, three seconds faster than my time of 4:54 set many years earlier when I was much younger and training specifically for shorter distances.

"One week later I ran the Sri Chinmoy 100-mile TAC/USA National Championship and established four new PR's for the 50-kilometer, 50-mile, 100-kilometer splits and 100-mile splits. My finishing time, good for the Masters title (my fourth in less than two years), was also a new PR. To top it off, my 13:15:50 was the sixth fastest ever run by a North American and set an American 40-44 age group record.

"As testimony to the Energy Drink mix, the morning of the race I consumed my usual 4 tablespoons with water. During the race I ate the breads that have taken me through these events in the past. I credit my new found nutritional aid with taking my 50-mile PR down 14 minutes and my 100-mile PR down 45 minutes. My 100-mile time was over an hour and twenty-two minutes faster than the previous year.

"To celebrate our victories, the leader Rae Clark went along with my idea of running the 10-kilometer race in Central Park the following day. For me it would be doubly special as it would be my 300th race since that day 8 years ago when the fat lady inspired this fat 32 year old to begin running!

"People were amazed we were doing a 10K just 12 hours after running the 100-mile race. Rae and I had challenged each other to see who could run the fastest last mile in the 100-mile race. Rae's 100th on Saturday was 6:50 and mine was 6:50:7. On Sunday we kept up a 6:50 per mile pace for the entire way, side by side, but Rae let me edge him out at the finish line because he said today was my special day. 300 races in 8 years!

"Now for the big one...the Spartathlon! In preparation for the race date of September 29th and 30th, 1989, I geared all my training towards distance. The miles added up quickly and the time seemed to fly past. I was running in excess of 100 miles per week, doing about 70 miles on the bicycle, 150 sit ups, and 50 pushups daily, and faithfully stretching after each run.

"Fortunately for me there was a trained naprapathic physician and massage therapist on staff at Natural Ovens, mainly for their employees. Paul suggested I use her services and I began weekly treatment sessions. I have to admit I was skeptical, as I had always believed in the philosophy, "if it ain't broke, don't fix it," and really had to force myself to return each week. Her fingers digging and probing left me sore at first. I gave it more time and to my astonishment I began enjoying the treatment at each weekly session, which now began leaving my body supple and relaxed.

"One thing I enjoy as much as running is racing. I planned my races carefully but never tapered off for any of them. I really didn't care what my performances were like. Mileage was the key ingredient in my training program and racing was just for fun.

"Much to my surprise my race performances were dramatically improved and I collected 16 new PR's in 1989, up to the week before Greece. A couple of them were raced during peak mileage weeks, and again there was no taper. The following day after the race I resumed my schedule of long miles. Fast recovery was a new ingredient that added spice to my training.

"Once my entry for the Spartathlon was confirmed by the USA liaison, Marvin Skagerberg, the excitement began. The stamp of approval came from the International Spartathlon Association, and I was on my way to run in the footsteps of Pheidippides along the route St. Paul had walked.

"Paul Stitt went with me as my handler to make sure my food and drink was ready at each check point. Seventy-eight runners representing 18 countries lined the steps leading to the stadium that set the stage for the revival of the Olympic tradition. A trumpet fanfare started the race, and we were off.

"I assumed the lead from the start, startled that no one was near. I felt good and ran easily in the lead through Old Corinth. At 75 kilometers I was passed by Patrick Macke of the United Kingdom, and Rune Larson of Sweden pulled alongside me. We ran together for 5 kilometers before he pulled ahead. They had established their finish order.

"The drama of the conditions of the Spartathlon was incredible. We started in Athens in 90 degree temperature through the smog that did not lift for several miles. Some wore masks.

"Then it turned cool and began raining heavily. By the time we reached the highest mountain, it was slippery, muddy and so dark that we all had to be guided by lights in order to keep on the trail. Then we went over the peak and headed down the mountain with just our penlights to guide us through the washed out pot holes in the trail. My sense of hearing and smell were keenly aware of the dogs dashing to the end of their chains, and the herds of goats along the way.

"Sunrise found me out of the mountain and heading toward Sparta. At 178 kilometers, I had been overtaken by a Japanese runner and he eventually finished in third place with me in fourth, six hours and twenty four minutes faster than any American had ever run the course!

"During the course of my 27 hours on the 155 miles of roads and trails between Athens and Sparta, Greece, I had time to reflect. It was important at the time to recall many of the things that had gotten me there. All the training and sacrifices were worth it to be able to be a part of the magnificent Spartathlon and be ranked as one of the top ultra-runners in the world.

"Somewhere between seeing that fat lady jogging a half mile to the restaurant for her sweet roll and back home, and touching the Statue of King Leonidas in Sparta, Greece, the fat man in me had finally escaped and had been replaced by a champion within.

"As this book goes to press, my preparations will have been completed for running the 1990 Spartathlon in September and I'm going to race for the gold."

10

WHAT ABOUT THE CHILDREN?

Each year the complaints mount up concerning decreased learning ability among our children, poorer physical fitness, inattentiveness and shorter attention span. Often forced to spend more time keeping order in the classroom than expanding our children's minds, many teachers feel as though they have been reduced to surrogate baby sitters. In general, teacher and student morale is disappointingly low.

Where have we gone wrong? Have we failed in passing along to our children the value of learning and education, or is our educational system at fault? While undoubtedly there are many causes and equally as many explanations, more and more people are beginning to examine our children's diet and how it may be working against the psychological, emotional, and mental conditioning needed to learn well.

In addition to confirming that fewer than 10% of the people in the U.S. eat adequate amounts of fruit and vegetables on a daily basis, the National Cancer Institute found that 22% never eat any vegetables or fruit at all. Now that is truly amazing! Nearly a quarter of the population—sixty million people—never expose their bodies to the nutrients in bananas, apples, oranges, pears, peaches, cherries, broccoli, cauliflower, beans, corn, peas, spinach, carrots, and on and on.

It is a fact, verified repeatedly in nutritional research throughout the world, that mental, emotional, and physical wellness are products of diet. Knowing this, is it any wonder that the children of America are not performing to their full capabilities in school?

The real picture becomes much clearer when we begin to look at the behavioral problems caused by various nutrient deficiencies. (This and other information used throughout this chapter was established in a review of nearly 400 scientific studies on the subject of diet and wellness.)

- **Thiamine (vitamin B-1) deficiency can result in confusion, poor coordination, depressed appetite, irritability, sleep disturbances, fatigue and general malaise.**

- **Riboflavin (vitamin B-2) deficiency can cause depression, hysteria, psychopathic behavior, lethargy, and general malaise.**

- **Niacin (vitamin B-3) deficiency can cause irritability, insomnia, weakness, mental depression, fatigue, and headaches.**

When we observe our children displaying symptoms of irritability, mental depression, fatigue and depressed appetite, how often do we associate these symptoms with B-vitamin deficiency? Moreover, how many of us would know where to go to in the market to get food rich in B-vitamins? For your information, B-vitamins are abundant in **whole grains**, such as wheat germ, wheat bran, and rice bran.

Now ask yourself how much rice your family consumes on a weekly basis—not the quick-cooking variety of white rice, which has most of its nutrients removed by the manufacturing process, but rather natural brown rice, which takes a little longer to prepare but is nutrient-rich. Also ask yourself how much whole grain bread your family consumes. The soft, white budget varieties don't count, as they have little to offer by way of nutrition.

If your answer to both questions is, "not much," then consider this. The consumption of sugar virtually negates vitamin B-1 and knocks it completely out of your system. Do your children eat a lot of sugar? Of course they do. Nearly everyone in the U.S. has a sweet tooth and consumes enormous amounts of sugar each year in dozens of different forms, from candy to chewing gum. Given our heavy sugar dependency, vitamin B-1 has little chance of staying around long in the body if in fact it ever gets in there in the first place.

Essentially, the nutrient needs of the human body have remained constant for thousands of years. And during that time, the human diet remained fairly stable and consistent, that is, until very recently. During the last 40 years, because of the speed at which society moves and increased needs for quickness and convenience, our diet has undergone dramatic changes. No longer are we eating the whole, natural foods that best sustain us. Rather we are relying on processed food and convenience food to get us by. And it's taking a heavy toll, perhaps most noticeably on our children.

Mimicking their parents, many of our children start the day without breakfast. Sure, they may eat a bowl of sugared cereal, a donut or sweet roll, or even a soda and candy bar. But as far as nutrition is concerned, that is not a breakfast. In other words, most of our children immediately begin the day with nutrient deficiency, which means they begin with the certain expectation of functioning inadequately, both emotionally and mentally. Whatever niacin they may have consumed in their cereal, if they ate any, has been completely obliterated by the cereal's sugar.

This is how the day goes without niacin, if we might borrow from research done by Dr. T.D. Spies, one of the first to study "sub-clinical pellagra," or niacin (vitamin B-3) deficiency:

> **Sub-clinical pellagrans are noted for the multiplicity of complaints. The most common of these are fatigue, insomnia, anorexia, vertigo, burning sensations in various parts of the body, numbness, headaches, forgetfulness, apprehension, palpitations, nervousness, a feeling of unrest and anxiety, and distractability. The conduct of a pellegran may be normal but he feels incapable of mental or physical effort.**

If all of this can result from the absence of only one essential nutrient from our diet, imagine the consequences of nutritional deficiency in general. Let's look at some other things our bodies and bodies of our children might be going without.

Vitamin B-5 (pantothenic acid)

Also known as vitamin B-5, pantothenic acid is found in small amounts in almost all plant life and is needed by every cell in the body. Dr. Roger Williams, a biochemist at the University of Texas, isolated vitamin B-5 from rice husks in 1939. Its nutritional importance and that of one of its main sources, rice (particularly natural brown rice), have been known, then, for over fifty years. However, approximately only 2-3% of our nation's children eat natural brown rice, which means that vitamin B-5 deficiency is common in this country.

Vitamin B-5 is important for several reasons. It helps to prevent fatigue and assists the adrenal glands in reducing the effects of stress. Through the manufacture of antibodies, B-5 also helps fight infection and aids the healing process. It even detoxifies the body by reducing the adverse effects of many antibiotics.

The adrenal glands are further assisted by vitamin B-5 in the conversion of protein into energy. When B-5 is in short supply, adrenal hormones cannot be produced, the conversion process is thwarted and energy levels plummet. Essentially, protein and fat cannot be turned into blood sugar. When this happens, hypoglycemia, another name for low blood sugar, causes frequent exhaustion, dizziness, nervousness, headaches, and, in severe cases, blackouts. This is why children (and adults) who have vitamin B-5 deficiency become exhausted so easily and appear generally listless.

Dr. Williams, who discovered vitamin B-5, also believed it to be directly connected to the prevention of mental illness. In his book *Nutrition Against Disease*, he described the vitamin as "essential to brain functioning." Prisoners placed on a diet deficient in pantothenic acid suffered profound mental depression as a result. He went on to say that a B-5 deficiency can even cause nerve degeneration, a finding he made when conducting tests on laboratory animals.

Vitamin B-5 is available from a variety of sources, including wheat germ and bran, whole grain breads, whole grain cereals, (brown rice & buckwheat), green vegetables, nuts, soy flour and tofu, eggs and poultry, legumes (beans, peas, lentils), and crude molasses. Unfortunately, there are not many from this list that play a strong part in our childrens' diets.

Iron

A deficiency of iron creates a number of problems related to mental, physical, and emotional wellness. One of them is that iron deficiency is difficult to recognize. By the time its primary symptom, anemia, becomes apparent, a great deal of damage can already have been done.

The following are a few of the many conclusions scientists have arrived at with regard to iron deficiency:

"Effects of Iron Deficiency on Attention and Learning Processes in Preschool Children. Bandung, Indonesia"
Soesmalijah Soewondo, M. Husaini, and Ernesto Pollitt.
University of Indonesia, Jakarta, Indonesia.

Pre and post-treatment psychological test data show that iron deficiency produces alterations in cognitive processes related to visual attention and concept acquisition, alterations reversed with iron treatment.

Am J Clin Nutr 1989;50:667-74

"Iron Deficiency and Behavior: Criteria for Testing Causality."
Molly Wilson Fairchild, Jere D. Haas, and Jean-Pierre Habicht
Cornell University, N.Y.

The association between iron deficiency and poor behavioral test performance is well established.

Am J Clin Nutr 1989;50:556-74

"Putative Biological Mechanisms of the Effect of Iron Deficiency on Brain Biochemistry and Behavior"
Moussa BH Youdim, Dorit Ben-Shachar, and Shlomo Yehuda.
Technion Medical School, Haifa, Israel.

An interference with iron metabolism at an early age can result in irreversible damage to developing dopamine neurons, with consequences that may manifest themselves in adult life.

Am J Clin Nutr 1989;50:607-17

Boron and Alertness

U.S. Department of Agriculture researchers found that people who have little boron in their diets are less mentally alert. James G. Penland, Ph.D., tested 15 people first on a low boron and then a low boron diet. When his subjects were put on low boron diet, it caused brain electrical activity to become sluggish, indicating a reduction in mental alertness. According to Dr. Penland, "Their brains produced more beta and delta waves which happens when you become drowsy." When switched to a high-boron diet (3 milligrams per day), Dr. Penland's subjects showed increased brainwave activity, confirming that boron definitely affects how well we can think.

Foods high in boron include nuts, flax, legumes (beans, peas, lentils); leafy vegetables, such as broccoli; and fruits, especially apples, pears, peaches and grapes.

Once again, because these are the very foods missing from our childrens' diets, it's no wonder we encounter headlines like the following from *Behavior Today*, June 17, 1986:

Shocker! 1 in 5 youngsters has a mental problem. As many as 12 million children under 18 — or 1 out of 5 American youngsters — suffer from mental health problems.

These mental health problems manifest themselves in other disturbances, both emotional and psychological, among our country's youth. Did you know that between 10% and 20% of America's adolescents are problem drinkers? Also, between 1980 and 1984, there was an estimated 350% increase in the number of adolescents admitted for psychiatric care.

This is really sad. But with volumes of data pointing to the contribution made by nutrient deficiency to the wellness problems of our youth, it should be obvious that we are taking the wrong approach legislating for higher drinking ages or increased spending on drug rehabilitation programs. We need to be educating our youth, and ourselves, in proper nutrition.

And we should be soliciting greater cooperation from food manufacturers and advertisers, who send out the wrong messages every Saturday morning in what might be called **the cartoon diet**. The cartoon diet consists of sugar, fat, artificial coloring, and caffeination. Given the attentiveness shown by children watching TV, what better opportunity could there be for "programming" this little captive audience with the right nutritional impulses? Then, rather than grabbing for a cola and a candy bar for a snack, they might reach for a glass of natural fruit juice and an apple.

What's Missing?

As we've alluded to previously in this book, the cause of nutrition deficiency lies not only in the food we don't eat but also in the food we do. By the time most of it reaches our mouths, whatever nutrition it once held has been processed out almost entirely. For example, let's look at what happens to a kernel of wheat:

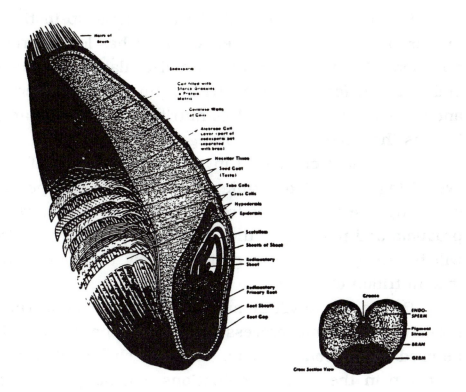

Essentially, what you're seeing here is not what you're getting in your daily bread:

BRAN MAY BE PRESENT IN 7 LAYERS, OR 14 1/2% OF THE KERNEL IS COMPOSED OF BRAN. WHILE INCLUDED IN WHOLE WHEAT FLOUR, MORE OFTEN IT IS *REMOVED AND USED IN ANIMAL OR POULTRY FEEDS.* THE BRAN, IN ADDITION TO THE INSOLUBLE FIBER, CONTAINS ABOUT:

86% Niacin	**73% Pyridoxine**
73% Pantothenic Acid	**42% Riboflavin**
33% Thiamine	**19% Protein**

By the time our kernel of wheat pops up in the morning toaster or pours out of the cereal box, it has lost nearly all of its nutritional identity. It has been milled, flaked, and likely salted and sugared (or sweetened with artificial sweetener), colored, and turned into something less nutritionally sound than pet food. Now, is that food fit for a growing child?

If you have children, I invite you to keep an informal log of everything they eat or drink during a seven day period. Then count up the number of fresh vegetables, fruits, whole grain products and pure water they have consumed. I promise you, it will be an eye-opening experience, now that you know where true nutrition comes from.

By the way, don't be mislead by those lists of "vitamins" on boxes of refined and processed cereals. Chances are they can't be used by the body anyway. As we've shown, vitamins need to be taken in the right combinations and supplied by the right whole foods in order for the human metabolism to process them.

On the subject of sugar, let's allow the American Dietetic Association to have the last word. Keep in mind that the ADA believed for many years that, as they put it, "sugar is good food." Here is their latest position, as of June of 1987:

" Eating a candy bar or other sugar source for quick energy is a common practice based on myth. The high fat content of the candy bar slows the rate of digestion, and the quickly assimilated sugar may cause an insulin overshoot, producing an adverse reaction. This practice can lead to a hypoglycemic state, causing premature fatigue and decreased performance, and should be avoided".

On the subject of treating drug addicts, in September 1990 the ADA had this to say,

"Improved nutritional status can make treatment more effective, while reducing drug and alcohol craving, thereby preventing relapse."

224

FOODS FOR A HEALTHFUL LIFE STYLE

If you're feeling overwhelmed or panicked about your child's diet at this point, here are a number of suggestions that will hopefully ease your mind:

VEGETABLES

Fresh are preferrable, frozen acceptable. Avoid using sauces. Vegetables should be eaten raw, or lightly steamed "al dente," which means they should be crisp and not over-cooked, to retain the most possible nutrients. Eat several servings of vegetables daily. 40 to 50% of a diet should be raw foods.

Suggestions: Artichokes, Asparagus, Avocado, Bamboo Shoots, Bean Sprouts, Beets, Broccoli, Brussel Sprouts, Green Beans, Cabbage, Carrots, Cauliflower, Celery, Cress, Chard, Cucumber, Collards, Corn, Endive, Escarole, Fennel, Garlic, ALL GREENS (beet, collard, dandelion, kale, mustard, turnip, spinach), Kohlrabi, Lambsquarter, Leeks, Lettuce (all varieties of dark green lettuce except Iceberg, due to its low fiber and nutrient content), Lima Beans, Okra, Onions, Parsley, Pumpkin, Green Peas, Radishes, Rutabaga, Sauerkraut, Snowpeas (pea pods), Soybeans, Sprouts of all kinds, Squash, Turnips, Water Cress.

Homemade soups can be made with the above vegetables and legumes. Grains can be used in the soups. Have two dark green and two yellow vegetables daily to keep the eyes shining.

225

FRUITS

Fresh are preferred, frozen acceptable. No sugar is added.
Suggestions: Apples, Apricots, Bananas, Berries,
Cherries, Fresh Coconut, Grapefruit, Kumquats, Lemons,
Limes, Mango, Melons, Papaya, Peaches, Pears,
Pineapple, Oranges, Tangerines, Pomegranate.

PROTEINS

Limit yourself to 2-3 ounces of concentrated, non-fibered
protein per day. Use meats as flavoring, not the main
dish.
Suggestions: Legumes (dried beans, peas, lentils) Whole
grains, Nuts (raw almonds, pecans, cashews, etc. — 6 to 8
as a snack); Fresh or Frozen, Baked or Boiled Fish, Turkey,
Chicken (organically grown if possible—check with your
health food store or co-op for sources), Lamb, Rabbit,
Wild Game, Eggs.

SNACKS

Raw and/or sprouted
Suggestions: Sunflower Seeds, Pumpkin Seeds, Almonds,
Popcorn (air popped or popped with olive or canola oil),
Granola (homemade or from the natural food section),
Berries, Cantaloupe, Avacado, Raw Nut Mix (peanuts
should be roasted), Fresh Fruits, or any of the Natural
Nut Butters, such as Almond, Cashew, or Sesame on
1/2 slice of Whole Grain Bread.

OMEGA-3

It's very important to supplement the diet with Omega-3, an essential fatty acid found abundantly in flax seed and to a lesser extent in fish, walnuts, olive oil, dark green leafy vegetables, and sea vegetables. Two products on the market that are very effective are Energy Drink mix (a combination of flax, oats and barley) and Stabilized Fortified Flax.

GRAINS

Eat whole, soaked or cooked.
Suggestions: Natural Brown Rice, Rolled or Steel Cut Oats, Rolled or Pearl Barley, Millet, Buckwheat, Cracked Wheat, etc. (Available in natural foods sections and health stores.)

BREAD

Whole grain breads free of dairy products and refined sugar, preservatives, and dough conditioners. If the bread is firm, it is likely nutritional. If it is soft, it likely is void of nutritional value.

MILKS

Make delicious nut milk by adding a heaping teaspoon of almond butter, cashew butter or pecan butter to a cup of water and blend for 15 to 20 seconds. Use this in any recipe that calls for milk. Soy milk is excellent and is usually available in natural food sections of your grocery.

OIL

Use virgin olive oil or canola oil for cooking or in salad dressing. Both of these are monounsaturated oils and contain Omega-3. Canola oil is now being offered by several cooking oil bottlers. It shouldn't be hard to find.

BEVERAGES

Drink 6-8 glasses of water daily, before, between, or after meals. Bottled spring or distilled water is best for the body. Start every day with a large glass of water with the juice of a quarter of fresh lemon or lime added, hot or cold. Herbal teas are refreshing. If you must have a soft drink, Fresca or club soda are the least harmful, BUT should not be consumed very often. You will find that if you drink enough water your body will not crave other less beneficial drinks.

WHAT TO AVOID

IT IS POSSIBLE FOR A PERSON TO BE ALLERGIC TO ANYTHING. WHEN A FOOD CAUSES IRRITABILITY, DEPRESSION, OR OTHER BAD REACTIONS, YOU SHOULD ELIMINATE IT FROM YOUR DIET IMMEDIATELY. VARY YOUR FOODS SO YOU DO NOT EAT THE SAME ONES EVERY DAY.

ALSO avoid refined or processed sugar, refined bleached flour, dairy products and drinks that contain caffeine.

Never use artificial sweeteners. Natural sweeteners which do not seem to trigger the desire to overeat are fresh or dried fruit, *real* maple syrup, black strap molasses, and fruit juices. Use less and less of these sweeteners to re-educate your taste buds.

SUPPLEMENTS

The following supplements have been found to be helpful:
B-Complex 50: 1 or 2 with each meal according to weight.
Vitamin C (complex with bioflavinoids) 500 mg:
1-2 with each meal according to weight.
Good Multiple Vitamin and Mineral: 1 daily.
Magnesium: 1 with breakfast and/or before bed.
Royal Jelly: 2 capsules each morning.

A SAMPLE DAY
FOR A HEALTHFUL LIFE STYLE

Wake up to a glass of warm pure water with fresh lemon or lime. For desired sweetness add 1 teaspoon of black strap molasses.

For breakfast:
• fresh melon, fruit or berries, together with one or two slices of whole grain bread, or a bowl of brown rice with a little real maple syrup or raisins and soy milk
• 8 ounces of pure water an hour or so later

Mid-morning:
• a pear or other fruit
• 8 ounces of pure water an hour or so later

For lunch:
• a fresh, crisp salad; or plate of raw vegetables, such as carrot or celery sticks, cucumber slices, broccoli and cauliflower florets on a bed of leaf lettuce, with whole grain pasta; chow mein-style vegetables with chicken or fish, and 1 or 2 slices of whole grain bread
• 8 ounces of water an hour or so later

Mid-afternoon:
• 6 to 8 unsalted raw almonds, a handful of sunflower seeds, a piece of fresh fruit, or vegetable sticks
• 8 ounces of pure water an hour or so later

Evening meal:

• This meal should be light. Enjoy a vegetable stir fry served on boiled potatoes (skin on) or with a bed of brown rice or whole grain bread; or perhaps a sandwich of whole grain bread, sliced tomato, avocado and sprouts (a thin slice of onion is optional) or any other vegetable desired. You'll be amazed at how satisfying this can be.

• For vegetable sandwiches, add a little hot sauce or coleslaw dressing on the toast or bread to give them some zip.   Top off with a dill pickle and lightly salted corn chips.

• Another satisfying supper is a bowl of lentil/vegetable soup (homemade, of course) served with a salad and 1 or 2 slices of whole grain bread.

NOTE: If you did not take a morning walk, or if you had a sedentary day, take a 20 - 30 minute walk and enjoy a restful night's sleep.

Because we don't want you to think you have to become a rabbit or "boring food freak" in order to reach sound nutrition and a more healthy lifestyle, we've assembled a number of superb recipes for you in Appendix A. Quickly leafing through them should show you that healthy people can indeed eat like "normal people." Enjoy!

FOR YOUR INTERST

As a parting note for this chapter, we'd like to share with you several interesting thoughts from the experts on the subject of nutrition and child wellness.

Rosetta Schuman, author of the book *Childrens' Lunchboxes and Party Snacks:*

It has now been clinically established beyond dispute that the conditions that bring on many diseases-arthritis, high blood pressure, arteriosclerosis, etc.-develop long before the symptoms become obvious. In fact, studies on children indicate the beginnings of these conditions generally associated with old age are in evidence at a very young age.

Ghandi linked diseased bodies with perverted tastes. When we allow our children to acquire a taste for sweets and other nutritionally unsatisfying foods, we interfere with their opportunity to choose a healthful diet. The consequences of these early indulgences will dog us at every step. Money is wasted on highly processed, enticingly packaged foods that have little value. Ultimately we fall easy prey to the medicine man.

Sir Robert McCarrison was an army doctor stationed in British India in the early part of this century. An astute observer of well people, he noted that in the kaleidoscope of ethnic subgroups inhabiting that country, some were generous in stature and robust; others were flagging in stature and generally sickly. McCarrison believed that differences in wellness were due, in large part, to the eating patterns of each group. He put ideas to the test by feeding groups of rats the same foods that the different groups of people ate. The growth, vigor, and resistance to disease shown in the rats paralleled exactly what he had observed in the corresponding ethnic group.

Despite such compelling evidence, McCarrison's work suffered total oblivion among his medical colleagues. Many practitioners still believe that nutrition, outside of the vitamin deficiency diseases, has no bearing on illness. If Dr. McCarrison were alive today, he would surely ask what the effects might be from eating fast food hamburgers, French fries, milkless milk shakes and cola drinks.

Lady Cilento, pediatrician, lecturer, writer, and author of the book, *Nutrition of the Child,* said:

Our biological heritage demands that we eat only the tissue and cells or plants and animals...Whether mothers allow their children sugar, refined, starchy foods, and the ever-present artifically colored and flavored junk foods, or whether they set the example to see that their children eat only wholesome, fresh foods will determine whether they have healthy, happy, cooperative, mentally alert children-in short, that they may eventually die young late in life.

Otherwise they should not feel aggrieved when they allow their children to go along with the crowd (eat what they like according to the TV advertisements), if their children catch every infection, are whining, naughty, slow to learn, and have poor concentration. They are laying the foundation for acne, anti-social behavior in adolescence, for cardiovascular and heart disease in middle life, and cancer as the years advance.

Cecelia Rosenfeld, M.D.

This statement is addressed to you with a sense of urgency. It bears on conditions which prevail in the eating habits of children today. There is abundant scientific evidence that suggests that many diseases of advancing age such as high blood pressure arthritis, abnormal heart conditions, arteriosclerosis, and other diseases do not begin mysteriously late in life, but have their origin in the bodies of young people who have not received correct nutritional guidance.

Dr. Joan Gussow of the Department of Nutrition, Columbia University:

It is now possible, to pick but a few recent examples, to buy chocolate chip cookie-shaped breakfast cereals, fruit-juiceless breakfast drink mixes, synthetic whipped cream, and hamburger sauce to make your homemade burger taste commercial. We have created a food supply from which it is extremely difficult for many people not to choose a poor diet.

234

Many years ago the University of California estimated that you are paying 92% more for your grains when you buy them in the form of boxed cereal in the supermarket. Recently we did some comparison shopping. We found a one-pound box of saltine crackers that sells for $1.19 is made of refined white flour, baking soda, salt, and has the nutrient value of only 10% of its whole grain counterpart. "Five cents' worth of junk food selling for more than a dollar a pound, and practically everything in it causes heart disease"-so says Dr. Nichols, founder and, for many years the president, of Natural Food Associates.

If a soda drink is part of your food dollar, then your food dollar is really taking a beating. A cola drink contains water, phosphoric acid, sugar, synthetic flavoring and coloring, caffeine and trace amounts of cocaine from de-cocainized cocoa leaves. The only food value is possibly some trace minerals in the water and food energy from the sugar. If there are any vitamins in this concoction, it is strictly by accident. In other words, you're paying an exorbitant price for sugar water.

The easiest way to retain the integrity of food is to eat it raw, or "unfired." Heat upsets the balances of food constituents. Some enzymes, essential for digestion and metabolism, are destroyed at 120 degrees; the balance are destroyed when 140 degrees is reached. Innumerable disorders and illnesses which afflict mankind can be healed by living on vital, uncooked food. A good seasonal balance is maintained by eating 50% unfired foods in winter and 60% in summer.

Dr. Fred Miller, who practiced preventive dentistry before the term "preventive medicine" came into use, would not keep a patient who did not practice good nutrition. According to Dr. Miller, author of *Open Door to Health*:

I believe mothers should help their children cultivate tastes for raw foods that appear naturally in many children. If older people must always have their peas, beets, cauliflower, etc., cooked, but children begin by liking them raw, why not give them their vegetables in a raw salad or as a pre-meal snack? Of course, it you have allowed your children's taste buds to become perverted by sweets, you may have a hard time in persuading them to eat vegetables at all.

The minerals in raw fruits and vegetables give them their desirable alkaline reaction. Most people suffer from over acidity as a result of their intake of processed, fragmented, adulterated carbohydrate foods. All successful dietary patterns utilize raw, leafy green vegetables. Greens are alkaline in their reaction in the body and contain up to 90% pure organic matter, unadulterated and living. Because they also contain certain bulk or fibrous materials, they become magnetized as they pass through the intestine, drawing up used tissue and cell wastes, acting as a broom and vacuum cleaner. When cooked, the action is more that of a wet mop.

"The doctor of the future will give no medicine,
but will interest his patient in the care of the human frame,
in diet and in the prevention of disease."

—Thomas A. Edison

11

ENLIGHTENMENT

Sometimes we find meaningful messages in the least likely places. Take the story of the three little pigs, for instance. As you well remember, the story centers around three pigs with an unusual penchant for building. One pig chooses straw for building materials. It's light and manageable and makes building quite easy. A second pig chooses sticks. They're somewhat more durable than straw but equally easy to use. The third pig, however, is an industrious little character who chooses to build with brick, an extremely labor-intensive method of construction. Of course, to complicate matters, there's a very windy wolf in the picture who has a real hankering for ham.

Upon finishing their houses quickly, the pigs who built with straw and sticks kick back and take their leisure as they watch the third pig sweat over his bricks in the hot sun. If my memory serves me, there may have been a few well-directed jeers at the foolish pig who chooses to make life difficult for himself. The wolf, however, doesn't see it this same way. The houses of straw and sticks are no contest. He blows them down, has a feast on fresh pork chops, then goes on to the brick house for a quick dessert. Little does he know about brick. After huffing and puffing and blowing himself out, the wolf eventually gives up and slinks away with a deflated ego. Though a little tired after a hard day's building, the third pig retires to enjoy the fruits of his labor.

I suppose there are many morals to this story, depending on how much you want to read into it. One might be that some pigs are just no match for a hungry, resourceful wolf. However, a little deeper interpretation might be that doing things the easy way—building with straw and sticks—is not the best and prudent way to build for the future. It may in fact cost you your life.

In many respects, the story of the three pigs can be applied to how Americans are accustomed to thinking about health maintenance. In the rush and haste of today's world, we neglect the most important element for a healthy tomorrow—**NUTRITION**. We all know that food (nutrition) is one of the three basic building blocks of life, the other two being water and shelter. Yet we have become accustomed to eating nutritionless food primarily because it is fast and convenient.

Because Americans are getting farther and farther from the whole-food diets Nature intended for us, we are getting dangerously close to a national health crisis. Many claim we are already in one. Our hospital staffs are overworked, the cost of health care is astronomical, and the incidence of degenerative disease is on the rapid incline.

Part of the problem is that our entire nation's health philosophy and health care system depends on the twisted premise that whatever goes wrong with our bodies can be fixed by modern medical wizardry. We have built for ourselves a bubble of security by intentionally remaining naive. First we delude ourselves by thinking the wolf will never bother our house. Then as a backup, we tell ourselves that we can always rebuild in the event the wolf does manage to blow our house down.

But a person can't rebuild a house when suffering from a debilitating, degenerative illness, such as cancer, premature senility, osteoporosis, or heart disease. The building materials have been weakened, damaged or totally destroyed; given the irreversible nature of degenerative disease, they're just never going to get stronger. Oh, maybe you can scrounge around the rubble and find enough to put up a meager shelter over your head. You may recover a portion of your health. But in the end, the shelter will collapse more easily with each new wind.

For the life of me, I can't understand why we spend millions of dollars annually on medical research just to preserve our thinly built illusions about curing degenerative diseases. It's such a waste! All the research in the world is not going to alter the fact that your house is built of straw and that a wolf is blowing at your door. If you haven't built a strong house of your body, eventually he's going to blow it down. He'll catch up with you as the consequence of excess sodium in your diet, harden your arteries, and tear your house down with high blood pressure and degenerative heart disease. He'll catch up with you as the consequence of having few anti-mutagens in your diet (whole foods of a wide variety), mutate a few cells in your pancreas, lungs or stomach, and tear your house down with degenerative cancer. There's so many ways the wolf can catch

240

up with you, and most of these are nutrition-related, as we've shown repeatedly throughout this book. It's just a matter of time.

The answer is to adopt a nation wide philosophy of preventive health care. Rather than fighting disease after it strikes, we should be doing things for ourselves which prevent disease in the first place. We should reverse our dietary trends and begin eating Nature's disease-preventive foods.

Such a change seems slow in coming. In the meantime, costs of health care in this country are skyrocketing. Research for cures is caught in an inflationary spiral that staggers the mind. Diagnostic costs are totally out of line. And hospitalization and treatment for degenerative diseases, which, by definition, have no "cure," can wipe out a family's lifelong savings over night.

Actually the present crisis in the cost of health care in this country should come as no surprise to anyone. It's a simple matter of economics—supply and demand. With a combination of increased population (the population of this country has essentially doubled in the last fifty years) and decreased national average health, there are more people in serious need of sickness care. Adding to the "downside" is the fact that the number of doctors and sickness care givers has not increased in proportion to the number of people needing care. It's the age-old problem of "too little food for too many mouths." As any business person can tell you, when you have a situation like this, the price of food is going to escalate—or in our case, the price of sickness care.

How do we stop these cost increases from continuing to spread like wildfire? **Preventive health maintenance**. That means eating whole foods which contain the molecules, chemicals, or "nutrients" proven to prevent degenerative disease and putting less faith in the ability of modern medical technology to bail us out when we get sick.

How often have you said or heard it said, "Isn't it a miracle what doctors can do these days?" Doesn't this attitude make it a little easier to sleep at night, or to have another cigarette, another beer or bag of french fries, knowing you have nothing to fear from abusing your body?

Now, consider how often you've said, "Isn't it a miracle what I can do?" If you're like most people, that's not very often. Therefore, isn't it conceivable that the magic of modern medical technology has managed to cause a flip-flop in our thinking about health? Has it allowed us to pass off what should be our own personal health care responsibility to modern medical specialists and their medical miracles?

It would indeed be hard to deny that these medical miracle workers are doing things as a matter of routine which we never dreamed possible half a century ago. They transplant organs, perform laser surgery on eyes, re-attach severed limbs, replace bones, even create life artificially. Yet there are some problems for which they have never found solutions. Outside of a few break-through immunizations, they have not figured out how to prevent diseases. Only you can do that.

The first principle of a preventive health maintenance philosophy is: **Disease prevention is a personal responsibility.** This responsibility begins with feeding your body the right food, getting the correct balance of nutrients and fueling yourself with life's natural disease fighters. All of the disease-preventive compounds needed to create a self-sustaining immune system against degenerative disease are contained in **whole foods.** That is how Nature set it up for us.

Unless we make significant changes in our attitudes toward disease prevention, the present crisis in health care is only going to get worse. We may end up doing what England has done. There, a person is not allowed to have kidney dialysis or heart bypass surgery after the age of 50. Why age 50? Because this is the point where most types of negligence toward one's health begin to show up. High blood pressure, cholesterol problems, arteriosclerosis—all of the problems associated with high sodium and fat intakes, as well as with smoking—surface right around the age of 50. England simply couldn't afford to pick up the medical bills for people who choose to ignore the risks and abuse their bodies in their early years. The message is loud and clear. If you want to dance, the piper has to be paid.

While the value system adopted by England may sound inhumane and pragmatic, from another perspective it makes a lot of sense. If we make choices to eat improperly, live irresponsibly and expose ourselves to a variety of diet-related diseases, then we have to pay the consequences of those choices. That's simply the way the world works for everyone but fools and babies.

Perhaps we need to remind ourselves that **actions have consequences** and stop expecting someone else to foot the bill for our deplorable eating habits—the government, Medicare, insurance companies, whomever.

Actually, there is a very simple solution. Each individual pays according to his or her "nutritional life style." If you're a smoker, the system will be happy to provide the necessary treatment for lung cancer, but it is not going to pick up the bill for you. Payment comes directly out of your own pocket. Likewise, if you drink and develop cirrhosis of the liver, the system will be happy to provide the necessary therapy, but you are the one who ultimately pays all the bills. Think about it. Isn't that what responsibility is.

I agree, this is a tough attitude. It's very tough. But it's also very necessary, as Canada recently found out. In response to escalating medical costs and a full-scale health care crisis, Canada decided that it was time to stop pampering irresponsible life styles. It cracked down on tobacco and alcohol users and got tough on nutrition-related disease.

Today in Canada, if you use tobacco, your health insurance premiums and hospitalization fees are adjusted accordingly. The same goes for people who abuse alcohol or suffer from ailments related to poor nutrition. As you might expect, Canadians are learning to be much more careful about their health, and average health care costs have dropped dramatically.

What is unique is that Canada is not advocating a system where people are denied the choice to drink, smoke, or eat non-nutritional food to their heart's content. Whatever you do with your life is your own business. What is being said, however, is that when it comes time to pay the consequences, no one is going to pay for you—not the government, not health insurers and not the company you work for. The buck stops here—with you!

What is also interesting about Canada's new health care program and attitude is the fact that medical malpractice suits are rapidly becoming a thing of the past. As hospitals become less burdened with degenerative disease related to poor nutrition, doctors' case loads are once again becoming manageable. Without the stress and haste created by case overloads, fewer errors are being made. This is bringing down the cost of medical malpractice insurance, which has an effect on the cost of sickness care in general.

This is something we in America should be taking a very hard look at, considering the malpractice issue has gotten completely out of hand. In the event of physician error, it is simply taken for granted that a malpractice suit will be initiated. Because attorneys' fees are often dependent upon the size of the malpractice settlement, the legal system must accept some responsibility for creating the nationwide desire to get rich quick off the system.

No matter what the cause, it's clear that each and every one of us is paying for this situation. The cost of malpractice insurance is going up. To compensate, physicians' fees and hospital costs are going up. The cost of health insurance is going up. And who ultimately foots the bill? You and I!

The truth of the matter is, this condition can be changed. By returning to the basics of nutrition, by embracing the concept of preventive medicine through nutritional wellness, and by taking personal responsibility for our own individual health care programs, we can lighten the medical case loads of our country's doctors. When this happens, human error will become negligible or even nonexistent, thus reducing the cost of sickness care on every front.

Throughout this book I have alluded to the fact that we're a nation infatuated with convenience. Periodically I've criticized the fast food giants, food manufacturers, and various bureaucratic research institutes and foundations for their contributions to America's nutrition problems. But in the final analysis, it is my belief that each one of us is ultimately responsible on a personal level for the nation's critical health condition. As soon as we accept this responsibility and put a halt to our nutritional negligence, many, if not all, of our problems will become self-correcting.

Provided we can embrace a new preventive health philosophy, the time of nutritional enlightenment will come. We'll be eating right, feeling better, working more effectively, playing harder, and paying less for sickness care. When that time arrives, presidents of the United States will feel obliged to make headlines putting out the word about disease control through whole foods: fortified flax, oat bran, carrots, whole grain bread, apples, peppers...Oh, and don't forget broccoli!

APPENDIX   A

RECIPES FOR A HEALTHFUL LIFESTYLE

SOUPS AND SALADS

BROCCOLI SOUP

1 cup broccoli flowerets
2 stalks celery, minced
sea salt

1-1/2 cups water
1/8 cup millet, uncooked

Place broccoli and celery in saucepan and cover with water. Add 1/2 teaspoon salt. Cover pan and bring to boil. Reduce heat and simmer for 25 minutes. Add millet and cook 20 minutes longer.

SEAFOOD BOUILLON

2 lbs. fish trimmings
2 quarts water
1 bay leaf
2 carrots, sliced
3 stalks celery, chopped

1 large onion, sliced
pinch thyme
3 sprigs parsley
2 t. salt

Boil together for 1 hour. Strain. A good basic stock. Can be made ahead and kept in a jar in the refrigerator for up to a week.

CURRIED LENTILS

4 cups lentils, cooked
1 large onion, sliced
2 T. oil
2 T. mild curry powder

1 cup carrots, sliced
2 cups rice, cooked
1-1/2 cups water
1 cup parsley, minced

Sauté onion in oil. Stir in curry powder. Add carrots and continue stirring. Gradually add water or broth. Simmer vegetables. Combine lentils with other vegetables. Sprinkle parsley on top before serving.

MINESTRONE

1/4 lb. white beans
3 cups bok choy or
 cauliflower, cut up
2 quarts water
4 T. leeks, chopped
1 shallot, crushed

1/4 lb. green string beans,
 cut in small pieces
1/2 lb. zucchini,
 peeled & diced
2 T. olive oil
salt and basil to taste

Pour boiling water over beans and let stand 2 hours. Drain. Put them in 2 quarts water and cook 4 hours. Saute leeks and zucchini in oil for 5 minutes and add to beans. Add rest of ingredients. Cover and cook over low heat 1 1/4 hours. Serve.

BARLEY OR RICE SOUP

1-3 lbs chicken, disjointed
8 cups cold water
1/2 cup onion, chopped

1 T. sea salt
1/2 cup barley or brown rice
1 cup celery, chopped

Place all ingredients in a large pan and cook over medium heat until done. Or may be cooked all day on low. Serves 4.

HOT AND SOUR SOUP

6 cups stock
1/4 cup turnips, in thin strips
1/4 cup string beans
1/2 cup water chestnuts
1 lb. tofu, cubed
1 T. lemon juice
1 t. honey
1T. corriander leaves, minced

1/4 t. cayenne
2 T. arrowroot
4 T. water
1 t. sesame oil
2 green onions, sliced
1 t. salt
1/2 t. pepper

Heat stock to boiling. Add next 4 ingredients. Turn down heat and simmer for 10 minutes. Mix lemon juice and salt. Add to soup. Dissolve arrowroot in water. Stir into soup until it thickens slightly. Add oil. Garnish with onions and corriander. Serve immediately.

CINCINNATI'S FAMOUS SPLIT PEA SOUP

2 cups dried peas
2 quarts water
2 cups celery and leaves
1 cup parsley, chopped

1 cup onions, chopped
1 leek (optional)
1/3 t. thyme
3 T. oil

Boil peas for 1 hour while skimming foam from top. Add rest of ingredients and simmer for 30 minutes. Add seasonings and oil and cook for 5 minutes. May be made with lentils. Serves 8.

BROCCOLI SOUP

Steam broccoli stems or cook covered, in small amount of boiling water until tender, about 10 minutes. Purée stems in blender or processor. Add chicken broth and thick nut or soy milk to desired consistency. Season with your favorite spices (tarragon, basil, or marjoram approximately 1/2 teaspoon). Heat gently, do not boil. Salt to taste. Serve hot or chilled.

TURKEY AND VEGETABLE SOUP

2 turkey legs
2 medium carrots, sliced
2 sliced celery stalks
1/4 cup whole wheat flour
1/2 t. dried basil leaves

1-1/2 quarts water
1 cup onion
oil
2 t. salt
1/4 t. pepper

Rinse turkey and place in 6 quart kettle. Add turkey, cover and bring to boil. Reduce heat and simmer 1 1/2 hours. Sauté onion in oil and add to soup. Add flour to soup, and simmer 1/2 hour. Garnish with parsley.

CHICKEN SOUP

2-1/2 lbs. of chicken pieces
1 -/2 quart water
4 medium carrots, sliced
2 cups fresh spinach
1 cup broccoli bits
1 T. salt

2 slices of ginger root
1/4 t. pepper
3 chicken bouillon cubes
4 celery stalks, sliced
   green beans, green onions
   fresh parsley, pea pods

Put chicken in a 4-quart saucepan, cover with water, and add all the rest of the ingredients but spinach. Bring to boil, reduce heat and simmer for 45 minutes. Remove chicken from broth and put it in a shallow pan. Let it cool for a few minutes. Then remove the skin and the bones from the meat, and cut meat into small chunks. Place the meat in the broth, and add spinach. Heat soup for another 5 minutes and serve. Serves 8.

TURKEY SALAD WITH RICE

1 cup cooked turkey, diced
1 cup celery, diced
1 medium clove garlic
2 T. pimiento, chopped

2 T. parsley, chopped
1/2 cup oil
1/3 cup lemon juice
1/2 t. curry
2 cups rice, chilled

Mix and chill all ingredients except last three. Chill. Combine oil, lemon juice and curry. Pour over chilled mixture. Toss and let stand for one hour. Pour over rice just before serving.

HEARTY SALAD

1/3 cup carrots, finely diced, cooked to barely tender
1/4 cup celery, diced
2-1/2 cups rice, cooked
4 T. oil
Pinch of thyme
Almonds, sunflower seeds, chopped nuts

2 T. parsley, minced
1/2 cup red onion, chopped
3 T. lemon juice
Salt to taste

Combine first 4 ingredients in large bowl. Add rice. Mix together. Combine oil, lemon juice, thyme and salt. Whisk until smooth. Pour over salad. Toss until everything is thoroughly combined. Chill for several hours. Decorate with any or a combination of seeds or nuts.

"USE YOUR BEAN" SALAD

2 cups kidney beans, cooked
2/3 cup cucumber, diced
1/2 cup celery, diced
2 hard cooked eggs, diced
1/4 t. salt

1/3 cup mayonnaise
1/8 t. pepper
1/4 cup onion, chopped
parsley for garnish

Mix all ingredients. Chill. Serve over crisp lettuce. Garnish with parsley. Serves 6.

CRAB MEAT AND AVOCADO SALAD

1/2 lb. crab meat	1/2 t. salt
1/3 cup celery, chopped	1/2 cup dressing
3 hard boiled eggs, chopped	3 large avocados
2 T. pimiento, chopped	Salt to taste
1 T. onion, chopped	1 t. oil
3 T. nuts, chopped	2 T. almonds, slivered

Mix together crab meat, celery, eggs, pimiento, onion, salt and dressing. Cut unpeeled avocados lengthwise in half. Remove pits. Brush halves with lemon juice and sprinkle lightly with salt. Fill avocados with crab meat mixture. Toss together nuts, oil and almonds. Spoon over crab meat. Place in a baking dish and bake in 400° F oven for 10 minutes. Remove from oven. Sprinkle with almonds and bake 5 minutes longer.

BEAN SPROUT SALAD

1 quart bean sprouts
3 green onions, cut diagonally
1/2 lb. green beans, sliced
4 radishes
1/3 cucumber, unpeeled, thinly sliced

Rinse sprouts. Blanch in boiling water for 3 minutes. Drain in colander. Immediately dip colander in large pan of ice water to stop cooking process. Stir gently with a fork. When cold, remove colander from water and let drain. Turn onto double-thickness of paper toweling and drain thoroughly. Mix sprouts with rest of ingredients. Chill. When ready to serve, toss with 2-3 tablespoons dressing, according to taste.

GALA SALAD

1 head leaf or bibb lettuce, separated into leaves
5-6 carrots, chopped
3-4 celery stalks, chopped
1 jicama*, peeled
2-4 jalapeno chiles, sliced
sprouts

Place lettuce on platter, mound rest of ingredients on top, alternating colors. Serve with dressing.
*Jicama (hee'kah'mah): Very crisp, juicy vegetable. Does not darken when cut. Great for water chestnut and potato replacement, since it stays crisp. Choose as you would a potato. Serve: Raw or in salads or with dips. Add to soups, stir-fry or stews. Store: In cool dry place. Refrigerate after peeling. Available: Mostly November to June.

GREEN GARDEN SALAD

3/4 cup frozen peas
boiling water
1 small head romaine lettuce
1 small head Boston lettuce
1 small head red-leaf lettuce
2 green onions, thinly sliced
1 small cucumber, sliced
1 celery stalk, sliced

1/2 small bunch watercress
1/4 cup oil
3 T. white wine vinegar
1 t. honey
1 T. chopped parsley
1/4 t. garlic salt
1/4 oregano leaves
dash of seasoned pepper

About 20 minutes before serving: Place frozen peas in a small bowl. Cover with boiling water and let stand 5 minutes to "cook" peas. Meanwhile, tear all lettuce leaves into bite sized pieces and put in large bowl. Drain peas and add to lettuce in bowl with green onions, cucumber, celery, and watercress. Prepare dressing in small bowl with fork, mix salad oil and remaining ingredients. Toss salad gently with dressing to coat. Serves 12.

BROWN RICE SALAD
(1 dish meal)

4 cups cooked & cooled brown rice
1-16 oz. kidney beans, drained and rinsed
1-16 oz. black beans, drained and rinsed
1 1/2 cups frozen green peas - thawed
1-4 oz cans mild green chiles or
      3/4 cup salsa verde (green chile salsa - not red)
1 cup chopped cilantro or fresh parsley
1/2 cup chopped red onion
1 cup chopped, unsalted nuts (walnuts, cashews or almonds)
1-16 oz. garlic Italian dressing (Newman's is excellent)

Mix all together, cover and chill in refrigerator 1-2 hours before serving on dark green lettuce leaves.

WALKING APPLE SALAD

Core small apple. Fill center with raisins and almond butter mixture.

CHINESE SALAD

2-8-oz. bunches spinach   1 oz. anchovy, mashed
1/4 cup oil   1/2 lb. small shrimp

Cook spinach. Rinse in ice-cold water. Chop. Combine rest of ingredients and add to spinach. Serve very cold.

ON THE SIDE

BASIC SALAD DRESSING

1 t. salt
1/4 t. black pepper
1 t. dry mustard

Dash of Tabasco
1/4 cup lemon juice
2/3 cup olive oil

Mix all ingredients and shake well. Shake again just before pouring over salad. Double or triple the recipe and store in refrigerator.

GREEN GODDESS DRESSING

8 anchovy fillets
1 scallion
handful parsley

8-10 tarragon leaves
3 cups basic dressing

Blend in the blender until smooth. Serve over firm lettuce.

FRENCH DRESSING

1 t. salt
1 t. honey
1/8 t. pepper
2/3 cup oil

1/2 t. dried herbs
1 t. zanthan
1/3 cup lemon juice

Combine all ingredients in jar with tight fitting cover. Shake vigorously, or mix in blender. Refrigerate. If desired, add garlic, onions, anchovies.

GUACAMOLE

1 large, ripe avocado, mashed   1/8 cup lime juice
1/4 t. salt   chili powder

Combine, and mix well. Good as a dip also.

NUT & SEED BUTTER, SPREADS & MILK

ALMONDS   PUMPKIN SEEDS
CASHEWS   SUNFLOWER SEEDS
MACADAMIA NUTS   SESAME SEEDS
PECANS   WALNUTS
PINE NUTS   PEANUTS & SOY
PISTACHIOS   BRAZIL NUTS

TO MAKE MILK: Blend 1 heaping teaspoon of the nut butter with 1 cup of water. Blend until smooth. Use with cereal or in any recipe calling for milk.

BROCCOLI WITH WALNUT BUTTER

Trim outer leaves and tough ends from broccoli. Separate top half into flowerets. Save stems for broccoli soup.

Steam flowerets or cook in small amount of boiling salted water in saucepan, covered, 10 minutes or until crisp-tender. Drain well. Turn into serving bowl. While broccoli is cooking, heat oil in small skillet over low heat. Add walnuts, cook slowly, stirring frequently until oil just begins to brown (watch carefully to prevent burning). Add lemon juice, salt and pepper, if desired. Pour over hot broccoli. Toss gently. Serve immediately.

BEANCAKES

1/4 cup stabilized Fortified Flax*	1/4 t. salt
3/4 cup water	1/2 t. soda
1/2 cup bean flour	1/2 cup nuts, chopped

Mix together flax seed and water, let stand 10 minutes. Combine dry ingredients and mix with wet ingredients. Let stand until mixture thickens. Cook on nonstick surface for best results. When done, transfer to warm platter, sprinkle with nuts.

For an even lighter cake, omit soda and mix the night before, then add soda just before cooking. Bean and other heavy flour yield a finer finished product the longer they soak. Freezing improves texture, also.

* Available in natural food stores.

BASIC STEAMED RICE

2 cups brown rice (Basmati rice is excellent.)

1 T. olive oil	4 cups water
4 T. soy grits	1 t. salt

Do not wash rice. Simply add water. Add the rest of ingredients. Cover pan tightly. Cook on high flame until boiling, then turn to active simmer. When done (about 40 minutes) there will be no liquid left at all, rice will stay firmly in place when you turn the pan sideways, and "clam holes" will show in top. You might also want to add 1 t. American saffron or Spanish saffron before cooking.

RICE PILAFF

1 cup brown rice
4 T. soy grits
4 T. olive oil
1 onion, chopped

2 cloves garlic, chopped
4 cups liquid
salt, pepper
pinch rosemary, thyme

Heat oil in heavy skillet. Sauté onion until wilted and golden. Add garlic. Cook briefly. Add rice and stir over high heat for about five minutes. When rice is slightly opaque, add boiling stock all at once. Then cover tightly and let cook about 20 minutes. Add salt, pepper and spices to taste, and more liquid if necessary. Cover again and simmer another 20 minutes.

THANKSGIVING DRESSING

3 cups whole wheat bread crumbs
3/4 cup mushrooms, chopped
3/4 cup carrots, shredded
3/4 cup celery, chopped
1-1/2 small onions, chopped

3/4 t. sage
1-1/2 cups tofu
3 eggs, beaten
4 1/2 T. oil

Make bread crumbs. Toast bread in the oven on both sides, hold 2-3 slices under warm water, squeeze gently and crumble into large bowl. Mix all ingredients together. If not moist enough, add a few tablespoons of soy milk or water.

Saute the mushrooms, carrots, celery, onions and diced tofu. Mix with the crumbled toast and add the sage, eggs and oil. Mix and place in oiled pan. Bake for 20-25 minutes in 350* oven.

MAIN DISHES

OATMEAL AND PEACHES

2 fresh peaches, sliced   sea salt to taste
1 serving oatmeal

Dice peaches. Prepare oatmeal according to package directions. Mix peaches and oatmeal together.

SCRAMBLED EGGS WITH MUSHROOMS

6 eggs   1 t. minced onion
1/2 cup mushrooms   2 T. olive oil
1/4 cup mushroom liquid

Beat eggs until frothy. Heat oil in heavy pan, add mushrooms and onion. Simmer for a few minutes. Add mushroom liquid and simmer for another minute. Pour in egg mixture, continue cooking at very low heat, scraping constantly from the bottom of the pan until desired texture is achieved. Serves 4-6.

HURRY UP HEARTY HASH

1/2 cup celery, chopped   1/2 t. salt
1/2 cup nuts, chopped   1 clove garlic, pressed
1/4 cup flour or egg   2 cups beans, cooked
2 T. oil   and mashed

Combine all ingredients. Fry patties in lightly oiled skillet until browned on both sides. Great for breakfast.

GREAT STEAMED VEGGIES

8 slices Sunny Millet Bread
1 medium onion, chopped
2 stalks celery, chopped
1 or 2 carrots, chopped
1 cup summer squash & zucchini

1 cup tofu, cubed
1 cup mushrooms, cut
 handful bean sprouts
1 cup broccoli, cut
2 T. tamari sauce

Sauté the onion, celery and carrots in a wok or large pan. Add all remaining vegetables except broccoli and sprouts. Cover wok or pan and steam vegetables for about 10 minutes. Stir occasionally. Add broccoli and sprouts and cook for 3 or 4 minutes. All the vegetables should remain crisp. Serve over Natural Ovens Sunny Millet bread. Serves 4.

RICE AND SHRIMP BARCELONA

2 lbs. shrimp
3/4 cup olive oil
1 t. salt
10 cloves garlic

1/2 cup fresh parsley
juice of 2 lemons
1/4 cup dry wine
2 cups cooked rice

Peel and devein shrimp. Heat oil in large skillet. Add garlic and heat until it begins to brown. Add shrimp and cook, turning frequently to cook all the shrimp, for about 5 minutes. Add remaining ingredients, saving parsley until just before serving. Serve over rice using garlic oil as a sauce.

BAKED STUFFED FISH

3-5 lb. whole fish: bass, cod, haddock, bluefish
1/2 cup chicken broth   1/4 cup oil
1/2 cup chopped celery   1 1/2 cups brown rice

Clean fish. Sauté celery in oil until lightly browned. Add rice and broth and blend together until well mixed. Stuff fish not more than 2/3 full. Close the opening with skewers or toothpicks laced together with string. Put on an oiled ovenproof platter or oiled unglazed paper or cooking parchment in a shallow baking pan. Cut 3-4 gashes through the skin on each side to keep the fish in shape during baking. Bake at 400° F for 30 to 45 minutes. Serves 6.

CUBAN-STYLE FISH

1-2/3 lbs. trout   1 small sliced onion
2 T. lemon juice   2/3 T. chopped parsley
1/8 cup oil   1/8 t. thyme
1/4 cup chopped almonds   2/3 bay leaf
1/4 cup chopped onion   1-1/3 T. hot water

Clean fish, sprinkle with 1 tablespoon lemon juice. In frying pan add 1-1/2 tablespoon oil, almonds, chopped onion, hot water, and parsley. Simmer all together for 5 minutes. In a roasting pan put the remaining oil, the sliced onion, thyme, and bay leaf. Place fish on top of this, cover with cooked mixture, sprinkle with remaining lemon juice. Bake at 350° F for 35-45 minutes. Baste often. Serves 6.

EASY CHICKEN AND RICE

3 lbs. frying chicken pieces
1 cup brown rice
2 cups water
Optional: onions, celery, nuts

1-1/2 T. oil
3 T. chopped parsley
1 t. salt

Place rice, water, salt, butter and parsley in 4-quart casserole. Stir and bring to a boil. Salt chicken and lay on top of rice. Lower heat to simmer. Cover tightly and cook 45 to 60 minutes until water is absorbed and chicken is tender.

CHICKEN AND BROCCOLI BAKE

1-10 oz. pkg. frozen broccoli
4 T. thickener
2 cups chicken broth

1 lb. cooked chicken
1/2 cup chopped nuts
2 small onions

Preheat oven to 375° F. Cook broccoli until just tender, according to package directions. Mix thickener and chicken broth in a shaker so it does not lump. Cook over medium heat until thickened and smooth. Season to taste. Place broccoli pieces in baking dish. Cover with chicken. Pour gravy mixture over chicken and broccoli. Combine nuts and onions, top chicken. Bake uncovered 20-25 minutes until bubbly and brown on top. Serves 6.

TUNA CASSEROLE

1/2 cup oil
1 leek, minced
2 T. flour

1-1/2 cups clam juice
4 cups vegetables, chopped
2 -7 oz. cans tuna

Sauté first 3 ingredients. Gradually work in flour to make a smooth mixture. Add slowly and stir until thick. Put vegetables in casserole bowl. Add tuna. Pour sauce over tuna in a casserole and top with cracker crumbs or chopped nuts. Bake at 350° F for 20 minutes.

SCALLOP STIR-FRY

2 T. oil
1 cup pea pods
1/2 lb. scallops

sea salt
ginger

Heat 1 tablespoon oil in wok till hot, add pea pods, salt, and pinch of ginger. Fry for 3 minutes. Remove and place second tablespoon oil in wok. Add scallops with salt & ginger. Stir fry and toss together. Serve hot.

STIR-FRIED CHICKEN AND VEGETABLES

3 boned chicken breasts
1 T. dry sherry (optional)
1 egg white, slightly beaten
4 t. cornstarch
2 t. soy sauce
5 T. oil

1 carrot, shredded
1 t. ginger, shredded
1 stalk scallion
1 t. honey
2 T. cold water

Slice chicken into thin horizontal pieces. Cut the slices into strips and place in bowl. Combine sherry, egg white, 2 teaspoons of cornstarch, and 1 teaspoon of soy sauce. Pour over the chicken slivers and let stand 30 minutes. Heat 1 tablespoon oil in skillet. Sauté carrot slivers 1 minute. Remove from skillet and set aside. In the same skillet, heat the remaining 4 tablespoon of oil and sauté ginger and scallion for 30 seconds. With a slotted spoon, remove chicken from the soy sauce mixture and add to skillet, cooking and stirring until it shreds and turns white. Add reserved vegetable mixture, honey and remaining soy sauce. Cook until heated through, then stir in remaining 2 teaspoons of cornstarch dissolved in 2 tablespoons of cold water. Cook briefly until all ingredients are coated with a clear glaze. Serve at once. Serves 6.

GINGER BROCCOLI STIR-FRY

1 bunch (1#) broccoli
1/2 cup almonds, chopped
3 T. oil
3 cloves garlic, thinly sliced

2 T. soy sauce
1/2 t. ginger root, ground
1 t. lemon juice

Cut broccoli into flowerets. Trim and peel stalks. Cut on diagonal into thin slices, reserve. Sauté almonds in oil 1 minute. Add broccoli and stir-fry until barely tender, about 3 minutes. Add garlic and stir-fry until tender, about 2 minutes. Stir in soy sauce and ginger. Continue stir-frying about 1 minute. Add lemon juice. Makes 4 servings.

ORIENTAL STIR-FRY

1 T. canola oil
1 stalk bok choy, chopped
1 lb. fresh bean sprouts
1/2 lb. fresh pea pods

1 can water chestnuts
1/4 lb. fresh spinach
salt and pepper
1 cup shrimp, cooked

Optional: mushrooms, bamboo shoots, and celery.

Heat oil in a large kettle or wok. Add bok choy and stir for a minute or two. Add remaining ingredients. Stir constantly over high heat until mixture is piping hot and vegetables are crisply tender. Serve immediately over rice or Chinese noodles. Garnish with slivered almonds, serves 4.

BEST CORN BREAD YOU'VE EVER EATEN!

1 cup high lysine or yellow corn meal
1 cup Oat Bran Plus (80% oat flour and 20% Fortified Flax)
2/3 t. soda
2/3 t. baking powder

Mix well.
Add and stir in 2/3 cup soy milk.

In cup first put 1/4 cup olive oil or canola oil, then add 1/4 cup real maple syrup. Add 1 or 2 eggs. Mix with other ingredients and stir well. Pour into an oiled 10" pan and bake in a 350 preheated oven for 25 minutes. Delicious with bean or pasta dishes.

Scrumptious Pancakes and Waffles

1-1/2 cups Oat Bran Plus Flax (80% oat flour/20% Fortified Flax)
2/3 t. baking soda
2/3 t. baking powder
2 T pecan bits (optional)

Mix well and add:
1-1/2 cups soy milk
2 eggs or 3 egg whites. Mix again.

Spoon into waffle iron or griddle, (add water if batter becomes too thick.)

Serve with real maple syrup, sliced bananas, strawberries or other fruit.

For blueberry pancakes or waffles, add 1/2 to 1 cup frozen or fresh blueberries and mix in.

Makes 4 Belgian waffles or 10, 4-inch pancakes.

SANDWICHES AND FILLINGS

Date filling: Grind 1 cup dates and 4 tablespoons nuts using fine knife or food-chopper. Add enough orange juice to make the mixture of spreading consistency. A little lemon juice added will take away the too-sweet taste.

Almond butter and vegetables: Combine grated or ground raw carrots, celery or onions with nut butter. Season to taste.

Tuna: Remove excess oil from tuna fish. Or better, buy tuna packed in water and drain. Flake fish and mix with 1/4 cup each of chopped celery and nuts, and moisten with lemon salad dressing.

Raw vegetables: Grind 1/4 cup raisins and 1/2 cup each shredded cabbage, carrots, and apples. Add 1 tablespoon lemon juice and season to taste. Moisten with desired dressing.

Vegetables: Thin slices of burmuda onion, tomato and avocado with sprouts and/or leaf lettuce. Spread thinly on the toast-cold slaw dressing and mild to medium salsa. Serve with a pickle and low salt chips. Great for a quick lunch or supper.

Chicken: To 1 cup chopped chicken, add desired amount of celery, cucumber, olives, and radishes chopped fine. Season to taste and moisten with mayonnaise.

JUST VEGGIES

MARINATED VEGGIES

1/3 cup lemon juice
1 or 2 cloves garlic, slivered
1 t. dried salad herbs

1 lb. vegetables
 or cooked beans
1/2 t. salt
1/2 cup olive

In small saucepan, mix together first 3 ingredients. Add oil and simmer very gently for about 5 minutes. Cover and set aside to steep. Cut vegetables into bite-sized pieces. Hard vegetables such as cauliflower, broccoli, or green beans may be lightly steamed first, while others such as cucumber, zucchini or sweet onion are best left raw. Bite-sized pieces of raw tofu are delicious marinated, as are large beans such as chick peas or kidney beans. Toss vegetables, etc. with salt in a good sized bowl. Some scallion or fresh herbs make a nice addition at this point. Pour on marinade evenly and toss again. Let sit at least an hour or so, or preferably overnight to develop full flavor. Toss from time to time to mix marinade with veggies, or marinate under pressure by placing a weighted dish on top of them. NOTE: Marinated veggies can be mixed into salads or served as pickles or as a side dish. They make a nice winter salad, and are a delicious accompaniment to grains, pasta, and non-vegetarian main dishes alike. Refrigerated, they will keep well for 10 days. FOR SEASONING: Any fresh or dried salad herbs such as parsley, basil, marjoram, or dill, or smaller amounts of lightly crushed aromatic seeds such a celery, fennel, or caraway, are good. Other possibilities include dulse or kelp flakes, bay leaf, peppercorns, or a bit of ginger, curry or cayenne.

SQUASH AND VEGETABLE SAUTE

3 T. oil	1/8 t. pepper
3 1/2 cups zucchini, thinly sliced	1/4 t. oregano, crushed
3 cups cabbage, coarsely chopped	1/4 t. thyme
3/4 t. salt	1 T. cider vinegar

Heat oil in skillet over medium-high heat. Add squash and cabbage. Toss to mix. Cover and cook over medium heat, about 5 minutes or until vegetables are crisp-tender. Add seasonings and cider vinegar. Continue cooking until vegetables are heated through, 3-4 minutes.

BLUSHED CAULIFLOWER

1 medium-size head cauliflower	dash white pepper
1 t. tarragon leaves, crumbled	1/2 t. salt

Wash cauliflower thoroughly. Remove outer leaves and core, keeping head intact. Place in 1-inch boiling water in a large saucepan. Add tarragon and white pepper. Add cauliflower and cook for 10 minutes basting frequently with tarragon flavored liquid. Cover, reduce heat and simmer 15-20 minutes longer or until tender. Carefully remove cauliflower to serving dish.

SWEET POTATO VEGETABLE MEDLEY

4 sweet potatoes	1 cup mushrooms, sliced
1 cup chicken broth	1 cup water chestnuts
2 cups fresh green beans	pepper to taste
1 small onion, chopped	

Steam potatoes 35-45 minutes or until just barely tender. Drain, cool, peel and slice. Place 1/2 cup of broth in large skillet; add beans and onions. Cover and steam about 8 minutes or until beans are tender. Add remaining broth. Fold in mushrooms, sweet potatoes and chestnuts. Heat over medium heat until vegetables are hot. Season with pepper.

DESSERT!

CUSTARD

4-6 eggs
1 quart soy milk
1/4 cup honey

1 t. vanilla
1/2 t. salt

Heat milk until bubbles show around edge of pan. Beat eggs, honey, and vanilla together. Beating constantly, add half of milk slowly, then the rest may be added more quickly. Pour egg and milk mixture into a mold or individual custard cups. Put molds in pan of boiling water in a 350° F oven for 25-45 minutes; when knife inserted in center comes out clean, custard is done. Serve with scrambled eggs and sprouts.

NUT LOAF

1/2 cup Brazil nuts
1 cup almonds
1 cup sunflower seeds
1/4 cup flax seed, ground
2 small onions, diced
1/2 cup fresh parsley
1/2 t. sage
1/2 t. thyme

1/2 t. salt
1/2 t. sweet basil
1/2 cup almonds, ground
2 cups water
2 T. arrowroot flour
2 T. oil
1/2 t. salt

Grind all nuts in blender. Mix flax seed with water until it reaches the consistency of an egg. Combine onions, parsley, sage, thyme, salt and basil. Place mixture in a well oiled loaf pan. Bake at 350° F for 25 minutes. Serve hot. Mix last 5 ingredients and stir over medium heat until thick. Pour over cooked loaf.

CHEWY CAROB BARS

12 oz. carob chips   2-1/2 cups rolled oats
3/4 cup peanut butter   1/2 cup granola

Combine carob chips and peanut butter in saucepan. Cook over low heat, stirring constantly until smooth. Remove from heat. Stir in oats and granola. Pour into oiled 8" x 9" pan. Chill and cut into 36 bars.

OATMEAL BARS

1/2 cup peanuts   1/2 cup rolled oats,
                                        uncooked
8 figs, chopped

Place peanuts and oats in food processor or blender. Process and add figs, process again. Press into 8-inch-square baking dish. Cover. Refrigerate for at least 2 hours. Cut into bars.

NUTTY FROZEN BANANAS

6 bananas, peeled   3/4 cup nuts, chopped
1 cup orange juice, freshly squeezed

Place bananas on waxed paper on cookie sheet. Coat each with 1 tablespoon orange juice. Freeze about 15 minutes, roll in nuts. Freeze till firm. Serve frozen.

YUM BALLS

1 cup plain peanut butter
2 cups coconut, shredded
1/4 cup cashews, chopped
1 T. orange juice

1/2 cup dates, chopped
1/2 cup sunflower seeds
1/4 cup real maple syrup

Combine all ingredients in a bowl. Mix well and roll into 1 inch balls. Place on ungreased cookie sheet and refrigerate until firm and store in air tight container in refrigerator.

APPLE IN A GLASS

Grate an apple, skin and all, mix with a pinch of cinnamon and a tablespoon each of chopped dates and sunflower seeds. Serve in a chilled, long-stemmed glass.

APPENDIX B

SCIENTIFIC RESEARCH ON BROCCOLI

This is an unusual appendix. It organizes most of the research work that has been done on the health benefits of broccoli. It was prepared by Dr. Christopher Beecher of the Department of Medicinal Chemistry and Pharmacognosy at the University of Illinois-Chicago. This appendix shows the tremendous importance of gathering together the published research results from all over the world. If these results are not collected in one place, many researchers would end up repeating what has already been done, and people like you and me, would never realize that this tremendous amount of information is available.

The first section is ethnomedical information. It tells where the work was done, the parts of the plant used, what biological effect was examined, information on concentration, and whether the material was biologically Active or Inactive. After the results is a code, e.g. W 2457. This is the literature reference. The last part of this appendix lists all of the references in alphabetical order. This allows you to find the primary reference for further study.

ETHNOMEDICAL INFORMATION

1. *BRASSICA OLERACEA* (CRUCIFERAE)

   a) PART NOT SPECIFIED

      i. EUROPE

         • USED TO INDUCE MENSES.
           TYPE EXT NOT STATED * ROUTE NOT GIVEN * HUMAN ADULT * FEMALE *
           A4537

2. *BRASSICA OLERACEA* VAR.BOTRYTIS (CRUCIFERAE)

   a) FRESH INFLORESCENCE

      i. USA

         • USED FOR SCURVY.
           HOT H2O EXT * ORAL * HUMAN ADULT * * W4177

         • USED AS A BLOOD PURIFIER.
           HOT H2O EXT * ORAL * HUMAN ADULT * * W4177

         • USED FOR ANTACID EFFECTS.
           HOT H2O EXT * ORAL * HUMAN ADULT * * W4177

   b) DRIED SEED

      i. EGYPT

         • USED AS A CONTRACEPTIVE BEFORE OR AFTER COITUS.

         • DATA OBTAINED AS A RESULT OF QUESTIONING 1200 PUERPERAL WOMEN
           ABOUT THEIR KNOWLEDGE OF BIRTH CONTROL METHODS. 52.3%
           PRACTICED A METHOD AND

         • 47.6% OF THESE DEPENDED ON INDIGENOUS METHODS AND/OR
           PROLONGED LACTATION. THEIR INFORMATION WAS OBTAINED FROM
           NEIGHBORS,FRIENDS,RELATIVES,TRADITIONAL BIRTH ATTENDANTS
           (DAYAS) OR HERB MEN.
           HOT H2O EXT * ORAL * HUMAN ADULT * FEMALE * W2811

3. *BRASSICA OLERACEA* VAR.CAPITATA (CRUCIFERAE)

   a) DRIED ENTIRE PLANT

      i. USA

         • USED FOR CANCER.
           TYPE EXT NOT STATED * ORAL * HUMAN ADULT * * T9386

   b) FRESH LEAF

      i. USA

         • USED FOR RHEUMATISM.
           HOT H2O EXT * ORAL * HUMAN ADULT * * W4177

         • USED FOR TUBERCULOSIS.

BRASSICA OLER* (3part query for [BEECHER.GROUP], 1-MAY-1990)

HOT H2O EXT * ORAL * HUMAN ADULT * * W4177

- USED FOR CANCER.
  HOT H2O EXT * ORAL * HUMAN ADULT * * W4177

- USED FOR GOUT.
  HOT H2O EXT * ORAL * HUMAN ADULT * * W4177

- USED FOR EYE DISEASES.
  HOT H2O EXT * OPHTHALMIC * HUMAN ADULT * * W4177

- USED FOR PYORRHEA, AS WELL AS FOR GANGRENE.
  HOT H2O EXT * ORAL * HUMAN ADULT * * W4177

- USED FOR ASTHMA.
  LEAVES * ROUTE NOT GIVEN * HUMAN ADULT * * W4177

- USED TO PREVENT TOOTH DECAY BECAUSE OF BENEFITS TO TOOTH
  ENAMEL.
  TYPE EXT NOT STATED * ORAL * HUMAN ADULT * * W4177

- USED TO PROMOTE HAIR GROWTH.
  HOT H2O EXT * EXTERNAL * HUMAN ADULT * * W4177

- USED AS A BLOOD PURIFIER. USED FOR DISEASES CAUSED BY CALCIUM
  DEFICIENCY AND INADEQUATE MINERAL INTAKE.
  HOT H2O EXT * ORAL * HUMAN ADULT * * W4177

c) DRIED SEED

   i. ARABIC COUNTRIES

- USED AS A CONTRACEPTIVE IN THE FORM OF A PESSARY IN UNANI
  MEDICINE
  SEEDS * VAGINAL * HUMAN ADULT * FEMALE * T6813

- USED AS AN ABORTIFACIENT IN UNANI MEDICINE
  HOT H2O EXT * ORAL * HUMAN(PREGNANT) * * T6813

- USED AS AN EMMENAGOGUE IN THE FORM OF A PESSARY IN UNANI
  MEDICINE
  SEEDS * VAGINAL * HUMAN ADULT * FEMALE * T6813

- USED AS AN EMMENAGOGUE IN UNANI MEDICINE BY FUMIGATION.
  SEEDS * INHALATION * HUMAN ADULT * FEMALE * T6813

   ii. EGYPT

- USED AS A CONTRACEPTIVE BEFORE OR AFTER COITUS.

- DATA OBTAINED AS A RESULT OF QUESTIONING 1200 PUERPERAL WOMEN
  ABOUT THEIR KNOWLEDGE OF BIRTH CONTROL METHODS. 52.3%
  PRACTICED A METHOD AND

- 47.6% OF THESE DEPENDED ON INDIGENOUS METHODS AND/OR
  PROLONGED LACTATION.

- THEIR INFORMATION WAS OBTAINED FROM
  NEIGHBORS,FRIENDS,RELATIVES,TRADITIONAL BIRTH ATTENDANTS
  (DAYAS) OR HERB MEN.

274

BIOLOGICAL ACTIVITIES FOR EXTRACTS

- *BRASSICA OLERACEA* (CRUCIFERAE) COMMERCIAL SAMPLE OF JAPAN

  a) ANTIMUTAGENIC ACTIVITY * AQUEOUS HIGH SPEED SUPERNATANT * * AGAR PLATE * * CONC USED 0.1 ML/PLATE * ACTIVE * * SALMONELLA TY PHIMURIUM TA98 * T12116

    1. METABOLIC ACTIVATION WAS REQUIRED FOR ACTIVITY.

- *BRASSICA OLERACEA* (CRUCIFERAE) AERIAL PARTS CZECHOSLOVAKIA

  a) OESTROGENIC EFFECT * ETOH(95%)EXT * SC * MOUSE(INFANT) * FEMALE * DOSE NOT STATED / * ACTIVE * * * A4667

  b) OESTROGENIC EFFECT * ETOH(95%)EXT * SC * RAT(OVARIECTOMIZED) * FEMALE * DOSE NOT STATED / * ACTIVE * * * A4667

- *BRASSICA OLERACEA* (CRUCIFERAE) AERIAL PARTS GERMANY(WEST)

  a) ANTIBACTERIAL ACTIVITY * ETOH(95%)EXT * * AGAR PLATE * * CONC USED VARIABLE / * ACTIVE * * BACILLUS SUBTILIS * A12151

  b) ANTIBACTERIAL ACTIVITY * ETOH(95%)EXT * * AGAR PLATE * * CONC USED VARIABLE / * ACTIVE * * ESCHERICHIA COLI * A12151

  c) ANTIBACTERIAL ACTIVITY * ETOH(95%)EXT * * AGAR PLATE * * CONC USED VARIABLE / * ACTIVE * * STAPHYLOCOCCUS AUREUS * A12151

- *BRASSICA OLERACEA* (CRUCIFERAE) DRIED AERIAL PARTS USSR

  a) ANTITUSSIVE ACTIVITY * HOT H2O EXT * ORAL * GUINEA PIG * * DOSE NOT STATED / * INACTIVE * * * W2509

    1. DATA INCOMPLETE - DERIVED FROM AN ABSTRACT.

- *BRASSICA OLERACEA* (CRUCIFERAE) INFLORESCENCE GERMANY(WEST)

  a) NADH OXIDASE INHIBITION * H2O EXT * * * DOSE NOT STATED / * ACTIVE * * * L0490

- *BRASSICA OLERACEA* (CRUCIFERAE) LEAF

  a) OESTROGENIC EFFECT * TYPE EXT NOT STATED * SC * MOUSE(OVARIECTOMIZED) * FEMALE * DOSE VARIABLE / * ACTIVE * * * T6788

    1. THESE DATA ARE FROM A REVIEW ARTICLE.

- *BRASSICA OLERACEA* (CRUCIFERAE) FREEZE-DRIED LEAF BELGIUM

  a) ANTIVIRAL ACTIVITY * ETOH(80%)EXT * * CELL CULTURE * * CONC USED VARIABLE / * EQUIVOCAL * * ADENOVIRUS(UNSPEC) * T6435

    1. VS.PLAQUE-INHIBITION.

  b) ANTIVIRAL ACTIVITY * ETOH(80%)EXT * * CELL CULTURE * * CONC USED VARIABLE / * EQUIVOCAL * * MEASLES VIRUS * T6435

    1. VS.PLAQUE-INHIBITION.

275

BRASSICA OLER* (3part query for [BEECHER.GROUP], 1-MAY-1990)

c) ANTIVIRAL ACTIVITY * ETOH(80%)EXT * * CELL CULTURE * * CONC USED VARIABLE / * INACTIVE * * COXSACKIE B2 VIRUS * T6435

    1. VS.PLAQUE-INHIBITION.

d) ANTIVIRAL ACTIVITY * ETOH(80%)EXT * * CELL CULTURE * * CONC USED VARIABLE / * INACTIVE * * HERPES VIRUS TYPE 1 * T6435

    1. VS.PLAQUE-INHIBITION.

e) ANTIVIRAL ACTIVITY * ETOH(80%)EXT * * CELL CULTURE * * CONC USED VARIABLE / * INACTIVE * * POLIOVIRUS I * T6435

    1. VS.PLAQUE-INHIBITION.

f) ANTIVIRAL ACTIVITY * ETOH(80%)EXT * * CELL CULTURE * * CONC USED VARIABLE / * INACTIVE * * SEMLICKI-FOREST VIRUS * T6435

    1. VS.PLAQUE-INHIBITION.

- *BRASSICA OLERACEA* (CRUCIFERAE) FRESH LEAF

    a) ANTITHYROID ACTIVITY * LEAVES * ORAL * HUMAN ADULT * * DOSE 380.0 GM/PERSON * ACTIVE * * * W4283

- *BRASSICA OLERACEA* (CRUCIFERAE) FRESH LEAF ENGLAND

    a) DERMATITIS PRODUCING EFFECT * LEAVES * PATCH TEST * HUMAN ADULT * * DOSE NOT STATED / * ACTIVE * * * M20732

- *BRASSICA OLERACEA* (CRUCIFERAE) SHADE DRIED LEAF PAKISTAN(CULT)

    a) ACID NEUTRALIZATION ACTIVITY * H2O EXT * * * * CONC USED 400.0 MG/SQ M * * * * M21921

    b) ACID NEUTRALIZATION ACTIVITY * MEOH EXT * * * * CONC USED 400.0 MG/ * ACTIVE * * * M21921

    c) ACID NEUTRALIZATION ACTIVITY * POWDER * * * * CONC USED 400.0 MG/ * WEAK ACTIVITY * * * M21921

    d) ANTIULCER ACTIVITY * H2O EXT * INTRAGASTRIC * RAT * * DOSE 4.0 GM/KG * STRONG ACTIVITY * * * M21921

        1. VS.ASPIRIN-INDUCED ULCERS.

    e) ANTIULCER ACTIVITY * MEOH EXT * INTRAGASTRIC * RAT * * DOSE 4.0 GM/KG * INACTIVE * * * M21921

        1. VS.ASPIRIN-INDUCED ULCERS.

    f) ANTIULCER ACTIVITY * POWDER * INTRAGASTRIC * RAT * * DOSE 4.0 GM/KG * INACTIVE * * * M21921

        1. VS.ASPIRIN-INDUCED ULCERS.

    g) GASTRIC SECRETORY INHIBITION * H2O EXT * INTRAGASTRIC * RAT * * DOSE 4.0 GM/KG * INACTIVE * * * M21921

        1. VS.ASPIRIN-INDUCED ULCERS.

276

h) GASTRIC SECRETORY INHIBITION * MEOH EXT * INTRAGASTRIC * RAT * * DOSE 4.0 GM/KG * INACTIVE * * * M21921

   1. VS.ASPIRIN-INDUCED ULCERS.

i) GASTRIC SECRETORY INHIBITION * POWDER * INTRAGASTRIC * RAT * * DOSE 4.0 GM/KG * INACTIVE * * * M21921

   1. VS.ASPIRIN-INDUCED ULCERS.

j) HEXOSAMINE SECRETION INHIBITION * H2O EXT * INTRAGASTRIC * RAT * * DOSE 4.0 GM/KG * INACTIVE * * * M21921

   1. VS.ASPIRIN-INDUCED ULCERS.

k) HEXOSAMINE SECRETION INHIBITION * MEOH EXT * INTRAGASTRIC * RAT * * DOSE 4.0 GM/KG * INACTIVE * * * M21921

   1. VS.ASPIRIN-INDUCED ULCERS.

l) HEXOSAMINE SECRETION INHIBITION * POWDER * INTRAGASTRIC * RAT * * DOSE 4.0 GM/KG * INACTIVE * * * M21921

   1. VS.ASPIRIN-INDUCED ULCERS.

m) PEPSIN BINDING * H2O EXT * * * * CONC USED 400.0 MG/ * ACTIVE * * * M21921

n) PEPSIN BINDING * MEOH EXT * * * * CONC USED 400.0 MG/ * WEAK ACTIVITY * * * M21921

o) PEPSIN BINDING * POWDER * * * * CONC USED 400.0 MG/ * WEAK ACTIVITY * * * M21921

p) PEPSIN SECRETION INHIBITION * H2O EXT * INTRAGASTRIC * RAT * * DOSE 4.0 GM/KG * STRONG ACTIVITY * * * M21921

   1. VS.ASPIRIN-INDUCED ULCERS.

q) PEPSIN SECRETION INHIBITION * MEOH EXT * INTRAGASTRIC * RAT * * DOSE 4.0 GM/KG * INACTIVE * * * M21921

   1. VS.ASPIRIN-INDUCED ULCERS.

r) PEPSIN SECRETION INHIBITION * POWDER * INTRAGASTRIC * RAT * * DOSE 4.0 GM/KG * INACTIVE * * * M21921

   1. VS.ASPIRIN-INDUCED ULCERS.

s) TOXIC EFFECT(GENERAL) * POWDER * INTRAGASTRIC * RAT * * DOSE 6.0 GM/KG * INACTIVE * * * M21921

- *BRASSICA OLERACEA* (CRUCIFERAE) ROOT

a) UTERINE STIMULANT EFFECT * PLANT * IN RATION * GUINEA PIG(PREGNANT) * * CONC USED 4.2 % OF DIET/ * ACTIVE * * UTERUS(PREG) * A0325

- *BRASSICA OLERACEA* (CRUCIFERAE) SEED GERMANY(WEST)

a) ANTIBACTERIAL ACTIVITY * ETOH(95%)EXT * * AGAR PLATE * * CONC USED VARIABLE / * ACTIVE * * BACILLUS SUBTILIS * A12151

BRASSICA OLER* (3part query for [BEECHER.GROUP], 1-MAY-1990)

b) ANTIBACTERIAL ACTIVITY * ETOH(95%)EXT * * AGAR PLATE * * CONC USED VARIABLE / * ACTIVE * * ESCHERICHIA COLI * A12151

c) ANTIBACTERIAL ACTIVITY * ETOH(95%)EXT * * AGAR PLATE * * CONC USED VARIABLE / * ACTIVE * * STAPHYLOCOCCUS AUREUS * A12151

- *BRASSICA OLERACEA* CV.EXCEL (CRUCIFERAE) FREEZE-DRIED AERIAL PARTS USA

  a) ANILINE HYDRASE INHIBITION * AERIAL PARTS * IN RATION * RAT * * DOSE 20.0 % OF DIET/ * ACTIVE * * * M6032

    1. EFFECTS MEASURED IN LIVER.

    2. RESULTS SIGNIFICANT AT P L0.05 LEVEL.

  b) ENZYME EFFECTS(UNSPECIFIED) * AERIAL PARTS * IN RATION * RAT * * DOSE 20.0 % OF DIET/ * ACTIVE * * * M6032

    1. EFFECTS MEASURED IN LIVER.

    2. RESULTS SIGNIFICANT AT P L0.05 LEVEL.

  c) ENZYME EFFECTS(UNSPECIFIED) * AERIAL PARTS * IN RATION * RAT * * DOSE 20.0 % OF DIET/ * ACTIVE * * * M6032

    1. EFFECTS MEASURED IN LIVER.

    2. RESULTS SIGNIFICANT AT P L0.05 LEVEL.

  d) NADPH-CYTOCHROME C REDUCTASE INHIBITION * AERIAL PARTS * IN RATION * RAT * * DOSE 20.0 % OF DIET/ * ACTIVE * * * M6032

    1. EFFECTS MEASURED IN LIVER.

    2. RESULTS SIGNIFICANT AT P L0.05 LEVEL.

  e) TOXIC EFFECT(GENERAL) * AERIAL PARTS * IN RATION * RAT * * DOSE 20.0 % OF DIET/ * ACTIVE * * * M6032

    1. HISTOPATHOLOGY DATA ARE PRESENTED AND DISCUSSED.

- *BRASSICA OLERACEA* CV.GEMMIFERA (CRUCIFERAE) FREEZE-DRIED FRUIT USA-CA

  a) ARYL HYDROCARBON HYDROXYLASE INDUCTION * ETOH(95%)EXT * IN RATION * MOUSE * FEMALE * DOSE 25.0 % OF DIET/ * ACTIVE * * * T15589

  b) CYTOCHROME P-450 INDUCTION * ETOH(95%)EXT * IN RATION * MOUSE * FEMALE * DOSE 25.0 % OF DIET/ * ACTIVE * * * T15589

  c) DNA BINDING EFFECT * ETOH(95%)EXT * IN RATION * MOUSE * FEMALE * DOSE 25.0 % OF DIET/ * INACTIVE * * * T15589

  d) EPOXIDE HYDRASE INDUCTION * ETOH(95%)EXT * IN RATION * MOUSE * MALE * DOSE 25.0 % OF DIET/ * ACTIVE * * * T15589

  e) ETHOXYCOUMARIN DEETHYLASE STIMULATION * ETOH(95%)EXT * IN RATION * MOUSE * * DOSE 25.0 % OF DIET/ * INACTIVE * * * T15589

  f) GLUTATHIONE-S-TRANSFERASE INDUCTION * ETOH(95%)EXT * IN RATION * MOUSE * * DOSE 25.0 % OF DIET/ * INACTIVE * * * T15589

278

BRASSICA OLER* (3part query for [BEECHER.GROUP], 1-MAY-1990)

g) MUTAGENIC ACTIVITY * ETOH(95%)EXT * IN RATION * MOUSE * FEMALE * DOSE 25.0 % OF DIET/ * INACTIVE * * * T15589

    1. METABOLIC ACTIVATION HAS NO EFFECT ON THE RESULTS.

- *BRASSICA OLERACEA* CV.JADE CROSS (CRUCIFERAE) LEAF USA-MN

a) ARYL HYDROCARBON HYDROXYLASE INDUCTION * PLANT * ORAL * RAT * * DOSE NOT STATED / * ACTIVE * * * K4324

- *BRASSICA OLERACEA* VAR CAPITATA (CRUCIFERAE) LEAF INDIA

a) ANTIHYPERGLYCEMIC ACTIVITY * ETOH(95%)EXT * SC * RAT * * DOSE 0.5 ML/ANIMAL * INACTIVE * * * W0260

b) HYPOGLYCEMIC ACTIVITY * ETOH(95%)EXT * SC * RAT * * DOSE 0.5 ML/ANIMAL * INACTIVE * * * W0260

- *BRASSICA OLERACEA* VAR.ACEPHALA (CRUCIFERAE) AERIAL PARTS SCOTLAND

a) TOXIC EFFECT(GENERAL) * PLANT * IN RATION * COW * * DOSE NOT STATED / * ACTIVE * * * N2289

- *BRASSICA OLERACEA* VAR.ACEPHALA (CRUCIFERAE) FRESH AERIAL PARTS USA-NC

a) ANTIMUTAGENIC ACTIVITY * ETOH(95%)EXT * * * * CONC USED NOT STATED / * ACTIVE * * * M15575

- *BRASSICA OLERACEA* VAR.ACEPHALA (CRUCIFERAE) FRESH LEAF USA

a) INTRAOCULAR PRESSURE REDUCTION * H2O EXT * IV * RABBIT * * DOSE 250.0 MCG/ANIMAL * ACTIVE * * * M21177

- *BRASSICA OLERACEA* VAR.ACEPHALA (CRUCIFERAE) FRESH LEAF JUICE TURKEY(CULT)

a) CYTOLYTIC ACTIVITY * CHROMATOGRAPHIC FRACTION * * * * CONC USED NOT STATED / * ACTIVE * * * T14715

- *BRASSICA OLERACEA* VAR.ACHEPHALA-CV.VATES (CRUCIFERAE) FRESH LEAF

a) GLUTATHIONE-S-TRANSFERASE INDUCTION * LEAVES * * * * CONC USED UNDILUTED / * ACTIVE * * SPODOPTERA FRUGIPERDA * T12014

- *BRASSICA OLERACEA* VAR.BOTRYTIS (CRUCIFERAE) BOILED AERIAL PARTS

a) ANTITHYROID ACTIVITY * AERIAL PARTS * ORAL * HUMAN ADULT * * DOSE 263.0 GM/PERSON * INACTIVE * * * W4283

- *BRASSICA OLERACEA* VAR.BOTRYTIS (CRUCIFERAE) DRIED AERIAL PARTS

a) ARYL HYDROCARBON HYDROXYLASE INDUCTION * ENTIRE PLANT * IN RATION * RAT * MALE * DOSE VARIABLE / * ACTIVE * * * N17332

b) CYTOCHROME P-450 INDUCTION * ENTIRE PLANT * IN RATION * RAT * MALE * DOSE VARIABLE / * ACTIVE * * * N17332

c) EPOXIDE HYDRASE INDUCTION * * IN RATION * RAT * MALE * DOSE VARIABLE / * ACTIVE * * * N17332

279

  d) GLUTATHIONE-S-TRANSFERASE INDUCTION * * IN RATION * RAT * MALE * DOSE VARIABLE / * ACTIVE * * * N17332

- *BRASSICA OLERACEA* VAR.BOTRYTIS (CRUCIFERAE) FREEZE-DRIED AERIAL PARTS USA-CA(CULT)

  a) MONOOXYGENASE INDUCTION * CHROMATOGRAPHIC FRACTION * IN RATION * RAT * * DOSE VARIABLE / * ACTIVE * * * M16212

  b) MONOOXYGENASE INDUCTION * PLANT * IN RATION * RAT * * DOSE 25 %/ * ACTIVE * * * M16212

- *BRASSICA OLERACEA* VAR.BOTRYTIS (CRUCIFERAE) FRESH AERIAL PARTS JAPAN

  a) ANTIMUTAGENIC ACTIVITY * H2O EXT * * AGAR PLATE * * DOSE 0.4 ML/PLATE * ACTIVE * * SALMONELLA TYPHIMURIUM TA100 * T14904

  b) TUMOR PROMOTION INHIBITION * MEOH EXT * * CELL CULTURE * * CONC USED 200.0 MCG/ * ACTIVE * * EPSTEIN-BARR VIRUS * T15279

- *BRASSICA OLERACEA* VAR.BOTRYTIS (CRUCIFERAE) FRESH FRUITJUICE(UNRIPE)

  a) ANTIMUTAGENIC ACTIVITY * JUICE * GASTRIC INTUBATION * MOUSE * MALE * DOSE 0.5 ML/ANIMAL * ACTIVE * * SCHIZOSACCHAROMYCES POMBE (P1) * T7559

      1. RESULTS SIGNIFICANT AT P L0.001 LEVEL.

- *BRASSICA OLERACEA* VAR.BOTRYTIS (CRUCIFERAE) FRESH FRUITJUICE(UNRIPE) JAPAN

  a) DESMUTAGENIC ACTIVITY * AQUEOUS HIGH SPEED SUPERNATANT * * AGAR PLATE * * CONC USED 0.5 ML/PLATE * ACTIVE * * SALMONELLA TYP HIMURIUM TA98 * T12543

  b) DESMUTAGENIC ACTIVITY * AQUEOUS HIGH SPEED SUPERNATANT * * AGAR PLATE * * CONC USED 0.5 ML/PLATE * ACTIVE * * SALMONELLA TYP HIMURIUM TA98 * T12543

- *BRASSICA OLERACEA* VAR.BOTRYTIS (CRUCIFERAE) FRESH LEAF JAPAN

  a) DESMUTAGENIC ACTIVITY * HOMOGENATES * * AGAR PLATE * * CONC USED 100.0 MICROLITERS/DISC * ACTIVE * * SALMONELLA TYPHIMURIUM TA100 * T12048

  b) DESMUTAGENIC ACTIVITY * HOMOGENATES * * AGAR PLATE * * CONC USED 100.0 MICROLITERS/DISC * ACTIVE * * SALMONELLA TYPHIMURIUM TA98 * T12048

- *BRASSICA OLERACEA* VAR.BOTRYTIS (CRUCIFERAE) FRESH PLANT JUICE JAPAN(CULT)

  a) CATALASE STIMULATION * JUICE * * * * CONC USED 0.5 ML/ * ACTIVE * * * T12593

  b) CATALASE STIMULATION * JUICE * * * * CONC USED 0.5 ML/ * WEAK ACTIVITY * * * T12593

  c) DESMUTAGENIC ACTIVITY * JUICE * * AGAR PLATE * * CONC USED 0.5 ML/PLATE * ACTIVE * * SALMONELLA TYPHIMURIUM TA98 * T12593

  d) DESMUTAGENIC ACTIVITY * JUICE * * AGAR PLATE * * CONC USED 0.5 ML/PLATE * ACTIVE * * SALMONELLA TYPHIMURIUM TA98 * T12593

BRASSICA OLER* (3part query for [BEECHER.GROUP], 1-MAY-1990)

i.

e) PEROXIDASE ACTIVITY * JUICE * * * * CONC USED 0.5 ML/ * ACTIVE * * * T12593

f) PEROXIDASE ACTIVITY * JUICE * * * * CONC USED 0.5 ML/ * WEAK ACTIVITY * * *
T12593

● *BRASSICA OLERACEA* VAR.BOTRYTIS CV.SNOWBALL (CRUCIFERAE) AERIAL PARTS
USA

a) ARYL HYDROCARBON HYDROXYLASE INDUCTION * ETOAC EXT * ORAL * RAT * * @
/ * ACTIVE * * * J3624

● *BRASSICA OLERACEA* VAR.BOTRYTIS-CAULIFLORA (CRUCIFERAE) BOILED AERIAL
PARTS

a) ANTITHYROID ACTIVITY * AERIAL PARTS * ORAL * HUMAN ADULT * * DOSE 560.0
GM/PERSON * INACTIVE * * * W4283

● *BRASSICA OLERACEA* VAR.BOTRYTIS-WALTHAM 29 (CRUCIFERAE) FRESH LEAF

a) GLUTATHIONE-S-TRANSFERASE INDUCTION * LEAVES * * * * CONC USED
UNDILUTED / * INACTIVE * * SPODOPTERA FRUGIPERDA * T12014

● *BRASSICA OLERACEA* VAR.CAPITATA (CRUCIFERAE) DRIED AERIAL PARTS CANADA

a) TUMOR INITIATING EFFECT * LEAVES * IN RATION * MOUSE * * DOSE 128.0 GM/KG
DIET * ACTIVE * * CA-ADENOCARCINOMA-COLON * T15228

b) TUMOR PROMOTION INHIBITION * LEAVES * IN RATION * MOUSE * * DOSE 128.0
GM/KG DIET * ACTIVE * * CA-ADENOCARCINOMA-COLON * T152 28

● *BRASSICA OLERACEA* VAR.CAPITATA (CRUCIFERAE) FREEZE-DRIED AERIAL PARTS
USA-CA

a) ANTIHEPATOTOXIC ACTIVITY * PLANT * IN RATION * RAT * * DOSE 25.0 %/ * ACTIVE
* * * T14913

b) ARYL HYDROCARBON HYDROXYLASE INDUCTION * PLANT * IN RATION * RAT * *
DOSE 25.0 %/ * ACTIVE * * INTESTINE * T14913

c) ARYL HYDROCARBON HYDROXYLASE INDUCTION * PLANT * IN RATION * RAT * *
DOSE 25.0 %/ * INACTIVE * * LIVER * T14913

d) EPOXIDE HYDRASE INDUCTION * PLANT * IN RATION * RAT * * DOSE 25.0 %/ *
ACTIVE * * INTESTINE * T14913

e) EPOXIDE HYDRASE INDUCTION * PLANT * IN RATION * RAT * * DOSE 25.0 %/ *
ACTIVE * * LIVER * T14913

f) ETHOXYCOUMARIN DEETHYLASE STIMULATION * PLANT * IN RATION * RAT * *
DOSE 25.0 %/ * ACTIVE * * INTESTINE * T14913

g) ETHOXYCOUMARIN DEETHYLASE STIMULATION * PLANT * IN RATION * RAT * *
DOSE 25.0 %/ * INACTIVE * * LIVER * T14913

h) GLUTATHIONE-S-TRANSFERASE INDUCTION * PLANT * IN RATION * RAT * * DOSE
25.0 %/ * ACTIVE * * INTESTINE * T14913

i) GLUTATHIONE-S-TRANSFERASE INDUCTION * PLANT * IN RATION * RAT * * DOSE
25.0 %/ * ACTIVE * * LIVER * T14913

281

BRASSICA OLER* (3part query for [BEECHER.GROUP], 1-MAY-1990)

- *BRASSICA OLERACEA* VAR.CAPITATA (CRUCIFERAE) FRESH AERIAL PARTS JAPAN

  a) TUMOR PROMOTION INHIBITION * ETOAC EXT * * CELL CULTURE * * CONC USED
     200.0 MCG/ * WEAK ACTIVITY * * EPSTEIN-BARR VIRUS * T1 5279

  b) TUMOR PROMOTION INHIBITION * MEOH EXT * * CELL CULTURE * * CONC USED
     200.0 MCG/ * INACTIVE * * EPSTEIN-BARR VIRUS * T15279

- *BRASSICA OLERACEA* VAR.CAPITATA (CRUCIFERAE) FRESH AERIAL PARTS THAILAND

  a) HYPOGLYCEMIC ACTIVITY * H2O EXT * GASTRIC INTUBATION * RABBIT * * DOSE
     NOT STATED / * ACTIVE * * * R0015

     1. DATA INCOMPLETE - DERIVED FROM AN ABSTRACT.

- *BRASSICA OLERACEA* VAR.CAPITATA (CRUCIFERAE) FIXED OIL NIGERIA

  a) ANTIHYPERLIPEMIC ACTIVITY * VEGETABLE OIL * ORAL * RAT * * DOSE 100 MG/KG
     * ACTIVE * * * T14157

- *BRASSICA OLERACEA* VAR.CAPITATA (CRUCIFERAE) FRESH FRUITJUICE(UNRIPE)
  JAPAN

  a) DESMUTAGENIC ACTIVITY * AQUEOUS HIGH SPEED SUPERNATANT * * AGAR
     PLATE * * CONC USED 0.5 ML/PLATE * ACTIVE * * SALMONELLA TYP HIMURIUM
     TA98 * T12543

  b) DESMUTAGENIC ACTIVITY * AQUEOUS HIGH SPEED SUPERNATANT * * AGAR
     PLATE * * CONC USED 0.5 ML/PLATE * INACTIVE * * SALMONELLA T YPHIMURIUM
     TA98 * T12543

- *BRASSICA OLERACEA* VAR.CAPITATA (CRUCIFERAE) DRIED LEAF

  a) BENZOPYRENE METABOLISM STIMULATION * LEAVES * IN RATION * MOUSE * *
     DOSE 20.0 % OF DIET/ANIMAL * INACTIVE * * LIVER * T15345

     1. DATA INCOMPLETE - DERIVED FROM AN ABSTRACT.

- *BRASSICA OLERACEA* VAR.CAPITATA (CRUCIFERAE) FRESH LEAF ENGLAND

  a) ANTIHYPERGLYCEMIC ACTIVITY * ETOH(70%)EXT * INTRAGASTRIC * RABBIT * *
     DOSE 1.0 KG/ANIMAL * ACTIVE * * * A14301

  b) HYPERGLYCEMIC ACTIVITY * ETOH(70%)EXT * INTRAGASTRIC * RABBIT * * DOSE
     1.0 KG/ANIMAL * ACTIVE * * * A14301

     1. DOSE EXPRESSED AS DRY WEIGHT OF PLANT.

  c) HYPOGLYCEMIC ACTIVITY * ETOH(70%)EXT * INTRAGASTRIC * DOG * * DOSE 3.0
     KG/ANIMAL * ACTIVE * * * A14301

     1. DOSE EXPRESSED AS DRY WEIGHT OF PLANT.

  d) HYPOGLYCEMIC ACTIVITY * ETOH(95%)EXT * INTRAGASTRIC * RABBIT * * DOSE
     NOT STATED / * INACTIVE * * * A14285

  e) HYPOGLYCEMIC ACTIVITY * ETOH(95%)EXT * SC * RABBIT * * DOSE NOT STATED / *
     INACTIVE * * * A14285

- *BRASSICA OLERACEA* VAR.CAPITATA (CRUCIFERAE) FRESH LEAF INDIA

BRASSICA OLER* (3part query for [BEECHER.GROUP], 1-MAY-1990)

a) ANTIULCER ACTIVITY * JUICE * * GUINEA PIG * * DOSE 10.0 ML/ANIMAL * ACTIVE *
   * * A11139

   1. HISTOPATHOLOGY DATA ARE PRESENTED AND DISCUSSED.

   2. VS.HISTAMINE-INDUCED ULCERS.

   3.

b) ANTIULCER ACTIVITY * JUICE * * GUINEA PIG * * DOSE 10.0 ML/ANIMAL * ACTIVE *
   * * A11139

   1. HISTOPATHOLOGY DATA ARE PRESENTED AND DISCUSSED.

   2.

   3. VS.PHENYLBUTAZONE-INDUCED ULCERS.

c) GOITROGENIC ACTIVITY * TYPE EXT NOT STATED * IN RATION * RAT * * DOSE 9.0
   GM/DAY * ACTIVE * * * T9416

- *BRASSICA OLERACEA* VAR.CAPITATA (CRUCIFERAE) FRESH LEAF JAPAN

   a) ANTIMUTAGENIC ACTIVITY * H2O EXT * * AGAR PLATE * * DOSE 0.4 ML/PLATE *
      ACTIVE * * SALMONELLA TYPHIMURIUM TA100 * T14904

   b) ANTIMUTAGENIC ACTIVITY * JUICE * * AGAR PLATE * * CONC USED 0.1 ML/ *
      ACTIVE * * SALMONELLA TYPHIMURIUM TA98 * T12477

   c) DESMUTAGENIC ACTIVITY * HOMOGENATES * * AGAR PLATE * * CONC USED 100.0
      MICROLITERS/DISC * ACTIVE * * SALMONELLA TYPHIMURIUM TA100 * T12048

   d) DESMUTAGENIC ACTIVITY * HOMOGENATES * * AGAR PLATE * * CONC USED 100.0
      MICROLITERS/DISC * ACTIVE * * SALMONELLA TYPHIMURIUM TA98 * T12048

- *BRASSICA OLERACEA* VAR.CAPITATA (CRUCIFERAE) FRESH LEAF PUERTO RICO

   a) CARCINOGENESIS INHIBITION * LEAF * IN RATION * MOUSE * * DOSE 13.0 % OF
      DIET/ * INACTIVE * * * T15737

- *BRASSICA OLERACEA* VAR.CAPITATA (CRUCIFERAE) FRESH LEAF JUICE JAPAN

   a) ANTIMUTAGENIC ACTIVITY * JUICE * * AGAR PLATE * * CONC USED UNDILUTED /
      * ACTIVE * * * T13252

- *BRASSICA OLERACEA* VAR.CAPITATA (CRUCIFERAE) FRESH LEAF JUICE
  TURKEY(CULT)

   a) CYTOLYTIC ACTIVITY * CHROMATOGRAPHIC FRACTION * * * * CONC USED NOT
      STATED / * ACTIVE * * * T14715

- *BRASSICA OLERACEA* VAR.CAPITATA (CRUCIFERAE) FRESH PLANT JUICE
  JAPAN(CULT;

   a) CATALASE STIMULATION * JUICE * * * * CONC USED 0.5 ML/ * WEAK ACTIVITY * *
      * T12593

   b) DESMUTAGENIC ACTIVITY * JUICE * * AGAR PLATE * * CONC USED 0.5 ML/PLATE *
      ACTIVE * * SALMONELLA TYPHIMURIUM TA98 * T12593

   c) PEROXIDASE ACTIVITY * JUICE * * * * CONC USED 0.5 ML/ * ACTIVE * * * T12593

BRASSICA OLER* (3part query for [BEECHER.GROUP], 1-MAY-1990)

- *BRASSICA OLERACEA* VAR.CAPITATA (CRUCIFERAE) FRESH SEED USA

    a) ANTITUBERCULOSIS ACTIVITY * H2O EXT * * * AGAR PLATE * * CONC USED NOT STATED / * WEAK ACTIVITY * * MYCOBACTERIUM TUBERCULOSIS * W1074

- *BRASSICA OLERACEA* VAR.CAPITATA CV.CHIEFTAN (CRUCIFERAE) AERIAL PARTS USA

    a) ARYL HYDROCARBON HYDROXYLASE INDUCTION * ETOAC EXT * ORAL * RAT * * @ / * ACTIVE * * * J3624

- *BRASSICA OLERACEA* VAR.CAPITATA CV.CHIEFTAN (CRUCIFERAE) FRESH LEAF USA-MN(CULT)

    a) MICROSOMAL METABOLIZING SYSTEM INDUCTION * PLANT * ORAL * HUMAN ADULT * * DOSE 100.0 GM/PERSON * ACTIVE * * * N2964

        1. STATISTICAL DATA IN REPORT INDICATING SIGNIFICANT RESULTS.

        2. EFFECTS DESCRIBED ARE FROM A MULTI-COMPONENT RX.

- *BRASSICA OLERACEA* VAR.CAPITATA CV.NAPPA (CRUCIFERAE) FRESH AERIAL PARTS USA

    a) INTRAOCULAR PRESSURE REDUCTION * H2O EXT * IV * RABBIT * * DOSE 250.0 MCG/ANIMAL * INACTIVE * * * M21177

- *BRASSICA OLERACEA* VAR.CAPITATA CV.RED (CRUCIFERAE) FROZEN FRUITJUICE(UNRIPE)

    a) MUTATION INHIBITION * JUICE * * AGAR PLATE * * CONC USED 0.1 ML/PLATE * ACTIVE * * SALMONELLA TYPHIMURIUM TA1538 * M14151

        1. METABOLIC ACTIVATION REQUIRED TO OBTAIN POSITIVE RESULTS.

- *BRASSICA OLERACEA* VAR.CAPITATA CV.RED CABBA (CRUCIFERAE) FRESH LEAF JAPAN

    a) DESMUTAGENIC ACTIVITY * HOMOGENATES * * AGAR PLATE * * CONC USED 100.0 MICROLITERS/DISC * ACTIVE * * SALMONELLA TYPHIMURIUM TA100 * T12048

    b) DESMUTAGENIC ACTIVITY * HOMOGENATES * * AGAR PLATE * * CONC USED 100.0 MICROLITERS/DISC * ACTIVE * * SALMONELLA TYPHIMURIUM TA98 * T12048

- *BRASSICA OLERACEA* VAR.CAPITATA CV.SAVOY (CRUCIFERAE) FRESH AERIAL PARTS USA

    a) INTRAOCULAR PRESSURE REDUCTION * H2O EXT * IV * RABBIT * * DOSE 250.0 MCG/ANIMAL * INACTIVE * * * M21177

- *BRASSICA OLERACEA* VAR.CAPITATA CV.WHITE (CRUCIFERAE) FROZEN FRUITJUICE(UNRIPE)

    a) MUTATION INHIBITION * JUICE * * AGAR PLATE * * CONC USED 0.1 ML/PLATE * ACTIVE * * SALMONELLA TYPHIMURIUM TA1538 * M14151

        1. METABOLIC ACTIVATION REQUIRED TO OBTAIN POSITIVE RESULTS.

- *BRASSICA OLERACEA* VAR.CAPITATA-CHARLESTON (CRUCIFERAE) FRESH LEAF

BRASSICA OLER* (3part query for [BEECHER.GROUP], 1-MAY-1990)

a) GLUTATHIONE-S-TRANSFERASE INDUCTION * LEAVES * * * * CONC USED UNDILUTED / * ACTIVE * * SPODOPTERA FRUGIPERDA * T12014

- *BRASSICA OLERACEA* VAR.GEMMIFERA (CRUCIFERAE) FREEZE-DRIED AERIAL PARTS USA(CULT)

  a) ANTITUMOR ACTIVITY * AERIAL PARTS * IN RATION * RAT * * DOSE 20 %/ * ACTIVE * * * T14498

- *BRASSICA OLERACEA* VAR.GEMMIFERA (CRUCIFERAE) FREEZE-DRIED BUDS ENGLAND

  a) MIXED FUNCTION OXIDASE ACTIVITY * BUDS * IN RATION * RAT * * DOSE 25.0 % OF DIET/ * STRONG ACTIVITY * * INTESTINE(LARGE) * M2 1684

  b) MIXED FUNCTION OXIDASE ACTIVITY * BUDS * IN RATION * RAT * * DOSE 25.0 % OF DIET/ * STRONG ACTIVITY * * INTESTINE(SMALL) * M2 1684

  c) MIXED FUNCTION OXIDASE ACTIVITY * BUDS * INTRAGASTRIC * RAT * * DOSE 25.0 % OF DIET/ * STRONG ACTIVITY * * LIVER * M21684

- *BRASSICA OLERACEA* VAR.GEMMIFERA (CRUCIFERAE) FREEZE-DRIED BUDS NETHERLANDS

  a) MUTAGENIC ACTIVITY * CHCL3 EXT * * AGAR PLATE * * CONC USED NOT STATED / * INACTIVE * * SALMONELLA TYPHIMURIUM TA100 * M5461

  b) MUTAGENIC ACTIVITY * CHCL3 EXT * * AGAR PLATE * * CONC USED NOT STATED / * INACTIVE * * SALMONELLA TYPHIMURIUM TA98 * M5461

  c) MUTAGENIC ACTIVITY * MEOH EXT * * AGAR PLATE * * CONC USED NOT STATED / * INACTIVE * * SALMONELLA TYPHIMURIUM TA100 * M5461

  d) MUTAGENIC ACTIVITY * MEOH EXT * * AGAR PLATE * * CONC USED NOT STATED / * INACTIVE * * SALMONELLA TYPHIMURIUM TA98 * M5461

  e) MUTAGENIC ACTIVITY * PET ETHER EXT * * AGAR PLATE * * CONC USED NOT STATED / * INACTIVE * * SALMONELLA TYPHIMURIUM TA100 * M 5461

  f) MUTAGENIC ACTIVITY * PET ETHER EXT * * AGAR PLATE * * CONC USED NOT STATED / * INACTIVE * * SALMONELLA TYPHIMURIUM TA98 * M5 461

- *BRASSICA OLERACEA* VAR.GEMMIFERA (CRUCIFERAE) FRESH BUDS

  1. RESULTS SIGNIFICANT AT P L0.05 LEVEL.

     a) GLUTATHIONE-S-TRANSFERASE INDUCTION * CHROMATOGRAPHIC FRACTION * IN RATION * RAT * * DOSE 20.0 % OF DIET/ * ACTIVE * * * T93 99

  2. RESULTS SIGNIFICANT AT P L0.05 LEVEL.

     a) GLUTATHIONE-S-TRANSFERASE INDUCTION * CHROMATOGRAPHIC FRACTION * IN RATION * RAT * * DOSE 20.0 % OF DIET/ * ACTIVE * * * T93 99

  3. RESULTS SIGNIFICANT AT P L0.05 LEVEL.

- *BRASSICA OLERACEA* VAR.GEMMIFERA (CRUCIFERAE) FROZEN FRUITJUICE(UNRIPE)

  a) MUTATION INHIBITION * JUICE * * AGAR PLATE * * CONC USED 0.1 ML/PLATE * ACTIVE * * SALMONELLA TYPHIMURIUM TA1538 * M14151

     1. METABOLIC ACTIVATION REQUIRED TO OBTAIN POSITIVE RESULTS.

BRASSICA OLER* (3part query for [BEECHER.GROUP], 1-MAY-1990)

● *BRASSICA OLERACEA* VAR.GEMMIFERA (CRUCIFERAE) DRIED LEAF

  a) BENZOPYRENE METABOLISM STIMULATION * LEAVES * IN RATION * MOUSE * *
  DOSE 20.0 % OF DIET/ANIMAL * INACTIVE * * LIVER * T15345

    1. DATA INCOMPLETE - DERIVED FROM AN ABSTRACT.

  b) EPOXIDE HYDRASE INDUCTION * LEAVES * IN RATION * MOUSE * * DOSE 20.0
  %/ANIMAL * ACTIVE * * * T15345

    1. DATA INCOMPLETE - DERIVED FROM AN ABSTRACT.

● *BRASSICA OLERACEA* VAR.GEMMIFERA (CRUCIFERAE) FREEZE-DRIED LEAF BUDS USA

  a) MICROSOMAL METABOLIZING SYSTEM INDUCTION * LEAVES * IN RATION * RAT * *
  DOSE 25.0 % OF DIET/ * ACTIVE * * * T9853

● *BRASSICA OLERACEA* VAR.GEMMIFERA CV.JADE CRO (CRUCIFERAE) AERIAL PARTS

  a) * * * * * @ / * * * * J3624

● *BRASSICA OLERACEA* VAR.GEMMIFERA CV.JADE CRO (CRUCIFERAE) FRESH SPROUTS
USA-MN(CULT)

  a) MICROSOMAL METABOLIZING SYSTEM INDUCTION * PLANT * ORAL * HUMAN
  ADULT * * DOSE 150.0 GM/PERSON * ACTIVE * * * N2964

    1. STATISTICAL DATA IN REPORT INDICATING SIGNIFICANT RESULTS.

    2. EFFECTS DESCRIBED ARE FROM A MULTI-COMPONENT RX.

● *BRASSICA OLERACEA* VAR.GONGYLODES (CRUCIFERAE) FRESH AERIAL PARTS USA

  a) INTRAOCULAR PRESSURE REDUCTION * H2O EXT * IV * RABBIT * * DOSE 250.0
  MCG/ANIMAL * ACTIVE * * * M21177

● *BRASSICA OLERACEA* VAR.GONGYLODES (CRUCIFERAE) FROZEN
FRUITJUICE(UNRIPE)

  a) MUTATION INHIBITION * JUICE * * AGAR PLATE * * CONC USED 0.1 ML/PLATE *
  ACTIVE * * SALMONELLA TYPHIMURIUM TA1538 * M14151

    1. METABOLIC ACTIVATION REQUIRED TO OBTAIN POSITIVE RESULTS.

● *BRASSICA OLERACEA* VAR.GONGYLODES (CRUCIFERAE) DRIED TUBER

  a) ANTIFUNGAL ACTIVITY * ESSENTIAL OIL * * AGAR PLATE * * CONC USED 1-10 / *
  ACTIVE * * SEVERAL FUNGI * A11825

  b) ANTIFUNGAL ACTIVITY(PLANT PATHOGENS) * ESSENTIAL OIL * * AGAR PLATE * *
  CONC USED 1-10 / * ACTIVE * * SEVERAL PLANT PATHOGEN IC FUNGI * A11825

  c) ANTIYEAST ACTIVITY * ESSENTIAL OIL * * AGAR PLATE * * CONC USED 1-10 / *
  ACTIVE * * SEVERAL YEASTS * A11825

● *BRASSICA OLERACEA* VAR.ITALICA (CRUCIFERAE) FRESH AERIAL PARTS JAPAN

  a) TUMOR PROMOTION INHIBITION * MEOH EXT * * CELL CULTURE * * CONC USED
  200.0 MCG/ * INACTIVE * * EPSTEIN-BARR VIRUS * T15279

● *BRASSICA OLERACEA* VAR.SAB☺AUDA(CRUCIFERAE) FRESH SEED USA

LITERATURE CITED

A0325   TRANSIENT OXYTOCIC DEPRESSION OF IMMATURE GUINEA PIG FED ON
          GRASS(BRACHIARIA PURPURASCENS).
          PEREIRA JR,J
          ENDOCRINOLOGY 50 : 124- (1952)

A11139   EFFECT OF BRASSICA OLERACEA VAR. CAPITATA IN THE PREVENTION AND
          HEALING OF EXPERIMENTAL PEPTIC ULCERATION.
          SINGH,GB: ZAIDE,SH: BAJPAL,RP:
          INDIAN J MED RES 50 : 741-749 (1962)

A11536   GLUCOSINOLATES IN SEED OF SWEDISH BRASSICA CROPS.
          JOSEFSSON,E: MUEHLENBERG,C:
          ACTA AGR SCAND 18 1-2: 97-100 (1968)

A11821   ISOTHIOCYANATES. XI. 4-METHYLTHIOBUTYL ISOTHIOCYANATE, A NEW
          NATURALLY OCCURRING MUSTARD OIL.
          KJAER,A: GMELIN,R:
          ACTA CHEM SCAND 9 : 542-544 (1955)

A11825   OCCURRENCE OF ANTIFUNGAL SUBSTANCES IN BRASSICA RAPA, BRASSICA
          OLERACEA AND BETA VULGARIS.
          GERRETSEN,FC: HAAGSMA,N:
          NATURE(LONDON) 168 : 659-. (1959)

A11973   FLAVONOLS AND FLAVONES OF VEGETABLES. 1. FLAVONOLS OF BRASSICA
          VARIETIES.
          WILDANGER,W: HERRMANN,K:
          Z LEBENSM-UNTERS FORSCH 152 : 134-137 (1973)

A12151   ANTIBIOTICS FROM HIGHER PLANTS. 9.
          WINTER,AG: HORNBOSTEL,M:
          NATURWISSENSCHAFTEN 40 : 489-490 (1953)

A12625   STUDIES ON ENDEMIC GOITER. I. THE IDENTIFICATION AND THEIR
          AGLUCONS IN WEED CONTAMINANTS OF PASTURES IN GOITROUS AREA S OF
          TASMANIA AND SOUTHERN QUEENSLAND.
          BACHELARD,HS: TRIKOJUS,VM:
          J BIOL SCI 16 : 147-165 (1963)

A13514   ISOLATION OF (-)-5-ALLYL-2-THIOOXAZOLIDONE FROM BRASSICA NAPUS L.
          TAPPER,BA: MAC GIBBON,DB:
          PHYTOCHEMISTRY 6 : 749-753 (1967)

A14057   THE ANTHOCYANINS OF RED CABBAGE (BRASSICA OLERACEA).
          TANCHEV,SS: TIMBERLAKE,CF:
          PHYTOCHEMISTRY 8 9: 1825-1827 (1969)

A14285   CABBAGE EXTRACTS AND INSULIN-LIKE ACTIVITY.
          LEWIS,JJ:
          BRIT J PHARMACOL 5 : 21-24 (1950)

A14301   EFFECTS OF CABBAGE EXTRACTS ON CARBOHYDRATE METABOLISM.
          MAC DONALD,AD: WISLICKI,L:
          J PHYSIOL 94 : 249-255 (1938)

BRASSICA OLER* (3part query for [BEECHER.GROUP], 1-MAY-1990)

A4442   ISOTHIOCYANATES. II. VOLATILE ISOTHIOCYANATES IN SEEDS AND ROOTS OF
         VARIOUS BRASSICAE.
         JENSEN,KA: CONTI,J: KJAER,A
         ACTA CHEM SCAND 7 : 1267- (1953)

A4537   MENSES-INDUCING DRUGS: THEIR ROLE IN ANTIQUE, MEDIEVAL AND
         RENAISSANCE GYNECOLOGY AND BIRTH CONTROL.
         JOCHLE,W:
         CONTRACEPTION 10 : 425-439 (1974)

A4667   PHYTOESTROGEN CONTENT OF PLANTS.
         CHURY,J
         EXPERIENTIA 16 : 194- (1960)

A5062   ALKALOID BEARING PLANTS AND THEIR CONTAINED ALKALOIDS.
         WILLAMAN,JJ: SCHUBERT,BG
         ARS,USDA,TECH BULL 1234,SUPT DOCUMENTS,GOVT PRINT OFF,WASHINGTON
         DC,1961. : - (1961)

A6599   STUDIES ON VITAMIN E IN FOODS OF EAST PAKISTAN.
         MANNAN,A: AHMAD,K
         PAK J BIOL AGR SCI 9 : 13- (1966)

A7316   AVAILABILITY OF CA IN LADY'S FINGER (HIBISCUS ESCULENTUS), CABBAGE
         (BRASSICA OLERACEA CAPITATA), DRUMSTICK (MORINGA O LEIFERA), AND
         AMARANTH TENDER (AMARANTHUS GANGETICUS). I. EXPERIMENTS.
         BASU,KP: GHOSH,D
         INDIAN J MED RES 31 : 29- (1943)

J3624   ARYL HYDROCARBON HYDROXYLASE INDUCTION IN RAT TISSUES BY
         NATURALLY OCCURRING INDOLES OF CRUCIFEROUS PLANTS.
         LOUB,WD: WATTENBERG,LW: DAVIS,DW
         J NAT CANCER INST 54 : 985-988 (1975)

J5247   ISOLATION AND CHARACTERIZATION OF A VIRUS INHIBITOR FROM CABBAGE
         (BRASSICA OLERACEA VAR. WIRSING) LEAVES.
         VARMA,JP
         INDIAN PHYTOPATHOL 26 : 712- (1973)

J6104   BRANCHED-CHAIN CONSTITUENTS OF BRUSSELS SPROUT WAX.
         BAKER,EA: HOLLOWAY,PJ
         PHYTOCHEMISTRY 14 : 2463- (1975)

J8408   ISOLATION OF A POLYSACCHARIDE FROM CABBAGE PLANTS AND ITS EFFECTS
         ON VIRUS INFECTION.
         WORMS,G: NIENHAUS,F
         PHYTOPATHOL Z 82 : 224- (1975)

J8745   1-CYANOEPITHIOALKANES: MAJOR PRODUCTS OF ALKENYLGLUCOSINOLATE
         HYDROLYSIS IN CERTAIN CRUCIFERAE.
         COLE,RA
         PHYTOCHEMISTRY 14 : 2293- (1975)

J8957 THE EFFECT OF MEMBRANE STABILIZERS ON PHYTOCHROME CONTROLLED
ANTHOCYANIN BIOSYNTHESIS IN BRASSICA OLERACEA.
BASSIM,TAH: PECKET,RC
PHYTOCHEMISTRY 14 : 731- (1975)

K1727 VOLATILE CONSTITUENTS FROM CAULIFLOWER AND OTHER CRUCIFERS.
WALLBANK,BE: WHEATLEY,GA
PHYTOCHEMISTRY 15 : 763- (1976)

K1811 COUMESTROL CONTENT OF FRACTIONS OBTAINED DURING WET PROCESSING
OF ALFALFA.
KNUCKLES,BE: DE FREMERY,D: KOHLER,GO
J AGR FOOD CHEM 24 : 1177- (1976)

K3469 DECANOIC ACID. NEW PRECURSOR FOR THE IN VITRO BIOSYNTHESIS OF
OLEIC ACID BY A PLANT SUBCELLULAR SYSTEM.
MAZLIAK,P: GROSBOIS,M: DECOTTE,AM:
BIOCHIMIE 57 : 943-. (1975)

K3507 N-METHYLPHENETHYLAMINE, AN INDIRECT SYMPATHICOMIMETIC AGENT IN
VEGETABLES.
MARQUARDT,P: CLASSEN,HG: SCHUMACHER,KA
ARZNEIM-FORSCH 26 : 2001-203 (1976)

K4324 STIMULATORY EFFECT OF VEGETABLES ON INTESTINAL DRUG METABOLISM
IN THE RAT.
PANTUCK,EJ: HSIAO,KC: LOUB,WD: WATTENBERG,LW: KUNTZMAN,R:
CONNEY,AH
J PHARMACOL EXP THER 198 : 278-282 (1976)

L0019 GLUCOSINOLATES AND DERIVED PRODUCTS IN CRUCIFEROUS VEGETABLES.
IDENTIFICATION OF ORGANIC NITRILES FROM CABBAGE.
DAXENBICHLER,ME: VAN ETTEN,CH: SPENCER,GF
J AGR FOOD CHEM 25 : 121- (1977)

L0490 A LOW-MOLECULAR ROTENONE-LIKE ACTING INHIBITOR OF THE NADH
OXIDASE SYSTEM IN CAULIFLOWER BUDS(BRASSICA OLERACEA).
SCHEWE,T: HIEBSCH,C: RAPOPORT,S:
ACTA BIOL MED GER 32 : 427-. (1974)

M10022 DISTRIBUTION OF QUERCETIN AND KAEMPFEROL IN LETTUCE, KALE, CHIVE,
GARLIC CHIVE, LEEK, HORSERADISH, RED RADISH, AND RE D CABBAGE
TISSUES.
BILYK,A: SAPERS,GM:
J AGR FOOD CHEM 33 2: 226-228 (1985)

M10145 CONSTITUENTS OF LOCAL PLANTS. PART 1. CHEMICAL INVESTIGATIONS ON
SOME CULTIVATED SAUDI ARABIAN PLANTS.
TAWFIK,NI: EL-TAWIL,BAH: EL-REFAI,AH: KHALAF,AA: KHALIL,AM:
QUAL PLANT PL FDS HUM NUTR 28 3: 203-210 (1978)

M10236 HPLC DETERMINATION OF CAROTENOIDS IN FRUITS AND VEGETABLES IN
THE UNITED STATES.
BUREAU,JL: BUSHWAY,RJ:
J FOOD SCI 51 1: 128-130 (1986)

M10340   OCCURRENCE OF THE PLANT GROWTH REGULATOR JASMONIC ACID IN
PLANTS.
MEYER,A: MIERSCH,O: BUTTNER,C: DATHE,W: SEMBDNER,G:
J PLANT GROWTH REGUL 3 : 1-8 (1984)

M10847   ORGANIC ACIDS OF VEGETABLES. I. BRASSICA SPECIES, LEAF AND BULBOUS
VEGETABLES, CARROTS, CELERY.
RUHL,I: HERRMANN,K:
Z LEBENSM-UNTERS FORSCH 180 : 215-220 (1985)

M12519   THE NATURAL DISTRIBUTION IN ANGIOSPERMS OF ANTHOCYANINS
ACYLATED WITH ALIPHATIC DICARBOXYLIC ACIDS.
HARBORNE,JB:
PHYTOCHEMISTRY 25 8: 1887-1894 (1986)

M12859   THE GLUCOSINOLATE CONTENT OF SOME FODDER BRASSICAS.
BRADSHAW,JE: HEANEY,RK: SMITH,WH: GOWERS,M: GEMMELL,S: FENWICK,DJ:
ROGER,G:
J SCI FOOD AGR 35 9: 977-981 (1984)

M13560   CONTRIBUTION TO THE CHEMICAL COMPOSITION OF SOME SORTS OF
CABBAGE PRODUCED IN THE REGION OF SKOPJE.
BAUER,O: DEMIROVSKA,V:
GOD ZB ZEMJOD FAK UNIV SKOPJE 30 : 55-59 (1982)

M14076   STRUCTURE OF MONOACYLATED ANTHOCYANINS ISOLATED FROM RED
CABBAGE, BRASSICA OLERACEA.
IDAKA,E: SUZUKI,K: YAMAKITA,H: OGAWA,T: KONDO,T: GOTO,T:
CHEM LETT 1987 1: 145-148 (1987)

M14151   MODIFYING ACTION OF VEGETABLE JUICE ON THE MUTAGENICITY OF BEEF
EXTRACT AND NITROSATED BEEF EXTRACT.
MUNZNER,R:
FOOD CHEM TOXICOL 24 8: 847-849 (1986)

M14545   STRUCTURE OF THREE DIACYLATED ANTHOCYANINS ISOLATED FROM RED
CABBAGE, BRASSICA OLERACEA.
IDAKA,E: YAMAKITA,H: OGAWA,T: KONDO,T: YAMAMOTO,M: GOTO,T:
CHEM LETT 1987 : 1213-1216 (1987)

M14575   DETERMINATION OF GREEN LEAF CAROTENOIDS BY HPLC.
TAKAGI,S:
AGR BIOL CHEM 49 4: 1211-1213 (1985)

M14606   HIGH-PERFORMANCE LIQUID CHROMATOGRAPHIC ANALYSIS OF
ANTICARCINOGENIC INDOLES IN BRASSICA OLERACEA.
BRADFIELD,CA: BJELDANES,LF:
J AGR FOOD CHEM 35 1: 46-49 (1987)

M15309   GLUCOSINOLATES OF WILD AND CULTIVATED BRASSICA SPECIES.
MITHEN,RF: LEWIS,BG: HEANEY,RK: FENWICK,GR:
PHYTOCHEMISTRY 26 7: 1969-1973 (1987)

M15365 ISOLATION AND PARTIAL CHARACTERIZATION OF THE TRYPSIN INHIBITOR
FROM THE SEEDS OF BRASSICA OLERACEA VAR.SABELLICA.
WILIMOWSKA-PELC,A:
ACTA BIOCHIM POLON 32 4: 351-361 (1985)

M15575 INDOLES IN EDIBLE MEMBERS OF THE CRUCIFERAE.
WALL,ME: TAYLOR,H: PERERA,P: WANI,MC:
J NAT PROD 51 1: 129-135 (1988)

M16212 DIETARY MODIFICATION OF XENOBIOTIC METABOLISM: CONTRIBUTION OF
INDOLYLIC COMPOUNDS PRESENT IN BRASSICA OLERACEA.
BRADFIELD,CA: BJELDANES,LF:
J AGR FOOD CHEM 35 6: 896-900 (1987)

M17999 OCCURENCE OF 1-O-HYDROXYCINNAMYL-BETA-D-GLUCOSES IN VEGETABLES
I. PHENOLIC ACID COMPOUNDS OF VEGETABLES.
RESCHKE,A: HERRMANN,K:
Z LEBENSM-UNTERS FORSCH 174 1: 5-8 (1982)

M19391 4-O-BETA-D-GLUCOSIDES OF HYDROXYBENZOIC AND HYDROXYCINNAMIC
ACIDS. THEIR SYNTHESIS AND DETERMINATION IN BERRY FRUIT A ND
VEGATABLE.
SCHUSTER,B: WINTER,M: HERRMANN,K:
Z NATURFORSCH SER C 41 5/6: 512-520 (1986)

M20277 FLAVONOIDS IN BRASSICA NIGRA (L.) KOCH, B. OLERACEA L., B, CAMPESTRIS L.
AND THEIR NATURAL AMPHIDIPLOIDS.
AGUINAGALDE,I:
BOT MAG TOKYO 101 : 55-60 (1988)

M20732 CONTACT SENSITIVITY TO LETTUCE IN A CHEF.
MITCHELL,D: BECK,MH: HAUSEN,BM:
CONTACT DERMATITIS 20 5: 398-399 (1989)

M20789 ISOLATION OF COMPOUNDS WITH ANTIMUTAGENIC ACTIVITY FROM SAVOY
CHIEFTAIN CABBAGE.
LAWSON,T: NUNNALLY,J: WALKER,B: BRESNICK,E: WHEELER,D: WHEELER,M:
J AGR FOOD CHEM 37 5: 1363-1367 (1989)

M21177 WATER SOLUBLE HIGH MOLECULAR WEIGHT COMPONENTS FROM PLANTS
WITH POTENT INTRAOCULAR PRESSURE LOWERING ACTIVITY.
DEUTSCH,HM: GREEN,K: ZALKOW,LH:
CURR EYE RES 6 7: 949-950 (1987)

M21684 THE EFFECT OF FEEDING BRASSICA VEGETABLES AND INTACT
GLUCOSINOLATES ON MIXED-FUNCTION-OXIDASE ACTIVITY IN THE LIVERS
AND INTESTINES OF RATS.
MC DANELL,R: MC LEAN,AEM: HANLEY,AB: HEANEY,RK: FENWICK,GR:
FOOD CHEM TOXICOL 27 5: 289-293 (1989)

M21921 EVALUATION OF THE GASTRIC ANTILUCEROGENIC EFFECTS OF SOLANUM
NIGRUM, BRASSICA OLERACEA AND OCIMUM BASILICUM IN RATS.
AKHTAR,MS: MUNIR,M:
J ETHNOPHARMACOL 27 1/2: 163-176 (1989)

BRASSICA OLER* (3part query for [BEECHER.GROUP], 1-MAY-1990)

M5461   VEGETABLE MUTAGENICITY.
ANON:
FOOD CHEM TOXICOL 22 9: 774-775 (1984)

M6032   HEPATIC POLYSUBSTRATE MONOOXYGENASE ACTIVITIES IN DIFFERENT
STRAINS OF RATS FED CABBAGE (BRASSICA OLEARACEA).
MILLER,KW: STOEWSAND,GS:
DRUG CHEM TOXICOL 6 1: 93-110 (1983)

M7086   DETERMINATION OF S-METHYL CYSTEINE SULFOXIDE IN BRASSICA
EXTRACTS BY HIGH-PERFORMANCE LIQUID CHROMATOGRAPHY.
GUSTINE,DL:
J CHROMATOGR 319 3: 450-453 (1985)

M9217   VITAMIN C CONTENT IN VEGETABLES AND FRUITS IN SHENYANG (CHINA)
MARKET DURING FOUR SEASONS.
YAO,G: LI,YJ: CHANG,XQ: LU,J:
YINGYANG XUEBAO 5 4: 373-379 (1983)

M9293   THE ISOLATION AND PURIFICATION OF INDOLE GLUCOSINOLATES FROM
BRASSICA SPECIES.
TRUSCOTT,RJW: MINCHINTON,I: SANG,J:
J SCI FOOD AGR 34 3: 247-254 (1983)

M9426   PHENOLIC ACID CONTENT OF FOOD PLANTS AND POSSIBLE NUTRITIONAL
IMPLICATIONS.
HUANG,HM: JOHANNING,GL: O'DELL,BL:
J AGR FOOD CHEM 34 1: 48-51 (1986)

M9762   SIMULTANEOUS DETERMINATION OF ABSCISIC ACID AND JASMONIC ACID IN
PLANT EXTRACTS USING HIGH-PERFORMANCE LIQUID CHROMAT OGRAPHY.
ANDERSON,JM:
J CHROMATOGR 330 : 347-355 (1985)

N14041   NEW RED NATURAL PIGMENT. RED CABBAGE PIGMENT,SUNRED ETC.
YASUDA,S:
SAN-EI NEWS 141 : 16-23 (1981)

N14322   THE CHARACTERIZATION OF A NOVEL HYDROXINDOLE GLUCOSINOLATE.
TRUSCOTT,RJW: BURKE,DG: MINCHINTON,IR:
BIOCHEM BIOPHYS RES COMMUN 107 : 1258-1264 (1982)

N14323   A NOVEL METHOXYINDOLE GLUCOSINOLATE.
TRUSCOTT,RJW: MINCHNTON,IR: BURKE,DG: SANG,JP:
BIOCHEM BIOPHYS RES COMMUN 107 : 1368-1375 (1982)

N14632   ANTHOCYANIN COMPOSITION OF BRASSICA OLERACEA CV. RED DANISH.
HRAZDINA,G: IREDALE,H: MATTICK,LR:
PHYTOCHEMISTRY 16 : 297-299 (1977)

N15014   TWO NATURAL INDOLE GLUCOSINOLATES FROM BRASSICACEAE.
GOETZ,JK: SCHRAUDOLF,H:
PHYTOCHEMISTRY 22 4: 905-907 (1983)

N17332 EFFECTS OF DIETARY BROCCOLI AND BUTYLATED HYDROXYANISOLE ON
LIVER-MEDIATED METABOLISM OF BENZO(A)PYRENE.
ASPRY,KE: BJELDANES,LF:
FOOD CHEM TOXICOL 21 2: 133-142 (1983)

N2289 KALE POISONING.
SMITH,RH
ARC RES REV 2 : 17-21 (1976)

N2336 THE DIFFERENT AMYRIN COMPOUNDS IN MITOCHONDRIAL AND MICROSOME
FRACTIONS OF CAULIFLOWER BUDS.
DOIREAU,P:
C R ACAD SCI SER D 286 : 1877-1889 (1978)

N2964 STIMULATORY EFFECT OF BRUSSELS SPROUTS AND CABBAGE ON HUMAN
DRUG METABOLISM.
PANTUCK,EJ: PANTUCK,CB: GARLAND,WA: WATTENBERG,LW: ANDERSON,KE:
KAPPAS,A: CONNEY,AH
CLIN PHARMACOL THER 25 : 88-95 (1979)

R0015 HYPOGLYCEMIC ACTIVITY OF CABBAGE WATER EXTRACT
SEEHACHOT,P: LAMTHONG,P: TUUCHINDA,A: TRIRAT,A:
UNDERGRAD SPECIAL PROJECT REPORT 1952 : 13PP-. (1952)

T12010 PURIFICATION AND PROPERTIES OF DESMUTAGENIC FACTOR FROM
BROCCOLI (BRASSICA OLERANCEA VAR. ITALICA PLENCK) FOR MUTAGEN IC
PRINCIPLE OF TRYPTOPHAN PYROLYSATE.
MORITA,K: YAMADA,H: IWAMOTO,S: SOTOMURA,M: SUZUKI,A:
J FOOD SAFETY 4 : 139-150 (1982)

T12014 INTERACTIONS OF ALLELOCHEMICALS WITH DETOXICATION ENZYMES OF
INSECTICIDE-SUSCEPTIBLE AND RESISTANT FALL ARMYWORMS.
YU,SJ:
PESTICIDE BIOCHEM & PHYSIOL 22 : 60-68 (1984)

T12048 DESMUTAGENIC ACTION OF FOOD COMONENTS ON MUTAGENS FORMED BY
THE SORBIC ACID NITRITE REACTION.
OSAWA,T: ISHIBASHI,H: NAMIKI,M: KADA,T: TSUJI,K:
AGR BIOL CHEM 50 8: 1971-1977 (1986)

T12116 ANTI-MUTAGENIC ACTION OF VEGETABLE FACTOR(S) ON THE MUTAGENIC
PRINCIPLE OF TRYPTOPHAN PYROLYSATE.
KADA,T: MORITA,K: INOUE,T:
MUTAT RES 53 : 351-353 (1978)

T12477 ANTI-MUTAGENIC ACTION OF VEGETABLE FACTOR(S) ON THE MUTAGENIC
PRINCIPLE OF TRYPTOPHAN PYROLYSATE.
KADA,T: MORITA,K: INOUE,T:
MUTAT RES 53 : 351-353 (1978)

T12543 STUDIES ON NATURAL DESMUTAGENS: SCREENING FOR VEGETABLE AND
FRUIT FACTORS ACTIVE IN INACTIVATION OF MUTAGENIC PYROLYS IS
PRODUCTS FROM AMINO ACIDS.
MORITA,K: HARA,M: KADA,T:
AGR BIOL CHEM 42 6: 1235-1238 (1978)

BRASSICA OLER* (3part query for [BEECHER.GROUP], 1-MAY-1990)

T15589   EFFECTS OF DIETARY SCHIZANDRA CHINENSIS, BRUSSELS SPROUTS AND ILLICIUM VERUM EXTRACTS ON CARCINOGEN METABOLISM SYSTEM S IN MOUSE LIVER.
HENDRICH,S: BJELDANES,LF:
FOOD CHEM TOXICOL 24 9: 903-912 (1989)

T15737   CABBAGE AND VITAMIN E: THEIR EFFECT ON COLON TUMOR FORMATION IN MICE.
TEMPLE,NJ: EL-KHATIB,SM:
CANCER LETT 35 1: 71-77 (1987)

T6435   SCREENING OF HIGHER PLANTS FOR BIOLOGICAL ACTIVITIES. II. ANTIVIRAL ACTIVITY.
VAN DEN BERGHE,DA: IEVEN,M: MERTENS,F: VLIETINCK,AJ: LAMMENS,E:
J NAT PROD 41 : 463-467 (1978)

T6788   EXPOSURE TO PHYTOESTROGENS MAY SURPASS DES RESIDUES.
HOELSCHER,M:
FEEDSTUFFS 51 : 54-68 (1979)

T6813   THE CONCEPT OF BIRTH CONTROL IN UNANI MEDICAL LITERATURE.
RAZZACK,HMA:
UNPUBLISHED MANUSCRIPT OF THE AUTHOR. 1980 : 64PP-. (1980)

T7559   VEGETABLES INHIBIT, IN VIVO, THE MUTAGENICITY OF NITRITE COMBINED WITH NITROSABLE COMPOUNDS.
BARALE,R: ZUCCONI,D: BERTANI,R: LOPRIENO,N:
MUTAT RES 120 2/3: 145-150 (1983)

T7979   PRIMARY AND SECONDARY AMINES IN THE HUMAN ENVIRONMENT.
NEURATH,GB: DUNGER,M: PEIN,FG: AMBROSIUS,D: SCHREIBER,O:
FOOD COSMET TOXICOL 15 : 275-282 (1977)

T9386   TUMOR INHIBITORS: ARE CLUES FROM HISTORY ANY BETTER THAN RANDOM SCREENING OF THE PLANT KINGDOM?
CRELLIN,JK: PHILPOTT,J:
ABSTR INTERNAT RES CONG NAT PROD, COLL PHARM, UNIV N CAROLINA, CHAPEL HILL, N CAROLINA, JULY 7-12, 1985 : ABSTR-149 (1985)

T9399   HEPATIC GLUTATHIONE S-TRANSFERASE ACTIVITY AND AFLATOXIN B-1-INDUCED ENZYME ALTERED FOCI IN RATS FED FRACTIONS OF BRU SSELS SPROUTS.
GODLEWSKI,CE: BOYD,JN: SHERMAN,WK: ANDERSON,JL: STOEWSAND,GS:
CANCER LETT 28 2: 151-157 (1985)

T9416   EFFECT OF COMMON VEGETABLES ON THYROID FUNCTION IN RATS - A PRELIMINARY STUDY.
SARKAR,SR: SINGH,LR: UNIYAL,BP: MUKHERJEE,SK: NAGPAL,KK:
DEF SCI J 33 4: 317-321 (1983)

T9853   THE EFFECTS OF DIETARY BRUSSELS SPROUTS AND SCHIZANDRA CHINENSIS ON THE XENOBIOTIC-METABOLIZING ENZYMES OF THE RAT SM ALL INTESTINE.
SALBE,AD: BJELDANES,LF:
FOOD CHEM TOXICOL 23 1: 57-65 (1985)

T12593 DESMUTAGENIC ACTIVITY OF PEROXIDASE ON AUTOXIDIZED LINOLENIC
ACID.
YAMAGUCHI,T: YAMASHITA,Y: ABE,T:
AGR BIOL CHEM 44 4: 959-961 (1980)

T13252 ANTI-MUTAGENIC ACTION OF VEGETABLE FACTOR(S) ON THE MUTAGENIC
PRINCIPLE OF TRYPTOPHAN PYROLYSATE.
KADA,T: MORITA,K: INOUE,T:
MUTAT RES 53 : 351-353 (1978)

T13598 DEXTRACTION OF ANTIMUTAGENIC PROTEINS FROM BROCCOLI.
MORITA,K: YAMADA,H: IWAMOTO,S: TONOMURA,M: SUZUKI,A:
PATENT-JAPAN TOKKYO KOHO-62 10,968 : 5PP-. (1987)

T13846 POPULAR MEDICINE OF THE CENTRAL PLATEAU OF HAITI. 2.
ETHNOPHARMACOLOGICAL INVENTORY.
WENIGER,B: ROUZIER,M: DAGUILH,R: HENRYS,D: HENRYS,JH: ANTON,R:
J ETHNOPHARMACOL 17 1: 13-30 (1986)

T14157 HYPOLIPIDERMIC ACTION OF CABBAGE OIL IN ETHANOL-FED RATS.
UMAR,I: AUGUSTI,KT: JOSEPH,PK:
INDIAN J BIOCHEM BIOPHYS 24 4: 241-243 (1987)

T14498 PROTECTIVE EFFECT OF DIETARY BRUSSELS SPROUTS AGAINST MAMMARY
CARCINOGENESIS IN SPRAGUE-DAWLEY RATS.
STOEWSAND,GS: ANDERSON,JL: MUNSON,L:
CANCER LETT 39 2: 199-207 (1988)

T14715 THE CYTOLYTIC EFFECT OF TWO BRASSICA SPECIES.
GURKAN,E: KOSAL,G:
FITOTERAPIA 59 1: 47-48 (1988)

T14904 ANTIMUTAGENICITY OF DIALYZATES OF VEGETABLES AND FRUITS.
SHINOHARA,K: KUROKI,S: MIWA,M: KONG,ZL: HOSODA,H:
AGR BIOL CHEM 52 6: 1369-1375 (1988)

T14913 THE EFFECTS OF DIETARY CABBAGE ON XENOBIOTIC-METABOLIZING
ENZYMES AND THE BINDING OF AFLATOXIN B-1 TO HEPATIC DNA IN RATS.
WHITTY,JP: BJELDANES,LF:
FOOD CHEM TOXICOL 25 8: 581-587 (1987)

T15228 SELENIUM AND CABBAGE AND COLON CARCINOGENESIS IN MICE.
TEMPLE,NJ: BASU,TK:
J NAT CANCER INST 79 5: 1131-1133 (1987)

T15279 SCREENING OF EDIBLE PLANTS AGAINST POSSIBLE ANTI-TUMOR PROMOTING
ACTIVITY.
KOSHIMIZU,K: OHIGASHI,H: TOKUDA,H: KONDO,A: YAMAGUCHI,K:
CANCER LETT 39 3: 247-257 (1988)

T15345 EFFECTS OF DIETARY CABBAGE, BRUSSELS SPROUTS, ILLICIUM VERUM,
SCHIZANDRA CHINENSIS AND ALFALFA ON THE BENZOPYRENE MET ABOLIC
SYSTEM IN MOUSE LIVER.
HENDRICH,S: BJELDANES,LF:
FOOD CHEM TOXICOL 21 4: 479-486 (1983)

BRASSICA OLER* (3part query for [BEECHER.GROUP], 1-MAY-1990)

W0260   THE ANTIDIABETIC EFFECT OF SOME PLANTS.
         SHARAF,AA: HUSSEIN,AM: MANSOUR,MY
         PLANTA MED 11 : 159- (1963)

W0744   MEVALONIC ACID CONCENTRATIONS IN FRUIT AND VEGETABLE TISSUES.
         WILLS,RBH: SCURR,EV:
         PHYTOCHEMISTRY 14 : 1643-. (1975)

W1074   THE OCCURRENCE OF ANTIBACTERIAL SUBSTANCES IN SEED PLANTS WITH
         SPECIAL REFERENCE TO MYCOBACTERIUM TUBERCULOSIS (THIRD
         REPORT)
         FRISBEY,A: ROBERTS,JM: JENNINGS,JC: GOTTSHALL,RY: LUCAS,EH
         MICH STATE UNIV AGR APPL SCI QUART BULL 35 : 392-404 (1953)

W2224   INCREASED ARYL HYDROCARBON HYDROXYLASE(AHH) ACTIVITY IN RAT
         TISSUES BY 3-INDOLYLACETONITRILE FROM BRUSSEL SPROUTS(BRA SSICA
         OLERACEA VAR.GEMMIFERA).
         LOUB,WD: WATTENBERG,LW
         LLOYDIA 36 : 436-C (1973)

W2509   ANTITUSSIVE PROPERTIES OF CERTAIN MEDICAL PLANTS.
         ANDRONOVA,LM
         RAST RESUR 8 : 588-591 (1972)

W2811   STUDY OF INDIGINOUS (FOLK WAYS) BIRTH CONTROL METHODS IN
         ALEXANDRIA.
         EL-DEAN MAHMOUD,AAG
         THESIS-MS-UNIVERSITY OF ALEXANDRIA-HIGHER INSTITUTE OF NURSING : -
         (1972)

W3361   SOME BIOLOGICALLY ACTIVE COMPOUNDS OF VEGETABLES.
         LUKOVNIKOVA,GA:
         PRIKL BIOKHIM I MIKROBIOL 1 : 594-597 (1965)

W3726   A QUALITATIVE TEST FOR DEHYDROASCORBIC ACID.
         TIPSON,RS:
         J AMER PHARM ASS 34 : 190-192 (1945)

W3729   ON THE OCCURRENCE OF CAFFEIC ACID AND CHLOROGENIC ACID IN FRUITS
         AND VEGETABLES.
         HERRMANN,K:
         NATURWISSENSCHAFTEN 43 : 109-. (1956)

W3831   OXIDATIVE ENZYMES AND PHENOLIC SUBSTRATE IN VEGETABLES AND
         FRUIT. I. HYDROXYCINNAMIC ACIDS.
         HERRMANN,K:
         Z LEBENSM-UNTERS FORSCH 106 : 341-348 (1957)

W4177   THERAPEUTIC EFFECTS OF VARIOUS FOOD ARTICLES.
         LIEBSTEIN,AM:
         AMER MED 33 : 33-38 (1927)

APPENDIX C

OUR RESEARCH ON ARTHRITIS

Last year we became greatly concerned about people suffering with arthritis and having heart trouble; seemingly their medication was not solving their problems. We chose 13 subjects for a study. Some had only one ailment; others had both. This was not designed as a "scientific" study in that we did not have a control group because no one was willing to be in the "unchanged" group. We could not use a placebo, because we were going to impose six changes on the participants at once. We did this because we felt that arthritis and heart trouble have multiple causes. Removing one of the causes probably would not make much difference to the condition of the participants, and so we decided to do what was best for them; even though it didn't make our experiment "pure science."

For six weeks, thirteen participants were urged to strictly follow the diet and exercise sheet shown on page 299. The diet followed was the Daily Healthful Lifestyle listed on page 225 of this book. The participants were allowed to eat as much as they liked. The noon meal was served five times a week for six weeks at Natural Ovens Bakery.

Participants were involved in a mild stretching and exercise program for 20 minutes each day and were urged to go on walks each evening if they felt able. They were also offered a massage therapy session once a week. The participants were under the supervision of a medical doctor during the entire experimental period (his letter is reprinted below) and lab results were from the local hospital laboratory. No significant changes were made in medication, except to lower the dose if the doctor and participant decided. Each subject served as his/her own control. The results were astounding as you can see in the following report.

The results showed an average drop in serum cholesterol of 38 points (15%), systolic blood pressure of 13.5 points (14%) and in weight of 5 pounds. There was no significant change in HDL or serum triglyceride levels.

Multiplying the systolic blood pressure times the diastolic pressure gives blood pressure product, a measure of the constant tension of the arteries. In this study, the blood pressure product decreased from 11,523 to 10,062, a decrease of 12.6%.

Average joint flexibility before the program started was 47 in affected joints. In the same joints, after being on the program for 6 weeks, joint flexibility in affected joints increased to 97%, more than doubling the range of motion.

In summary, the patients showed dramatic impovement in joint flexibility and a dramatic decrease in heart risk factors in six weeks while on the diet. The study should be repeated with more testing being done before and after and a separate group should be used for a control group.

FLAX DIET PROGRAM CONSISTED OF:

(1)   **Mild Stretching and Exercise Program.**
(2)   **Moderate Protein Level in Diet.**
(3)   **Exclusion of all Dairy Products.**
(4)   **Consumption of 20 Grams/Day of Stabilized Flax.**
(5)   **Exclusive Use of Canola Oil in Diet.**
(6)   **Exclusion of Alcohol and Sucrose From Diet.**

CHANGE IN JOINT FLEXIBILITY

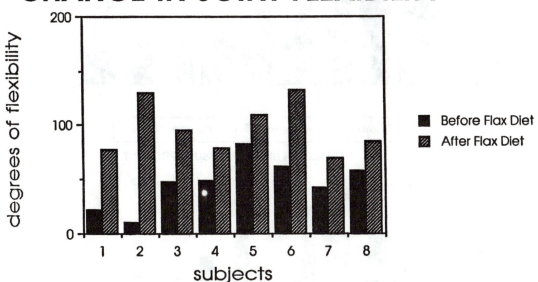

CHANGE IN DIASTOLIC BLOOD PRESSURE

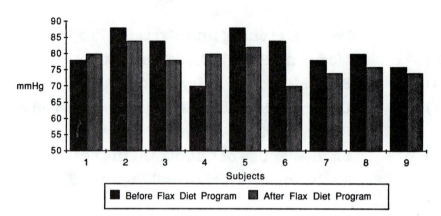

mmHg

Subjects

■ Before Flax Diet Program ▨ After Flax Diet Program

CHANGE IN SYSTOLIC BLOOD PRESSURE

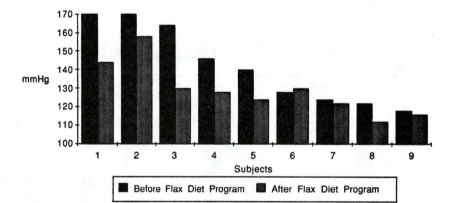

mmHg

Subjects

■ Before Flax Diet Program ▨ After Flax Diet Program

CHANGE IN BLOOD PRESSURE PRODUCT

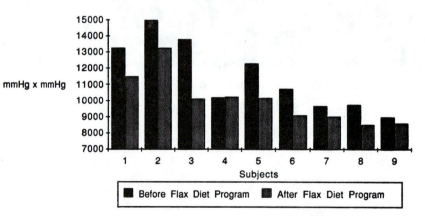

mmHg x mmHg

Subjects

■ Before Flax Diet Program ▨ After Flax Diet Program

CHANGE IN LDL

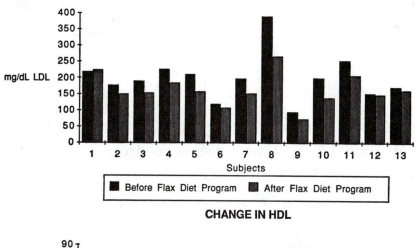

CHANGE IN HDL

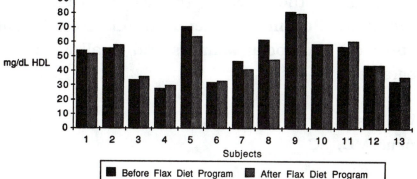

CHANGE IN TOTAL CHOLESTEROL

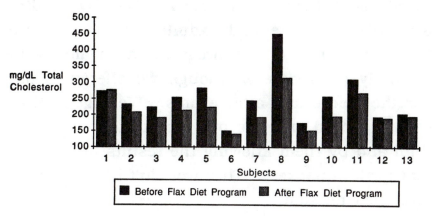

INTERNAL MEDICINE and
PREVENTIVE CARE

J. L. Stoune, M.D., S.C.

April 5, 1989

1000 Maritime Drive

Manitowoc, WI

54220   (414-682-1000)

Dear Paul,

Natural Ovens first study group absolutely amazed me. Improvement was 100%, blood pressure dropped, arthritis and arthralgias improved or disappeared, back aches improved, headaches disappeared. They all lost weight and felt better about themselves.

This group has the potential to make massive differences in our community. I commit our center to this group's continual spiritual, physical and social wellness and to all Natural Ovens future programs.

Yours in Wellness,

Dr. J. L. Stoune, MD, SC

The results were so good that we called our state University and asked them to become involved by sending an arthritis specialist to come and examine the next group of people before they started on the program and again six weeks later. They flatly refused, even though we offered to pay all expenses for the before and after exams. We argued that the state University should examine our results to keep our work 100% truthful and by them knowing the results firsthand, they could prevent health quackery. They wouldn't budge. They said that it wasn't "their mission."

APPENDIX D

WELLNESS TIPS

The labels in our breads contain newsletters. Many customers have suggested they would make a marvelous book, so the next 90 pages have been reprinted directly from our newsletters.

Japanese Brain Factor

Can certain foods make you smarter?

Biochemists around the world have been trying to determine if there is a **"brain factor"** in food which can account for differences in human intelligence. Nowhere is this being studied more vigorously than in Japan.

Early Studies

The "brain factor" was first studied in England by Sinclair and Crawford in the early 1970's.[1] Using archeological records, they determined that about the time mankind first domesticated wild animals, the size of the human brain decreased by 25%. Sinclair and Crawford theorized that the change in diet from animals to go without some nutrient related to brain power. The animals then passed on this loss of the "brain factor" to people who ate them for meat.

Israeli researcher Pierre Budowski discovered that chickens that tended to have brain development problems were deprived of the "brain factor.".[2]

Canadian researchers Lamptey and Walker discovered that rats suffered diminished learning capacity and difficulty in distinguishing between bright and dim lights when deprived of the "brain factor".[3]

Bourre and others in France found very significant biochemical changes in structures within the brains of rats when the "brain factor" was missing in their diets.[4]

Japanese Studies

The largest group of researchers in the world studying the "brain factor" is found in Japan, headed by H. Okuyama. This group used several tests to measure the intelligence of rats.

One test measured the amount of time needed for rats to discover a slightly submerged island in a swimming pool. How quickly a rat found rest on the island became a measure of its intelligence. The rats fed the "brain factor" tended to find the island much more quickly.[5]

Reaction to Changes

Another test required the rats to press a lever when a light flashed.[6] When the lever was pressed, a door to a food source opened. Again, rats fed the "brain factor" learned to perform much more quickly.

304

Then the rules were changed. No reward was given for correctly opening the door. The rats deprived of the "brain factor" continued to push the lever every time the light flashed, whereas the rats given the "brain factor" learned quickly that it no longer paid to push the lever.

A Brainy Heritage

The Japanese researchers also found that each progressive generation of rats fed the "brain factor" seemed to be smarter than the one before. Further, they found that each generation deprived of the "brain factor" seemed less intelligent than the one before.

What is the "Brain Factor"?

The "brain factor" is an essential fatty acid called alpha-linolenic acid (ALENA). Once consumed and digested, it becomes an integral part of brain tissue. It also becomes a part of the neural hormones that direct the manner in which brain structures are put together.

Where can you find this "brain factor"? It is present at a level of about 1% in green leafy vegetables, walnuts and cold water fish. (Fish, as you may recall, is often referred to as "brain food".) It is also present in canola oil, a new oil from Canada similar to olive oil. A particularly rich source of the "brain factor" is ground, fortified flaxseed, which contains a whopping 16% to 22% ALENA.

"Brain Factor's" Enemy

During their research the Japanese also found a compound that works against the "brain factor." It's called linoleic acid, otherwise known as polyunsaturated fat. High levels of linoleic acid are found in corn, safflower and soybean oils.

1. Crawford, M.A. and A. J. Sinclair. Nutritional influences in the evolution of the mammalian brain. Elsvier CIBA Symposium: Lipid Malnutrition and Developing Brain, 1972.
2. Budowski,P., M.J. Leighfield and M.A. Crawford. Nutritional encephalomalacia in the chick: an exposure of the vulverable period for cerebellar development and the possible need for both n-6 and n-3 fatty acids. *British Journal of Nutrition* 1987; 58:511-520.
3. Lamptey, M.S. and B.L. Walker. A possible essential role for dietary linolenic acid in the development of the young rat. *J. Nutrition* 1976;106: 86-93.
4. Bourre, J.M.,, *ea*. Effect of polyunsaturated fatty acids on fetal mouse brain cells in culture in a chemically defined medium. *Journal of Neurochemistry* 1983; 5:1234-1242.
5. Yamamoto N., M. Saitoh, A. Moriuchi, M, Nomura, and H. Okuyama. Effect of dietary alpha-linolenate/linoleate balance on breain lipid compositions and learning ability of rats. *J. Lipid Res.* 1987;28: 144-151.
6. Okuyama, H. ea. Effect of the dietary alpha-linolenate/linoleate balance on lipid compositions and learning ability of rats. II. Discrimination process, extinction process. and glycolipid compositions. *Journal of Lipid Research* 1988; 29: 1013-1021.

Studies give 'stinking rose' high marks for preventing, battling many dieases.

—By Jane E. Brody
1990 The New York Times

Can a clove or two of garlic a day keep the doctor away? After 4,000 years of folklore extolling garlic as a preserver and restorer of health and youth, modern scientists have begun to define the complex condiment's medically important effects and substantiate several of its reputed benefits.

Early results of studies reported here last week suggest that ancient herbalists and traditional healers were on to a food that can help prevent if not cure a host of modern ailments, including heart disease, several types of cancer and cell damage caused by pollutants, radiation and aging.

The studies suggest that garlic, a chemically unstable bulb containing more than 200 different compounds, has biological activities that can favorably influence the course of many diseases.

For example, garlic preparations have been shown in laboratory studies, and in some cases in patients, to suppress the formation and growth of cancer cells and to counter blood conditions that foster atherosclerosis, heart attacks and strokes.

No less prestigious a research center than the National Cancer Institute is planning a study of its possible role as a cancer-preventing agent.

The scientists reported that in laboratory animals garlic or one or more of its active ingredients can do these things:

• Suppress cholesterol synthesis by the liver, lowering total serum cholesterol by reducing only the harmful LDL cholesterol and leaving the protective HDL cholesterol at normal levels.

• Lower levels of triglycerides, another blood fat that has been linked to an increased risk of heart attacks.

• Reduce the tendency of the blood to clot, more effectively even than asprin, and help the body dissolve existing clots, effects that may ward off heart attacks and strokes.

• Promote regression of fatty deposits in blood vessels and perhaps reverse arterial blockages caused by atherosclerosis.

• Block the ability of chemical carcinogens to transform normal cells into cancer cells and in some cases inhibit the early growth of transformed cells.

• Stimulate various immunological factors that may help the body combat cancer as well as stubborn fungal infections, like Candida albicans, a yeast that plagues millions.

• Protect cells against damage by oxidizing agents and heavy metals that are widespread in modern industrial environments.

But even more intriguing were the findings of a few studies in people, which lent support to the laboratory observations and aroused the interest of organizations like the National Cancer Institute.

Dr. William J. Blot of the institute said recent large studies of people in China and Italy produced the unexpected finding that eating a lot of garlic and related vegetables like scallions and onions was associated with low rates of stomach cancer.

Large differences in cancer rates were seen between regions of high and low consumption of these allium vegetables. Those living in high-consumption of other fresh vegetables and fruits was also linked to a reduced cancer risk, garlic seemed to multiply the benefit, providing even more protection than would be expected from simply adding on its separate benefits.

One possible explanation for the observed benefit is garlic's ability to block the formation of nitrosamines, a class of potent carcinogens, in the digestive tract.

Dr. Jinzhou Liu, a Chinese scientist now studying at Pennsylvania State University, reported that garlic extract was "much more effective than vitamin C" in blocking nitrosamine formation in the laboratory and in people.

While scientists continue to sort out the benefits and risk of garlic and its constituents, Lin and other reseachers suggest that those who can tolerate garlic would be wise to eat it at least every other day in cooked form.

An alternative for those wishing to avoid garlic breath is regular use of aged garlic extract, a deodorized supplement sold in health-food stores under the trade name Kyolic.

To date, Lin said, aged garlic extract has been shown to possess the same benefits of fresh garlic but far fewer of the toxic drawbacks.

NUTRITION

Building Better Kids

by Lisa Plescia, M.S., R.D.

Young or old, large or small, healthy eating habits can enhance the performance of any athlete. On a daily basis we are bombarded with nutritional information and claims of the specific effects of dietary products on our health- as adults. What about our children? The young athletes we encourage to take up our beloved sport need good nutrition, too. Here are some guidelines for making sure your tri-kid eats right.

HIGH CARBOHYDRATE FOODS IN A FAST FOOD WORLD

Athletes of all ages require a low-fat high-carbohydrate diet, but may have difficulty eating the right foods because of limited time and access. To com-pound matters, the young athlete may be experiencing a rapid growth which increases demands for adequate calories and essential nutrients (e.g. iron, vitamin C, B-vitamins and calcium). While eating *enough* is often a problem with the growing athlete, it is probably more important to know *what* to eat. A diet which is deficient in nutrients and excessive in fat will not only adversely affect athletic performance, but will inhibit growth and promote deposition of body fat.

A look at a typical day for an adolescent reveals a diet full of snacks, fast foods and eating on the run. To suggest eating fresh vegetables and three home cooked meals a day would be equivalent to asking the government to reduce taxation. (It sounds wonderful, but don't hold your breath trying.) Instead, take a positive approach. The chart at the end lists high-carbohydrate, low-fat food items for each meal.

PROPER HYDRATION

What would happen if you forgot to put water into your car radiator? Right! It would overheat. Water acts as a temperature regulator. The heat which is produced by the working engine (the young athlete's body) is carried to the skin's surface by water where the heat escapes into the environment.

Since a young athlete has a high percentage of weight as body water and a smaller body surface area, he or she is at greater risk of dehydration. Even the slightest reduction of body water will impede performance.

Tips for proper hydration:
• encourage liberal fluid intake
• consume two cups of water one hour prior to exercise
• consume a half cup of fluid (water and/or fluid replacer) every 15 minutes during exercise
• drink one pint of water for every pound lost (weigh yourself before and after exercise)
• limit activity if temperature is greater than 85 degrees and humidity is greater than 75 percent.

MINERAL AND VITAMIN NEEDS

No one can expect a young athlete to consume a well balanced diet 100 percent of the time. However, due to their enormous caloric requirements (we should all be so lucky!) most athletes are able to meet the minimum vitamin and mineral requirements with their diets. Still, there is the potential for vitamin or mineral deficiencies, especially in a society where the most readily available food is also most lacking in nutrients. An understanding of the basics of good nutrition can help both of you develop a diet that keeps your young athlete at his or her best.

Regardless of socioeconomic status, deficiencies in vitamin C, thiamine, (B vitamin), calcium and iron are common in teens. A young athlete may require more thiamine than his or her more sedentary friends, and should be aware of personal needs. Thiamine, is essential in the meta-bolism of carbohydrates. Fortunately, the best sources of thiamine include whole-grain and enriched breads and cereals (complex carbohydrates). Since these products are traditionally consumed in the athlete's diet, there is rarely need for supplementation of thiamine.

Similarly, most young athletes can obtain sufficient amounts of vitamin C through his or her food selections. The daily requirement of vitamin C for a child 11 to 14 is 50 mg/day and 15 to 18 is 60 mg/day. This is equivalent to one orange, a half cup of orange juice or one large baked potato. If you child's physician recommends a vitamin C supplement, limit the dose to less than 100 mg. per day (available in a multivitamin/mineral supplement).

Iron deficiency is a major cause of anemia among teenage girls and boys in the early years of adolescence. The body's need for iron is especially high for the young endurance athlete (greater than 10 hours per week) and increases after menstruation. Both boys and girls are advised to consume 18 mg. of iron per day. Since the body absorbs approximately 10 percent of the iron digested, young adolescents may not be obtaining adequate iron from food sources.

With the advice of your physician, iron supplemen-tation (found in an adult multi-vitamin/mineral supplement) may be recommended during the adolescent years. To enhance iron absorption and avoid gastric irritation, consume the supplement with a meal and a vitamin C-rich food.

NOTE: In extremely high doses, iron can be toxic, particularly in children. Do not exceed the recommended dosage.

Since 1965, vitamin and mineral intake has risen for adolescents-with the exception of calcium. The requirement for calcium, an essential mineral found in bones and teeth and essential for muscle contraction, is higher in adolescence than any other time in life (with the exception of pregnancy and lactation). Vegetable are also excellent sources of calcium.

The young female athlete is at greatest risk for developing a calcium deficiency, the leading cause of osteoporosis. Adequate calcium intake and weight bearing exercise (running) which is associated with increased bone density, the young athlete who does not consume the recommended daily calcium intake is at risk for developing osteoporosis.

In addition, carbonated beverages, and meat (the mainstay of any teenager's diet) contain phosphorus, a mineral which causes a calcium deficiency by increasing the calcium lost in urine. A typical multi-vitamin/mineral supplement does not contain adequate amounts of calcium for the young athlete. If your physician recommends calcium supplementation, choose a source containing calcium carbonate or calcium lactate. remember, these are supplements and should not take the place of food sources.

Factors which influence vitamin absorption include:

Vitamin Loss in Sweat

Athletes who lose a considerable amount of body water as sweat may have an increased need for Vitamin C and the B-vitamins. These vitamins can be replaced by consuming high carbohydrate foods,, citrus fruits and orange/yellow vegetables.

Dieting

Many athletes equate a low body fat with improved performance. Demands from coaches to "make weight" without providing sound nutritional information quite often leads young athletes to use quick weight loss methods I.E. very low calorie diets, diuretics, vomiting and laxatives to reduce body weight. Unfortunately, these methods only lead to losses of body water or muscle, which hinders rather than enhances performance.

Due to constraints on caloric intake, the young athlete may not be able to obtain the necessary vitamins and minerals from the diet, especially calcium and iron. If necessary, include a multi-vitamin/mineral supplement in addition to a well balanced diet with no less than 1,700 calories for the female and 2,000 for the male.

Asprin

Routine asprin use may increase the athletes need for iron, vitamin C and folacin. These vitamins and minerals can be obtained from meats, citrus products and green leafy vegetables. Asprin use may also cause internal bleeding.

Your young athlete may never be excited about steamed vegetables and tofu, and you may never successfully veto the late-night burgers and fries. But with a good understanding of the nutritional and caloric needs of your child, you can work together to help him or her stay fit and healthy.

Above all, be careful; you might find some of this rubbing off on you.

Lisa Plescia, M.S., R.D. is the director/owner of Positive Eating Practices, a sports nutrition consulting firm based in New Jersey.

BREAKFAST
- Bagels with jelly
- graham crackers, any grain)
- matzoh, saltines, pancakes, waffles (now microwaveable)
- non-fat fruit muffins
- Fruit — the banana even comes in its own package!

LUNCH/DINNER
- Sandwiches or submarines with tuna, chicken, turkey, or boiled ham. Encourage mustard or ketchup in place of mayo.
- Fast food establishments -do not have roast beef, grilled chicken sandwiches or chili. Order baked potatoes and fix them up at the salad bars.
- Encourage juice and water Chinese food with extra rice is always a favorite!
- Quick and easy high carb meals include pasta with tomato sauce, rice or a "nuked" potato.

310

- Try a "healthy" microwave meal. Add extra carbs (pastas, rice, grains, potato) or whole wheat bread with a piece of fruit.

HEALTHY SNACKS

Between practices, after school activities and an active social life, the young athlete has little time or desire to sit down to three well balanced meals a day. In addition, it is virtually impossible to meet the caloric requirements without eating between meals. Healthy snacking (a.k.a. grazing) is encouraged for the young athlete. The following is a list of high-carbohydrate, low-fat foods which should be kept on hand to supplement the young athlete's training diet.

SNACKS

Pretzels, popcorn, crackers, vanilla wafers, graham crackers, fig or fruit bars, fruit roll-ups, or fresh fruit. Frozen fruit bars, bagel chips, angel food or sponge cake, or any snack food with less than three grams of fat per 100 calories.

Calcium the Killer

By Sherry A. Rogers, M.D.

Hard to believe, but true. The way in which many are supplementing their diets with calcium is killing them. They are actually accelerating the arteriosclerotic process. They are speeding up the aging process as well as the occurrence of the many degenerative diseases that accompany it like hypertension, diabetes, heart disease, arthritis, and yes, don't forget cancer.

"How can this be? I thought we all needed extra calcium to stave off osteoporosis," you say. But we forgot to stop and figure out why people get osteoporosis. First you need to understand what osteoporosis is.

Calcium and other precious minerals are normally absorbed from our foods and incorporated into the bones. However, if any of the minerals like magnesium, boron, zinc, manganese, etc., are missing, the calcium does not get put into the bone. When the bone is deficient in calcium, we have osteoporosis, or weak bones that can fracture so easily that they do so even without a fall, or as we say, spontaneously. Or the bone can slowly collapse or shrink over time, leaving a shorter person in its wake, often with a great deal of bone pain. One of the first bones to show signs of osteoporosis is the jaw bone; this results in the shifting of teeth and eventual loss of bone and teeth it supports.

And so what happens when one is deficient enough in trace minerals to cause osteoporosis and takes extra calcium in attempt to correct the problem? The extra calcium, still not accompanied by the missing trace minerals that allow it to be laid down in the bone has to find a home somewhere. And it does find a home. It lays down in areas of inflammation where the body wishes to put a patch to stop a leak: the blood vessels of the heart and brain. We call this calcification of blood vessels *arteriosclerosis*.

Since the government has published the fact that it is estimated that the average American diet supplies only 40% of the recommended daily amount of magnesium; this makes it rather likely that the average person taking calcium will be contributing to his arteriosclerosis rather than to his bones.

Osteoporosis occurs for any of five reasons. Either the person does not ingest enough calcium, he cannot absorb it well, he cannot incorporate it into the bone, he gets rid of too much calcium in the urine, or he actually pulls it out of the bones. Let's look at some common factors that contribute to each of those reasons for osteoporosis.

First, many processed foods do not contain enough calcium. Did you know that 2 cups of greens contain more calcium than even a glass of milk? Plus the greens also have the correct ratio of other minerals so the calcium can actually be incorporated into the bone. In terms of absorbing calcium, antacids and medications like cimetidine to suppress the acid secretion of the stomach cut down on the ionization of calcium so that less is absorbed. More importantly, phosphates in processed foods markedly inhibit the absorption of calcium. Where are phosphates found? Hidden in nearly every food that comes in a bag, jar, can or box. They are often not even on the label or disguised as unrecognizable names. They are buffers, stabilizers, inhibit phase separation, dough conditioners, acidifers and much more. They are particularly high, for example, in soft drinks.

You already know that most people are low in magnesium, in fact, leading magnesium authorities suggest that it is such an unrecognized problem that 80% of the population is deficient. And that's not all they are low in. Many are low in zinc, boron, manganese, and many other trace minerals. Why? Because processing of foods to extend their shelf life removes these minerals. Often the soils on which the foods are grown are also depleted of some of these minerals, and this leads to a further decline.

Some medications can cause the loss of calcium in the urine, like diuretics or high doses of vitamin C. But how do we pull calcium out of the bone once it has already been put there? Calcium is one of the major buffers of the blood. So when the blood gets too acid and has to be buffered, the body steals calcium from the bone to do it. How does the body get too acid? One way is to eat a diet high in meat (amino acids) or sugars.

So a person who likes a lot of meat, eats processed foods or eats out frequently, has a number of soft drinks each day, or takes medication for indigestion and high blood pressure is at a high risk for osteoporosis, and no amount of merely taking calcium is going to help him; in fact, it will help him add to his troubles by calcifying his vessels and speeding his development of arteriosclerosis. This could lead to coronary artery disease, senility, hypertension, and more.

So how does one stave off osteoporosis? First, you need a nutritionally trained physician who will do a magnesium loading test to see if you have enough magnesium. This urine test is necessary, because there is no blood test that can rule out a magnesium deficiency at this point in time. He will also check other minerals like an RBC or erythrocyte zinc (again, because a serum zinc test is inadequate for diagnosis), copper, and other vitamins (like D3 and B6), and minerals commonly found low in the average person and necessary for incorporation of calcium in the bone.

Once your nutrient dificiencies have been identified and corrected, you want to be sure that you will remain in balance and playing with a full deck. The best way to do this is by eating as organic or chemically less-contaminated foods as possible. And more importantly, you want to eat as nutritionally dense foods as possible; in other words, foods that give you the highest nutrient yield (vitamins, minerals, essential fatty acids). This is accomplished by eating whole grains and fresh vegetables as the predominant part of your daily meals.

But whatever you do, don't let someone sell you the idea that you just need to take calcium and your worries are over. For with calcium as the instigator of degenerative diseases, your problems will be just beginning.

—Dr. Sherry Rogers has lectured in over six countries, has published over half a dozen scientific papers in four medical journals, and has taught advanced courses throughout the United states for physicians learning these new techniques.

When Is A Calorie MORE Than A Calorie?

Dieters tend to believe that "a calorie is a calorie is a calorie." However, new studies suggest that different types of foods may act in very different ways once they have entered the body. In fact, the "rules" of dieting may be undergoing a dramatic—and intriguing—change.

It's well known that different foods have different "densities" of calorie content. For example, a gram of protein or carbohydrate has 4 calories; a gram of alcohol has 7; a gram of fat has 9.

But here's another consideration. Researchers arrived at the 4-7-9 rule by measuring the heat given off when they burned proteins, carbohydrates or fats in a closed metal box. But new research indicates that the body's response to foods is quite different from what one would expect from these tests.

How the body responds

"From a physical and chemical point of view, a fat calorie may equal a carbohydrate calorie, but not in humans," says Erick Jequier of the University of Lausanne in Switzerland. "There is a marked difference in the body's response to fat and carbohydrate feeding."

One difference is obvious. It's easier and more direct to turn food fat into body fat than it is to turn carbohydrate into body fat.

"Handling and storage"

"In the case of carbohydrates, you pay a greater cost for handling and storage," explains Jean-Pierre Flatt of the University of Massachusetts Medical School in Worcester.

According to Flatt, the estimated "handling" costs for various food types are:
- 3% to store fat as fat
- 7% to store carbohydrates as carbohydrate (in a form called glycogen), and

- 23% to convert carbohydrate to fat (Bray, G.A., *Recent Advances in Obesity Research 2:* 221, 1978).

Not only is it "expensive" to convert carbohydrates into fat, the body seems reluctant to do it.

How much is "too much?"

In one study, Flatt, Jequier, and co-workers fed healthy young people 700 grams of carbohydrate—that's 2,800 calories. "The whole thing was accommodated as glycogen [carbohydrate] storage," notes Jequier. "We had to give an enormous amount of carbohydrate to see a net increase in fat deposition."

According to current "diet wisdom," if you eat too much carbohydrate, you store the excess as fat. But how much is "too much?" Really massive amounts, according to the *American Journal of Physiology* (*246:* E62, 1984) and the *American Journal of Clinical Nutrition* (*48:* 240, 1988).

However, don't rush to your refrigerator to stuff yourself with sherbet, sodas, and other carbohydrate-rich foods and still expect to lose weight. Overweight people often have problems handling carbohydrates, especially sugars. And you still have to eat fewer calories than you expend in order to lose weight.

However, this study does imply that you should include filling, nutirious foods such as whole grain breads from Natural Ovens in your diet. Bread is a satisfying, wholesome food, and it will take an awful lot to add an ounce of fat to your hips.

Separate but NOT equal

In another of his studies, Flatt fed young men a low-fat breakfast of bread, jam and dried meat. On another day, they were

fed the same breakfast, with an extra 10 pats of margarine. On the margarine day, it was noted that their bodies did not adjust by burning a greater proportion of fat. (*J. Clin. Invest. 76:* 1019, 1985).

"You have to watch out for fat calories more than carbohydrate calories, because the body maintains carbohydrate and protein balance automatically," Flatt explains. "But it doesn't control fat as well."

Confirming studies

Eric Ravussin, a former co-worker with Flatt, is now at the National Institute of Diabetes and Digestive and Kidney Diseases in Phoenix. Ravussin has just completed a study that supports the earlier findings (*American Journal of Physiology. 255:* E332, 1988).

"The body is able to cope with excess protein and carbohydrate, but not excess fat," says Ravussin.

"I can tell you right now, the people in our clinic who are taught to keep fat out of their diet do better at keeping the weight off," says Elliot Danforth of the University of Vermont. "But no one will believe it unless we keep 100 people or so in a locked ward or dormitory for two-to-three years. That's a mega-expensive study."

A low-fat diet is not a magic wand that will eradicate obesity. Clearly, genes and exercise influence your chances of controling those pounds. But eating less fat, more carbohydrates, can help.

So don't hesitate—fill those cravings with healthful, carbohydrate-rich, whole-grain products from Natural Ovens. Letters from our customers attest that our breads, muffins and other products have helped many dieters lose wieght and keep it off—and feel healthy and energetic in the bargain!

Watch for Part Two of this article in an upcoming newsletter!

When Is A Calorie MORE Than A Calorie?
(*conclusion*)

It's discouraging to think that, even after you've fought the "battle of the bulge" and lost excess weight, your body may be primed to sabotage all your good work.

Studies suggest that people who have lost weight may be especially "hungry" for the fatty foods that are the worst for weight maintenance. What's worse, their bodies may be "programmed" to store every bit of incoming fat, rather than burn it for energy.

Not created equal

Why do some people stay trim and others get plump on virtually the same diet? Obviously, not everyone on a typical, high-fat American diet develops a high-fat American body.

Animal studies illustrate this point. When albino mice are fed low-fat diets, almost all stay slim (*International Journal of Obesity. 9*:443, 1985). The more fat—and the less complex carbohydrates—they're fed, the less uniform they look. Some grow fat, others stay slim. Just like humans.

It seems obvious from these studies that genetics plays a role in obesity. Genes may determine how well or how poorly your body handles fat.

Why are people who have lost weight so likely to regain it? This is one of the toughest questions in obesity research.

Trudy Yost of the University of Colorado Health Sciences Center in Denver has been studying women who have lost weight and kept if off for at least a few months.

Under scrutiny is a compound called liproprotein lipase (LPL). Among other things, this enzyme is responsible for loading fat into adi-pose (fat) cells. Apparently, the LPL in formerly-obese women behaves differently from LPL in others.

"If a normal person eats fat, the body's response is to [lower its LPL level]," says Yost. "The normal body attempts to use fat as energy before loading it into fat cells."

Yost found that formerly-obese women have unusually high levels of LPL. And when they ate fats, their LPL levels soared even higher (*J. Clin. End. Met. 67*: 259, 1988).

"If you present fat calories to a formerly-obese body, the first thing that happens is the fat is packed into cells."

Is LPL the answer?

Maybe, maybe not. Research shows that only some, not all genetically obese animals have high LPL levels. Yost's goal is to find out what can go wrong with LPL and "fix" it. But in the meantime the only solution is to not provide the fat calories.

"We used to say that if you eat a 1,500 calorie per day diet, it doesn't matter if it's fat, protein, or carbohydrate. For the formerly-obese, that isn't true. Fat calories are going to be metabolized differently than other calories," Yost states.

Spectacular results

At Laval University in Quebec, Canada, Claude Bouchard and colleagues ran a program where eight overweight women exercised five times a week for two years. The women lost weight, but then the losses leveled off.

However, when the women tried a 20 percent low-fat diet, "their weight loss was spectacular," says Bouchard. "Some lost 50 to 60 pounds."

But the women in Bouchard's program might have eaten fewer calories on the low-fat diet. The question is: will a 1,000 calorie low-fat diet lead to thinner bodies than a 1,000-calorie high fat diet? So far, no one knows.

A taste for fat

"If it tastes good, it must be fattening." Unfortunately, it may be true—especailly for dieters.

Recent studies suggest that the fatter people are, the more they prefer the taste of fat:

• When given a choice of milkshakes made with varying amounts of cream and sugar, overweight people chose fattier shakes than their lean counterparts (*Physiol. Behav. 35*: 617, 1985).

• Overweight people report eating no more calories than others, but more of those calories come from fat. (*Am. J. Clin. Nutr. 47*: 406, 995, 1988).

These studies suggest that whatever makes people fat also makes them crave fatty foods. What can you do about it?

Think carbohydrates

"If a formerly-obese woman eats 1,500 calories of fat, she's sunk," says Yost. "If she eats 200 calories of protein, 100 calories of fat, and 1,200 calories of complex carbohydrates, she has a chance."

The best defense against regaining weight you've already lost seems to be developing a taste for complex carbohydrates. As we stated before, that doesn't mean you can gorge yourself on high-sugar, low-nutrition snacks. However, there are many nourishing, whole-grain products rich in complex carbohydrates. Natural Ovens breads, muffins, cookies and granola are, we think, among the best.

So when you're hungry, think of Natural Ovens products—low in fat, high in health!

Experts Say Excess Fiber Intake Unlikely For Most Americans

By now, the dietary recommendation to eat more fiber is a familiar one. The reason? High-fiber diets may help prevent cancer, lower cholesterol and control blood sugar levels in diabetics. Unfortunately, most Americans still don't have enough fiber in their diets. But with all the fuss about fiber, the question also has arisen: are some people at risk of getting too much? And if so, how much is too much?

Fiber and Minerals. One of the questions nutritionists raise is," What effect do large amounts of dietary fiber have on mineral absorption?" Insoluble fiber like wheat bran, for example, decreases absorption of calcium, zinc and iron.

However, according to Peter Van Soest Ph.D., a prominent fiber researcher at Cornell University, "The negative effects on mineral absorption are not large." And most experts agree that while dietary fiber decreases absorption of minerals, the effect of 20 to 35 grams of fiber a day from a variety of foods is insignificant.

"Most of the studies which show a decrease in mineral absorption are short-term," explains Elaine Lanza, Ph.D. from the National Cancer Institute, "and there is evidence that humans adapt to very high fiber intakes over a period of time."

Though excessive fiber intake is possible, none of the experts we spoke with was willing to pinpoint exactly where a person crosses the line from a high-fiber to an excessive-fiber diet. Fiber intakes that seem excessive to most Americans (up to 70 grams a day) are common among vegetarians, Chinese and Africans. And they don't appear to suffer ill effects like mineral deficiencies.

Effects on Vitamins. With so much attention focused on minerals, less is known about fiber's influence on vitamin absorption. But according to David Klurfeld, Ph.D., Associate Professor at the Wistar Institute in Philadelphia, there's little reason to believe that vitamin absorption is affected.

Worth noting, however, is a recent study published in the *Journal of the American Dietetic Association*.

Researchers found that people who consumed fiber supplements containing psyllium gum suffered a significant reduction in their absorption of riboflavin, a vitamin necessary for energy production. Psyllium gum is the principle ingredient in many laxatives, including *Metamucil* and *Fiberall Wafers*. Clearly, more long-term research in this area is needed.

Dietary Fiber Content of Some Foods

A healthy person should consume roughly 20 to 35 grams of fiber daily. The chart below is a useful guide to foods and the amount of fiber they provide. A person on a diet of 1200 to 1500 calories per day should find 20 grams of fiber sufficient. As food intake increases, so should fiber.

Food	Serving Size	Fiber (grams per serving)
Natural Ovens Bread		
Nutty Wheat	1 slice	5.1
100% Whole Grain	1 slice	5.4
Raisin Bran Muffin	1	6.7
Bread, Pasta and Rice:		
Spaghetti, whole wheat	1 cup	3.9
Bran muffin	1	2.5
Bread, whole wheat	1 slice	1.4
Spaghetti, regular	1 cup	1.1
Rice, brown	1/2 cup	1.0
Bread, white	1 slice	0.4
Rice, white	1/2 cup	0.2
Fruits:		
Prunes	3	4.65
Banana	1 average	4.05
Strawberries	1 cup	3.42
Apple with skin	1 average	3.03
Raisins	1/4 cup	2.88
Orange	1 average	2.62
Cantaloupe	1/4 melon	1.33
Grapes	1/2 cup	0.72
Grapefruit	1/2 average	0.59
Legumes:		
Baked beans	1/2 cup	8.8
Kidney beans, cooked	1/2 cup	7.3
Lima beans, cooked	1/2 cup	4.5
Vegetables, cooked:		
Corn	1/2 cup	4.62
Broccoli	1/2 cup	3.18
Potato with skin	1 average	3.11
Carrots	1/2 cup	2.33
Vegetables, raw:		
Tomato	1 average	2.46
Cucumber with peel	1 average	1.21
Lettuce, iceberg	1 cup	0.82

All data taken from *Journal of the American Dietetic Association*, June 1986, pp. 732-740 and *Nutrients in Foods*, Leveille, Zabik and Morgan, The Nutrition Guild, Cambridge, Massachusetts, 1983. — EXCEPT FOR THE ADDED NATURAL OVENS PRODUCTS.

ENVIRONMENTAL NUTRITION

315

The good news about complex carbohydrates

Just how much carbohydrate should Americans be eating to maintain health? Nutritionists generally agree that 50 to 60 percent of total calories should be derived from this source, mostly in the form of starch. Currently, people in the United States are eating only about 45 percent of their calories as carbohydrates, of which approximately half are of the desirable starchy, "complex" variety. The other half comes from the sweet-tasting simple carbohydrates known as sugar, which is found in fruits but also in high concentrations in foods of minimal nutritional value such as soft drinks, candies, cakes, and pastries (many of which contain a good deal of fat).

The starch/sugar relationship

The reason sugar and starch are grouped together under the carbohydrates category is that they have a chemical likeness. That probably has much to do with the fact that a number of people still think *starch* is a dirty word. But that misunderstanding can easily be cleared up.

All carbohydrates—simple or complex—are actually made up of one or more simple sugars, the three most prominent of which are glucose, fructose, and galactose. By themselves, the simple sugars are monosaccharides. Two monosaccharides bonded together, known as a *disaccharide*, also constitutes a simple sugar. The monosaccharide glucose connected to fructose forms the disaccharide sucrose commonly referred to as table sugar. Glucose bonded to galactose creates lactose, the simple sugar found in milk. And two glucose molecules together make maltose, which is sometimes referred to as malt sugar and is found in malt liquor.

When more than two glucose molecules are "hooked up," a *polysaccharide*, or complex carbohydrate, is formed. Complex carbohydrates may contain anywhere from 300 to 1,000 or more glucose units linked together, and the nature of the links determines whether a complex carbohydrate is a starch or some other substance, such as cellulose. (The links are also what stops these multisugars from tasting sweet. That is, the part of the sugar molecule that normally bonds to taste receptors on the tongue to give the sensation of sweetness is bound instead to another sugar molecule.)

The human body uses both the sugars and the starches—specifically, the simple sugars they contain—for energy. In fact, glucose, the most common, which the body extracts from poly-, di-, and monosaccharides (even fructose by itself can be converted to glucose in the liver) is usually the sole source of energy for the brain and nervous system. Glucose (alternately known as blood sugar) also helps to maintain body temperature and to provide energy for such processes as muscle movement, digestion, respiration, tissue repair, and maintenance of the immune system. Some of the glucose we take in when we eat a meal, whether as starch or sugar, is stored in the liver and muscles as a complex carbohydrate called glycogen (animal starch) and is drawn upon for energy as needed until it is used up and more food is eaten. Excess carbohydrate is converted to fat.

If glucose itself performs all these vital functions, why does it matter whether it is provided by simple or complex carbohydrates, that is, sugar or starch? The answer lies partly in the different ways starch and simple sugars are packaged. Remember, the sweet foods that contain simple sugars often have a lot of fat, which most Americans eat in excess. In addition, many varieties of cookies, candy bars, and the like are almost always extremely low in vitamins and minerals—especially in proportion to their large number of calories. A number of starchy foods, on the other hand, are nutrient dense. That is, for the number of calories in starchy foods, there are usually plenty of vitamins and minerals as well as a fair amount of protein. (And they lend themselves to being eaten with other nutritious foods as part of a meal.)

To illustrate, let's compare a small baked potato to a third of a typical candy bar, both of which contain from 85 to 100 calories. The potato, rich in glucose in the form of starch, provides plenty of vitamin C along with small amounts of protein, B vitamins, about a half dozen minerals, and fiber. The third of a candy bar, whose glucose is contributed as the simple sugar sucrose, supplies the same amount of energy but several times the fat and little or no fiber. Clearly, while starch and sugar both contain glucose, the foods they come in may be very different nutritionally.

It should be mentioned that the sweetest-tasting of the simple sugars—fructose—is the sugar in fruits; fruit does not contain any starch. Does that make it a nutritionally undesirable food? Not at all. Since fruit is mostly water (91 percent of a watermelon is water), its fructose concentration is relatively low and therefore does not drive up the number of calories or make it taste overly sweet. And fruit is generally fat-free. Moreover, like starchy foods, many fruits come packed with vitamins A and C. Some contain minerals. Bananas, for instance, are a rich source of potassium, and oranges contain potassium, too.

To be continued.

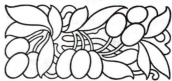

316

The good news about complex carbohydrates

(Part Two of the series. Watch for the concluding section.)

Are starchy foods fattening?

In the past, when someone wanted to lose weight he or she would follow, however grudgingly, the generally accepted advice to swear off bread, pasta, rice, and potatoes. In short, starchy foods. Today, these foods—minus the attendant butter, sour cream, and other fatty toppings—are considered the sort of fare a potential weight loser should include in a diet. The reason is simple: Starch has no more calories than protein; both contain just 4 calories per gram. In addition, most starchy foods are almost fat-free, whereas high-protein foods like meat and dairy products can contain plenty of fat, which contains a full 9 calories per gram.

Despite the facts, old habits die hard. Even though general consumption of complex carbohydrates is on the rise, a goodly number of Americans still see starchy foods as pound-adding "fillers." (Of course, the high-fat sauces and toppings many people put on these foods colors their perception.) More than 35 percent of those responding to a national survey conducted by the Good Housekeeping Institute a few years ago said they consider starch fattening. A 1983 Nielson survey found that close to 30 percent of the respondents avoided cereals and grains, both of which are rich in complex carbohydrates, because they were "fattening" or had "too much sugar." And half the people queried by the Wheat Industry Council that same year said that to control their weight they should eat less starch.

For the person who remains skeptical about converting to a diet high in starch for fear that it will not be conducive to weight control, consider the following: Several years ago, overweight students at Michigan State University who were fed 12 slices of bread a day for eight weeks, and were instructed to eat whatever else they wanted, lost an average of 14 pounds each. More recently at New York City's Hunter College, subjects who ate eight slices of bread a day for 10 weeks—plus whatever else they wanted—each lost about nine pounds. It's true that the subjects may have been making a special effort to cut back on their food intake because they wanted to insure that their weight-loss efforts would be successful. Still, like other starchy foods, bread has a stick-to-the-ribs quality about it that satisfies as well as satiates.

But there's more to why starch is good for weight control. It appears that the process of digestion "spends" more energy metabolizing carbohydrate than fat, so more calories are used up when starch is eaten than when fat is consumed. In fact, evidence is emerging from a host of recent studies conducted by Jean-Pierre Flatt, PhD, a professor of biochemistry at the University of Massachusetts Medical School, that as many as 25 percent

of the excess calories we take in as carbohydrate are used to convert the carbohydrate to body fat, which means only about 75 percent of the extra carbohydrate calories are "added on" as body weight. However, since only 3 percent of excess fat calories are needed to convert that dietary fat to body fat, a full 97 percent of extra fat calories actually wind up "on the body."

The average person, says Dr. Flatt, would have to eat a full 4,000 calories a day for many days before the carbohydrates in such a high-calorie regimen would be converted to fat. "You don't get fat from overeating carbohydrates," he adds, "but from the fats you eat." That does not mean, of course, that you can eat all the complex carbohydrate you wish and still not gain weight, but it does mean that if you are going to overeat, you're better off overdoing it on starch than on fat.

In addition to using more calories than fat in the conversion to body fat, carbohydrates increase the thermic effect of food (the small amount of heat given off by the body when food is eaten). As a result, more heat—and calories—are given off upon consumption of carbohydrates than on consumption of fats.

Carbohydrates may play a major role in weight control in still another way. It seems that they may be better than fats at informing the body that it has been fed and, when appropriate, that it has had enough. The reason is that unlike fat, carbohydrates trigger the release of the hormone insulin. And insulin, according to Elliot Danforth, Jr., MD, professor of medicine at the University of Vermont, may be the chemical that best informs the body when food has been consumed.

When risk factors synergize

If you smoke and drink, you are worse off than if you only smoke or only drink. Alcohol seems to multiply the cancer-causing effects of smoking—a phenomenon called synergism. A person who has one drink per day but doesn't smoke has a 60% higher risk of oral cancer than a nonsmoking teetotaler. A person who smokes up to a pack of cigarettes a day and doesn't drink has a 52% higher risk than a nonsmoking teetotaler. But the risk for a moderate smoker and drinker (a pack or less a day and one drink a day) is four times greater than that for a total abstainer. For a heavy smoker (two packs) and drinker (more than a drink a day), the risk is 15 times greater. No one knows exactly why these risks synergize in this instance. However, if you both smoke and drink and decide you'll give up one of these habits, quit smoking. Overall, it's the more harmful of the two.

UNIVERSITY OF CALIFORNIA,
BERKELEY WELLNESS LETTER

The good news about complex carbohydrates

(Part Three. The Conclusion.)

The fiber factor

As already noted, the nature of the links between glucose molecules in a polysaccharide determines whether that polysaccharide is a starch. If the links do not make for the formation of starch, they may be set up in such a way as to create substances like cellulose and hemicellulose, both of which are better known as fiber. Not all fibers are made up of glucose molecules. Pectins and lignin are types of fiber that have completely different biochemical and physical properties. What all fibers have in common, however, is that the human digestive system does not have the ability to break apart fiber's constituent units. Thus, fiber cannot be absorbed and cannot contribute any calories. Nonetheless, getting enough fiber is of major importance to health.

One reason is that it attracts water to the digestive tract, thereby softening the stool and helping to prevent constipation. Water-insoluble fibers, found in high concentrations in wheat bran, appear to be particularly effective at this task. They also exercise the muscles of the digestive system, which in turn keeps the intestines toned up and resistant to diverticulosis. (Some professionals think an adequate amount of fiber in the diet protects against colon cancer by pushing food through the gut faster and giving potential carcinogens in the food less time to irritate the colon wall.

People with diabetes can benefit by adding fiber to the diet because it appears to modulate levels of blood sugar after eating. Indeed, James Anderson, MD, of the University of Kentucky, has been able to lower the insulin requirements of diabetes victims from 40 to 98 percent by making sure they take in more fiber. And the American Dietetic Association has stressed the importance of fiber in its latest Diabetes Exchange Lists, which help guide people with the disease to the foods that will best keep their blood sugar on an even keel.

Soluble fiber, the kind found in oats, beans, and many vegetables and fruits (fruit has plenty of fiber even though it does not contain starch) has proven effective in lowering both cholesterol and triglyceride levels in the blood, thereby reducing the risk of heart disease. And all kinds of fiber, of course, may be of some value in weight control because this calorie-lacking substance makes food take longer to chew and adds bulk to a meal, both of which help a dieter to feel full. In the "bread" studies conducted at Michigan State University and Hunter College, in fact, those who ate high-fiber bread lost considerably more weight than those who did not. (The way to make sure you're buying high-fiber breads is to choose those that are made from whole wheat.)

Obviously, both starchy *and* fibrous foods have numerous health benefits. Fortunately, they are often one and the same. Whole-grain breads, cereals, rice, and pasta as well as beans (particularly high in protein for a plant food) and vegetables all contain substantial amounts of these two forms of complex carbohydrates. Fruits have no starch but are loaded with fiber. Keeping these few facts in mind makes it easier to remember that there's really nothing complex about complex carbohydrates at all. And because they come packaged in foods that most people already like, following the advice to eat more of them shouldn't be difficult.

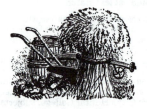

FLAXSEED UPDATE

Dr. Patricia Johnston at the Burnside Research Laboratory, University of Illinois has found that the type of Omega-3 found in flax seed can prevent tumor growth. Omega 3 is an essential fatty acid that is converted into the human body's specialized cellular hormones which in turn control cell growth.

The type of Omega-3 found in flaxseed is a tremendous advantage because it appears to counteract the affect of other dietary fats that seem to promote the growth of cancers. Moreover, it accomplishes this without drastically lowering the overall fat level in the diet. Omega-3's ability to counteract dietary fats is crucial. Afterall, researchers have found that people on a high fat diet tend to develop cancer more often than those on a low fat diet.

This is an important break-through for Americans because, even though they have been told for years to cut the overall fat levels in their diet, only a very small change has been made. More research is continually being done in this area. It is surely to become a future nutritional phenomenan.

Dr. Patricia Johnston recommends that people consume the flax in baked goods. Natural Ovens is one of the few bakeries in the United States that uses significant levels of flax in baked goods.

In the News

Vitamin Supplements May Aid Children's IQ Scores

Researchers in England studied 90 children ages twelve and thirteen and found those given a single daily multivitamin/mineral tablet for nine months scored significantly higher on intelligence tests than those whose diets were not supplemented. All the children consumed adequate diets prior to supplementation, with the exception of folic acid (a B vitamin) and vitamin D.

These preliminary findings raise new questions about so called "sub-clinical" deficiencies in which no signs of nutrient deficiencies exist, but subtle symptoms appear that go unrecognized. Clearly more research is needed.

Lancet, January 23, 1988, pp.140-143

ENVIRONMENTAL NUTRITION

☐ **A slow jog** burns only about 10% fewer calories than a fast run over the same distance. *Example:* A 160-pound runner burns 99 calories covering a mile in 10 minutes and 40 seconds, and 110 calories if he finishes in five minutes and 20 seconds.

Nutrition Education for the Patient by Lynn Caldwell, George F. Stickley Co., 210 W. Washington Square, Philadelphia 19106. $17.50.

☐ **Winter walking guidelines:** Slow down if the wind is strong or the snow is wet and heavy. You'll still be doing the same amount of work. Walk *into* the wind when you leave home and with the wind at your back when you return. Reschedule your walk (afternoon is usually best) if the wind-chill factor is extreme. *Important:* Protect your skin —face, neck, hands—as much as possible from the weather.

Dr. Henry Gong Jr., associate professor of medicine, UCLA Medical Center, quoted in *Prevention*, 33 E. Minor St., Emmaus, PA 18098. Monthly. $12.97/yr.

Bottom Line PERSONAL

It is one of the most beautiful compensations of this life that no man can sincerely try to help another without helping himself.
–Ralph Waldo Emerson

Vitamin C and the Common Cold: More Evidence

Researchers at the University of Wisconsin's Vital Research Center found direct evidence in support of the value of vitamin C in fighting the common cold. People who were given regular vitamin C has less severe cold symptoms and were less contagious. Coughing was twice as bad in the non-vitamin C group.

Source: *New Scientist*, November 19, 1987.

Q & As

I am not sure about the difference between crude fiber and dietary fiber. Which one is protective against heart disease? And which one stabilizes the blood sugar? Any light you can throw on this would be most helpful.

Answer: The crude/dietary fiber distinction is often confused with the soluble/insoluble fiber content of foods.

The crude fiber content is the amount of fiber left after the food is chemically broken down in the laboratory, using very strong chemicals. This usually includes only cellulose and lignin, two of the seven types of fiber.

The term *dietary fiber* refers to the fiber content remaining after the food is experimentally broken down using the same types of enzymes present in the human digestive tract, so it is a far more accurate figure—and can be from 5 to 20 times higher than the crude fiber analysis shows.

Your question, however, actually refers to the soluble/insoluble distinction in fiber types. The soluble fibers, including gums and pectins from fruits, vegetables, legumes, oats, and seeds, help stabilize blood sugar and low cholesterol.

The insoluble fibers, including wheat bran, are helpful in speeding the bowel transit time and thus relieving constipation and preventing bowel disease, including colon cancer, and possibly facilitating excretion of toxins and bile acids which promote other cancers.

There is some conflicting evidence saying that wheat bran also helps stabilize blood glucose. Consequently, it is best to encourage the use of whole foods rather than fiber supplements to insure that all types of fiber are amply represented in the diet. ☐

THE NUTRITION & DIETARY CONSULTANT

Skin Scan:
An Inside Look At The Outside Of Your Body

The outside surface of your body serves an amazing number of functions, from air conditioning and waste disposal, to communicating the tender blush of love. This newsletter is devoted to examining some of the fascinating facts about skin, and looking at some ways we can do more to take care of it.

Vital Statistics

The skin of an average adult weighs about seven pounds and has a surface area of some 20 square feet.

An average square inch of skin has:
- about 65 hairs
- 100 sebaceous glands
- 650 sweat glands
- 78 heat sensors
- 13 cold sensors
- 1300 nerve endings
- almost 10,000 cells
- 19 yards of blood vessels
- 165 separate structures to perceive pressure

Function AND Beauty

The skin is an amazing complex of interconnected microscopic structures. Its tiny pumps, pipes, sensing devices, reservoirs, electrical circuits and communication network busily carry on the business of the body's interface with the outside world. Every second your skin is buzzing with activity as blood is moved, oil is secreted, wastes are excreted, cells are fed, and messages are sent to the brain.

Your skin can also be a wonderfully expressive communication tool. Its color and temperature tell about your health and emotional state.

We've all felt the warmth of embarrassment or anger creep up our necks, coloring our cheeks and ears bright red. A body at war with foreign microbes signals its distress with the heat of fever on the skin. A healthy person's skin, on the other hand, seems to glow as if lit from within.

How Your Skin Works

Your skin consists of three layers, the outer layer or epidermis, the inner layer or dermis, and the subcutaneous layer. (See illustration.)

Most of the activity takes place in the dermis or "true skin." This part of the skin is packed with blood vessels,

AN INSIDE LOOK AT SKIN

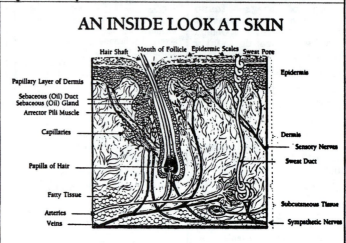

nerves, sweat and oil glands, hair follicles, muscle and connective tissue.

Blood vessels serve as food delivery system, delivering oxygen and nutrients. They also become larger or smaller as needed to help regulate body temperature.

Nerve endings are the body's alarm system. They trigger instant reactions to heat, irritation, cold and pressure. They also somehow absorb healing energy and pleasurable sensations. This mechanism is not well understood. It's theorized that nerves in the skin produce far-reaching hormonal and nervous system reactions that can affect everything from our moods to the strength of our immune systems.

The Care and Feeding of Skin

Healthy skin is important for both health and beauty. Of course, eating the right foods has a major effect on your overall health, and on the beauty of your skin.

A major function of the skin is waste elimination. You can help that, and all major functions of the body by drinking enough fluids. Six to eight glasses of water every day help the skin perform this function efficiently, and keep it clear of blemishes that can occur when the system gets "clogged."

Alpha-Linolenic Acid

Research has found that the essential fatty acid Omega-3 has an extremely beneficial effect on the skin. In one study, infants with red, inflamed skin found almost instant relief when flax oil was smoothed on.

Flax seed contains alpha-linolenic acid, which the body metabolizes into Omega-3. Studies with fortified flax seed have shown improvements in skin health and softness.

Natural Ovens uses flax seed and canola oil in our baked products—both excellent sources of alpha-linolenic acid.

So keep your skin working for you; drink plenty of water, and eat good, whole foods—including Natural Ovens breads!

320

Staying Healthy and Losing Weight with Fiber

One of the beautiful advantages of fiber is that it must be chewed. Your mouth cannot give the same treatment to a brussels sprout that it can to a forkful of creamed spinach. It takes time to chew fibrous foods and chewing is the first step towards weight control. Here's how it works:

Consider the difference between munching an apple and drinking a bottle of cola. It takes time to chew the natural-sugar fruit, but only a minute or two to quench your thirst with a sugar-laden soda. Because the refined concentration of sugar in the cola is easily absorbed into the intestines, your body is receiving all the calories it has to offer. But eating an apple, like all high fiber foods, means you can eat more and yet get less calories from it. Bulk foods pass through the digestive tract faster so that the digestive juices don't get a chance to break them down into absorbable form. Therefore, less calories enter the bloodstream than enter the stomach or intestines.

PUTTING THE BLAME WHERE IT DOESN'T BELONG

Overweighters blame overeating for their problem as they "compulsively" try to satiate their empty stomachs. But overeating zeros in on the wrong target. Vegetarians are rarely overweight because they consume only high fiber foods. Even lacto-vegetarians who eat eggs and cheese, are usually trim, healthy people. Animals in the wild aren't fat even when food is plentiful and, contrary to what you may think, most of them are quite sedentary creatures — so it's not exercise that keeps them fit. Obesity is caused by eating a high proportion of refined or processed — foods from which fiber has been removed and are high in carbohydrates.

When wheat is milled, almost all the fiber (or bran) is removed. From 0.7 grams the fiber is reduced to a mere trace in the starchy endosperm that remains. When sugar is extracted from the beet or the cane, it also is stripped of fiber, and the refined granules are put into almost every kind of processed food.

Refining changes the physical form of carbohydrates so that, when they enter the body they are quickly absorbed by the intestines and give a temporary feeling of having eaten enough. But soon the stomach is growling and demanding more food because it has been fooled into a false feeling of well-being.

Since the whole process of better health and weight control begins with chewing the fibrous foods, it should be emphasized again how important this function is. Remember that fiber has almost no nutritive value, yet it provides the body with all the natural sugar and starches it needs. Because of its bulk, it fills the stomach and then passes through the intestines quickly so that it cannot supply the body with too many calories. Finally, when it is excreted it carries with it fats, calories and nitrogens — all factors related to weight gain. Now, what happens when you eat brussels sprouts, apples, or whole grain bread?

1. You have to *chew* them and chewing takes time. It takes longer to eat a slice of whole wheat bread than it does a slice of white bread. Try it. This experiment was conducted among two groups of young women. One group took 45 minutes to consume a loaf of whole grain bread; the other group took 32 minutes to consume a loaf white bread.

2. Because chewing takes time, it is more satisfying and works as a natural control of the appetite. Nutritionists urge overweight person to stop gulping down their food because the stomach doesn't have time to signal the brain that it's full.

3. Chewing stimulates the saliva and gastric juices, along with drinking fluids, that are absorbed by fiber so the food becomes heavier. The the stomach is *honestly* filled and satisfied with few calories.

4. Bulky moisture-filled fiber passes through the digestive tract faster than low fiber food, reducing the intestinal absorption of calories and excreting excess body fat.

5. Finally, you will be freed from that demon constipation. You cannot be constipated on a high fiber diet. At last you'll be able to empty your medicine chest of addictive laxatives as yur body regains its natural health balance.

Can you imagine losing weight on a diet by *adding* food instead of taking it away? A diet that satisfies your hunger and doesn't leave you feeling deprived and starved? One of the main reasons you're always hungry on a typical low caloie diet is that the recommended foods like juices, eggs, milk, fish, meat and poultry are all fiberless foods. There's no bulk to fill your stomach and, because they can tend to keep you constipated, your body retains many of the fattening calories. You can maintain a 1200-calorie per day diet, but you must stay away from super-refined foods, add fibrous foods, drink plenty of fluids, and exercise. If you want to maintain the weight you're most happy with, you can stay on this diet for the rest of your life.

—High Fiber Weight Loss Diet, R. Fagen

Tips for Getting the Most Nutrition From Foods

It seems as if a new list of foods that people shouldn't eat surfaces every day. Well, amidst all the "don'ts" there are some "dos." Here are tips to get the most nutrition from foods.

When Shopping

- Stock up on bread, pasta and potatoes. Relatively low in calories, they provide little or no fat.
- If buying fresh produce isn't practical opt for frozen. It's the next best choice.
- Take advantage of fruits and vegetables in season. Know when they are available and plan recipes and menus around them to maximize nutrition.
- Choose dark green leaf lettuce over pale iceberg. The darker the color, the greater the beta-carotene content.
- Choose whole grain breads and cereals over refined ones. Not only do they provide more fiber, but they are also higher in vitamins and minerals.
- For a change, purchase protein foods that contain little or no saturated fat or cholesterol such as tofu, beans and dried peas.
- Keep plenty of fruit and vegetable juices on hand as an alternative to soft drinks. Fruit and vegetable juices are packed with vitamins. Soft drinks, on the other hand, provide little or no vitamins — only calories.
- Maximize the nutrient value and minimize the fat of desserts by choosing fresh fruits instead of rich cakes, cookies or ice creams.

When Storing

- Place fresh produce in covered containers and use as quickly as possible. Precious vitamins are lost during storage in the refrigerator.
- The same is true for the freezer. Cover and wrap foods tightly before storing in the freezer. Exposure to air accelerates nutrient loss. Use frozen foods with six to eight months of freezing for additional assurance against nutrient losses, espicially vitamin C.

- Wait until just before serving to chop or dice fruits and vegtables for salads. Vitamin losses are minimized this way.

When Preparing

- Miximize the nutritional value of vegetables by steaming or blanching. These cooking methods, rather than cooking in large amounts of water, save more vitamins from destruction.
- Plan to have an iron-containing non-meat food such as legumes, dried beans and peas along with food sources of vitamin C such as citrus fruits, canteloupe or tomatoes. The vitamin C enhances the body's ability to absorb iron from the plant foods.
- Use cooking water from vegetables to prepare soups and gravies. Vitamins and minerals that leech out into the cooking water are then recaptured. Or freeze the liquid in ice cube trays for later use.
- Make pasta, rice, vegetables and legumes the focus of meals instead of meat. Fat, cholesterol and calories in the meal drop and the nutrient and fiber content increase.
- Plan for five servings of fruits and vegetables each day as the National Academy of Sciences recommends for optimal nutrition.

—*Laura Conway, M.S.,R.D.*
ENVIRONMENTAL NUTRITION
TO SUBSCRIBE: 2112 BROADWAY, SUITE 200, NEW YORK, NY 10023

What is a Healthy Diet for a Child?

If you desire to prepare healthy foods for your children, but don't feel you know enough about nutrition, or where to look for recipes and ideas, try your local library or book store. The following books are just two of many excellent menu planning books available for infants through preteens.

Once Upon a Recipe, written by Karen Greene, contains over 50 fast and easy recipes that will delight and nourish children of all ages. It is brimming with nutritional information and unique pictures that you will want to treasure.

No Nonsense Nutrition for Kids, written by Annette Natow and JoAnn Heslini offers a daily food guide that suggests the number of serving sizes for 4 age groups: infancy, toddler, preschooler and the school-ager to preteen. It is packed with nutritional information.

—*Natural Food & Farming*

SUMMER PICKINS

Tomatillos when ripened are firm and dry with close-fitting husks that show no blackness or mold. They should be yellow or only slightly green in color. Tomatillos are a fair source of vitamin C and provide vitamin A. When preparing tomatillos remove the husks and wash in lukewarm water. They can be eaten raw, but usually are cooked and used in sauces or salsa.

Tomatillos

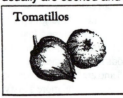

To cook, barely cover with cold water and poach gently until tender (2 to 15 minutes, depending on their size).

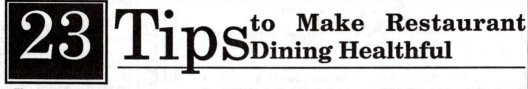

23 Tips to Make Restaurant Dining Healthful

The American appetite for restaurant dining is growing. We're eating out more than ever — an average of about four times a week, according to the National Restaurant Association. And a recent survey of 2000 households shows that Americans' eating habits when eating out differ radically from at home. It found that homebodies tend to make more healthful mealtime choices, while restaurant diners typically consume more calories, and the meals they select often have more fat and less nutrients than foods eaten at home.

For tips on healthy eating out read on.

Detouring Diet Disasters.

If controlling calories is the main concern, consider these strategies:

• Steer clear of buffets, smorgasbords, all-you can-eat specials, and *prix fixe* menus.

• Frequent restaurants that offer a wide variety of choices, with "a'la carte" selections.

• Request that butter, chips, salsa and other tempting pre-meal munchies be removed from the table.

• Ask for an extra plate and split an entree with a friend.

• Eat only half of what's served and ask for a doggie bag. Wrap it before temptation hits, and use it for tomorrow's lunch.

• Control the amount of calories added to the meal by asking that salad dressings, sauces and baked potato toppings be served on the side.

• Forget the so-called "diet plate" and typical chef's salad. Slimmer selections can be found on the menu.

• Avoid appetizers that are deep-fried or cheese-smothered. Try shrimp cocktail, smoked salmon, seafood salad, crudites or vegetable terrine instead.

• Control premeal hunger pangs and willpower by eating a piece of fruit or drinking a glass of tomato juice before arriving at the restaurant.

• When reaching for the bread basket, pick hard rolls, bread sticks, french bread or whole-wheat buns. Pass on the biscuits, croissants or muffins.

Slashing Fat.

A few lessons in menu-decoding will help raise red flags:

• "Breaded, " "batter-dipped," and "tempura," all mean fried and the coating acts like a grease sponge. Look instead for lower-fat "grilled," broiled," and "flame cooked." Other good choices include entrees that are steamed, poached, roasted, baked or cooked in their own juices.

• "Flaky," "puffed," and "crispy" — there's only one way this is achieved…with fat. Avoid croissants, biscuits, entrees *en croute*, Beef Wellington, pot pies, quiches and pastries.

• Avoid "hollandaise," "bearnaise," "bechamel," *beurre blanc* or anything that sounds creamy. For sauces, stick to wine, or thin, stock-based sauces. Also, skip the gravy.

• "Escalloped," "au gratin," and "parmigiana" also mean added fat.

• With pasta, opt for red sauces like "marinara" rather than cream sauces like "alfredo."

Upping Nutrient Value.

Restaurant meals — particularly from fast-food establishments — tend to be shy certain nutrients. Here are ideas to factor in more nutrition when ordering fast food:

• Choose salads made with nutrient-rich dark greens like spinach and romaine. Pale iceberg lettuce falls short in comparison.

• Order a side dish of steamed or marinated vegetables.

• Don't overlook the garnish. That wedge of melon, slice of orange or sprig of parsley is a good source of vitamin C.

• Bypass fat-laden desserts and enjoy a bowl of fresh fruit instead.

• Opt for a plain baked potato instead of french fries.

• Request whole grain bread or bun and brown rice, where they're available.

• Request lettuce, tomatoes, onions and mustard on sandwiches, but skip the mayonnaise and special sauces.

• Order a glass of orange juice with the meal. The vitamin C it contains will help boost iron absorption from vegetables and grains.

—Janet Helm, M.S., R.D.
Environmental Nutrition

Q. Dear Mrs. Stitt:

I tried using the apple and milk mask for wrinkles and my skin felt really good and taut. However, how do you keep it from falling off your face and neck?

A.O.,
Chicago, IL

A. Dear Mrs. O.,

Put the mixture in the blender for a few seconds on high, and you'll find it makes a wonderful mask that won't fall off. By putting it in a covered cup or small bowl, the mixture will keep nicely in the refrigerator for a week to ten days. You may find you'll enjoy the refreshing mask one to three times weekly, according to your own skin needs.

The recipe is simple: Core and chop one small apple, cover it with milk and on low heat cook until the apple is soft. Allow to cool a bit then blend to a smooth texture. Apply a thin layer to your clean face and neck. Allow to dry for 15 to 30 minutes. Splash with warm water then rinse off completely with cold water. Apply a moisturizer and enjoy the cool, taut, refreshing feeling.

Barbara Stitt

Aging

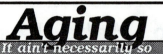

It ain't necessarily so

Middle age and old age, or at least our image of them, are not what they used to be. More often than not it is factors extrinsic to aging that bring on "middle-age spread," brittle bones, forgetfulness, loss of muscle strength.

When "maturity" includes an openness to healthful life-style changes, many of the physical and mental ills once blamed completely on aging can be alleviated or postponed.

One of the most important factors is exercise. A new report from the Medical College of Pennsylvania cites "growing evidence" that older people can start on an exercise program at almost any age and have short-term physiological benefits as well as a reduced incidence of chronic disease. In light of this report and a host of other studies, it seems clear that a long-term exercise program can make a substantial difference for both body and mind. When aging is accompanied by inactivity, it can result in declines on the following scale:

- By middle age, blood vessels typically narrow by 29%. Between the ages of 25 and 60, the circulation of blood from arms to legs slows down by as much as 60%.
- Muscle fiber is lost at the rate of 3 to 5% a decade after age 30, leading to a 30% loss of muscle power by the age of 60.
- The speed at which messages travel from brain to nerve endings decreases 10 to 15% by the age of 70.

Regular exercise has been shown to inhibit, arrest, or even reverse most such declines. Some experts estimate that *half the functional losses that set in between the ages of 30 and 70 are in fact attributable to lack of exercise.* Just consider: researchers have found that three weeks of complete inactivity (total bed rest) can result in the kind of physical decline typically seen after 30 years of sedentary aging. Fortunately, as you turn 40, 50, 60, or for that matter 70 or 80, there is always something you can do to slow down or reverse this decline. A long-term regimen of three or four brisk 30-minute walks each week, for instance, may not only add years to your life, but also life to your years.

It's never too late to start exercising; improvements in health don't depend on having trained vigorously in youth. Here are a few areas particularly sensitive to the rejuvenating effects of exercise:

Carbohydrate metabolism. Aging has been linked to increased difficulty in metabolizing glucose and thus to the onset of diabetes. But such glucose or carbohydrate intolerance isn't necessarily caused by biological aging. Studies suggest that improved diet and exercise habits can substantially increase tolerance.

Osteoporosis. Aging is associated in both men and women with a severe decline in bone density — and if bones become too light and porous, they're likely to break. However, studies have shown that inactivity can play a large part in promoting bone loss. Weight-bearing exercise, such as walking or lifting light weights, is vital in slowing the loss. Other steps you can take include abandoning habits that reduce bone density, such as smoking and high alcohol consumption.

Brain function. The Baltimore Longitudinal Study of Aging and other studies have found that many mental capacities are actually surprisingly stable with age. Comparisons of the mental agility of younger people and healthy older individuals who exercise at about the same level show that the elders react about as fast as their juniors — and significantly faster than their sedentary peers. Memory does change with age, though these changes don't necessarily constitute a decline. Regular aerobic exercise seems not only to help preserve neurological functioning into old age, but also potentially to enhance it in older people who have been sedentary.

"There is no drug in current or prospective use that holds as much promise for sustained health as a lifetime program of physical exercise." That statement appeared in the *Journal of the American Medical Association* in 1982, and it's likely to hold true for many years to come.

—*University of California, Berkeley Wellness Letter*

SUMMER PICKINS

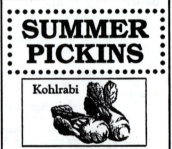

Kohlrabi

KOHLRABI When selecting a fresh, ripe kohlrabi, choose bulbs about two inches in diameter. Kohlrabi are an excellent source of potassium and vitamin C.

Eat peeled, raw or cooked. To cook, peel and cut up bulb. Then, steam in salted boiling water until tender. Season with lemon or lime juice. Cook the tops like any greens.

Sometimes it's not what food you select but how you prepare it. Bake a potato and you'll end up with a mere 0.2 grams of fat; turn it into half a cup of hash browns and you'll have 45 times more fat.

ONE-MINUTE HEALTH TIPS

From head to toe, several effective healing techniques that can be done in a flash

GOOD 'N QUICK CARE FOR SKIN

Moisturizing skin Add a glasssful of ordinary milk to your bath water to soothe dry skin. Proteins in milk help soften and moisturize. (Bathing in water with a cupful of salt water afterward.) Apply lotion after bathing while the skin is still damp.

Beating bug bites To relieve the itch of mosquito or other insect bites, apply a paste of baking soda and water. The alkaline moisture soothes irritation.

Slipping out slivers A little vegetable oil can help you remove painful splinters. Just pat some on and wait a moment for it to seep around and into the puncture. Then gently remove the splinter with tweezers. The "lube job" should help it slide right out.

Peeling away micro-splinters Splinters that are too small to get with tweezers can be removed with white glue or facial mask gel. Pour a thin layer of glue or gel over the skin and let it dry. Then peel the dried glue/mask off. The splinters go with it! This trick has worked for wood splinters, fiberglass fragments, and even cactus spines.

Taking the burn out of sunburn Soothe away sunburn pain with a cool or tepid oatmeal bath. There are several commercial brands of oatmeal bath soaks in the drugstore. Don't use your breakfast oatmeal — the flakes are too large.

Treating a broken blister The best way to treat an ordinary blister is to leave it alone. It it breaks on its own, wash the area with soap and water and cover with a bandage. Minor burn blisters should be flushed with cold water. The fresh juice of an aloe-vera plant can help speed healing. (For burns that cover a large area, see a doctor.)

Washing away poison ivy To prevent a rash from developing after exposure to poison oak, ivy or sumac, run lots of cold water over the area that was exposed. This works especially well within three minutes or so after contact. There's no need to use soap, but a rubbing-alcohol rinse before using water is ideal. (Wash clothes that touched the plants, too.)

Pickling athlete's foot Fight chronic athlete's foot with this one-minute-to-prepare soak. Fill a basin with warm water and add half a cup of white vinegar. This lowers the pH balance of your skin, making life uncomfortable for fungi and bacteria.

ANTIDOTES FOR ACHES AND PAINS

Curing a charley horse Calf cramps can be massaged away: Grasp your toes and gently pull them toward you. Use your other hand to rub lengthwise along the calf, from the back of the knee to the ankle. Always rub *with* the muscle, never across it.

Icing hurt muscles Ice is the best emergency treatment for sprains and pulled muscles. But most of us don't have ice packs, and makeshift packs fall apart as the ice melts. Simple solution: Use a bag of frozen peas or other small vegetable. Bang it on the counter to break the peas apart, and it will conform to the contours of the injured area. Wrap it in a towel and leave on for no more than 20 minutes at a time.

Halting a spasm Overworked runners sometimes get side stitches, painful cramps probably caused by spasms of the diaphragm. The best way to get rid of these spasms is to slow down your pace and take slow, rhythmic breaths.

Beating banged-finger syndrome Ouch! Reduce the trauma by quickly immersing your finger in cold water. The pain is reduced almost immediately. It also helps keep swelling down, for less discomfort later.

Treating a hangnail Hangnails are not really slivers hanging nail, but dried out and split skin along the nail's edge. And they can smart a lot. But rubbing a little petroleum jelly over and around them before you go to bed will ease the pain. How? The jelly will trap moisture and soften the dry skin underneath.

Rubbing away sinus pain Massaging the area just under your eyebrows (and above the eyes) can help reduce or relieve some attacks of sinus pain. Make firm, slow circles with your thumbs or fingertips.

EYE AID

Cooling down itchy eyes Close your eyes and cover them with cool cucumber slices for a few moments. A cool, wet washcloth can have the same effect.

Getting the specks out If you get a speck in your eye, you may be able to wash it out with your own tears. Simply pull your upper lid downward, slightly over the lower lid. This will cause tears to flow. If that doesn't work, try flushing the eye with water. If irritation persists, see a doctor. These measures, of course, are effective only for time, movable specks. If the object is embedded in the eye, skip the self-care and get medical help right away.

Deterring nausea Powdered ginger may be more effective than Dramamine in preventing nausea and motion sickness. A study rported in *Lancet* (March 20, 1982) tested the antinausea effect of three different treatments: two capsules of powdered ginger (940 milligrams total): a standard dose of Dramamine (100mg): and two capsules of an inactive herb. The six test subjects who took ginger were able to stay in a revolving chair an average of 50 percent longer than the six on the drug. (The inactive-herb group fared much worse: Three of the six threw up.) Ginger is safe: You can take two 450 mg capsules (available in many health-food stores) about 10 minutes before your flight or cruise, and two more again if you feel queasy.

Easy occasional constipation* Drink plain, hot water when you get up in the morning. The hot water seems to stimulate the natural movement of the intestinal tract. Since the intestines are usually active in the morning anyway, this remedy often works immediately. Constipation that lasts more than five days, however, should be reported to your doctor.

—These tips were listed in the July issue of PREVENTION magazine

---

**Another great way to relieve constipation* is to add 1 tablespoon of Fortified Flax to 5 ounces of your favorite juice. Stir or blend for a few seconds, allow to sit for 15-20 minutes then stir or blend again. Drink slowly, chewing with each mouthful of liquid. Delicious and it contains a bonus of Omega-3 and soluble fiber for added energy. Fortified Flax is in health food stores. (Natural Ovens *Energy Drink*, also high in flax, can be found in your favorite grocery store.)

Vitamin E may help elderly resist diseases

New studies suggest that depressed immune functions in elderly people can be partially improved with vitamin E supplements. These findings were reported by Dr. Simin Nikbin Meydani, an assistant professor at the U.S. Department of Agriculture's Human Nutrition Research Center on Aging at Tufts University in Boston.

As humans age, their ability to resist disease tends to decline because the immune system becomes less effective. Dr. Meydani said her group has found that some dietary antioxidants — particularly vitamin E and a substance called glutathione — can reverse some of the declines in immunity which occur during aging, and therefore should make it easier for the elderly to fight off disease. Based on her results, which she believes are the first for human trials, she said that dietary requirements for vitamin E may be greater than currently recommended.

Dr. Meydani's findings with vitamin E were first observed in animal studies. How these antioxidants work is not known, admits Dr. Meydani. However, the studies using vitamin E showed increases in interleukin-2, a substance that promotes the growth of white blood cells. They also showed a decrease in prostanglandin E2, a substance that suppresses white blood cells and which the body seems to produce more of as a person ages. —*source unknown*

To stretch or not to stretch?

A recent development in the sports medicine circle is a reversal of the thinking regarding stretching before exercising. The old logic was that we should stretch prior to exercise in order for the muscles to be loose and decrease the risk of strains or sprain to the soft tissues (muscles and ligaments). The new thinking is based on clinical experience of orthopedists, physical therapists and other sports medicine professionals. This experience seems to indicate that people who stretch before exercise do indeed experience a lower incidence of strain and sprain injuries to the soft tissues but at the same time experience an increased incidence of joint injuries. The logic is that after stretching the muscles are loose and provide less protection and support to the joints which they surround.

While neither injury is desirable, the recovery from a joint injury is far more complicated, hence the change in medical advice. The new advice, therefore, is to warm up before exercise and stretch afterward.
—*Thereapy Review, March 1989*

This will mow you over.
Sales of old-fashioned manual lawn mowers have risen during the past two years. Not only are they less expensive and less likely to break down, but they don't pollute the air. They also provide good exercise: pushing a manual mower burns between 420 and 480 calories an hour — as many as an hour of tennis.

The T-Factor Diet

Martin Katahn, Ph.D., author of *The T-Factor Diet* says that if fat is severely restricted in the diet, a person will lose weight regardless of how many calories he eats. The natural reaction to such news is, "You mean I can eat all I want as long as I cut down on fat?" According to Dr. Katahn, the answer is yes, if you eat whole foods.

He cites recent research which suggests two reasons why low-fat diets are important for weight loss.

1. The body is quite efficient at converting dietary fat into body fat, but sadly inefficient at converting high fibered dietary complex carbohydrates into body fat.

2. Regardless of the diet's fat content, the body still burns the same amount of fat after a meal, so that if the diet is low in fat, the body turns to fatty deposits for fuel. The Appendix offers a more detailed discussion of the scientific basis for Dr. Katahn's diet, as well as 13 references to back up his statements.

—*Environmental Nutrition June, 1989*

Dear Natural Ovens:

I am just writing to comment you on your excellent Blueberry-Oat Muffins.

They are moist, very tasteful and low in calories. I expecially like the part that on the ingredients, it says "egg whites" not just "eggs." I haven't yet tried the Raisin Bran Muffins but am anxious to! THANK YOU for a very good product! And, it's made locally, too!

R.O.,
Slinger, WI

Eating Your Way To Beauty

Nutrition plays a very important role in the formation of healthy skin, hair, nails and overall appearance. Diet and supplementation can help overcome many common problems, including rough skin, dull hair, premature greying, whiteheads, brittle nails and dandruff.

What foods can be eaten to promote overall improvements in appearance?

The role of food in one's appearance is directly related to the quality and quantity of vitamins, minerals and enzymes contained in the foodstuffs.

Beautifying veggies

Carrots, for instance, reportedly cause improvements in troubled complexions due to their high content of beta carotene.

Raw vegetable juice, high in minerals, vitamins, trace elements and enzymes, is said to help regenerate skin cells. Green vegetables such as romaine lettuce, high in chlorophyll, can act as powerful alkalinizers and blood purifiers, thus working as beauty rejuvenizers.

Other goodies

Brewer's yeast is said to affect skin and hair, due to a high RNA/DNA and B vitamin content. Other foods have been recommended for overall beauty and appearance improvements. They include flax seed, sprouts, tofu, yogurt, miso, sea vegetables, wheat germ, cold-pressed unsaturated vegetable oil, wheatgrass, whole grains, nuts and seeds, and beans. Foods that are discouraged include fried foods, meat, sugar and high butterfat foods.

Supplements

Which nutritional supplements have the most benefit toward one's appearance?

In general, adequate amounts of all vitamins and minerals are necessary to promote overall health and appearance. However, certain nutrients are recommended for specific problems.

Antioxidants

Vitamins E and C are said to be of particular importance. Vitamin E is an antioxidant, and a deficiency is said to lead to sagging facial muscles. It is described as an overall "rejuvenating" vitamin. Vitamin C, another antioxidant, reportedly helps prevent wrinkling due to its role in collagen production.

Beauty nutrients

If you have hair, skin and/or nail problems, you may have one or more nutritional deficiencies that should be addressed. In many cases, the source of appearance problems could be more than just "skin deep."

Start with your diet. Eat lots of whole foods, including fruits, vegetables, and whole grain breads (from Natural Ovens, of course). Drink plenty of water to keep your body running smoothly. Get enough rest and exercise. And watch the glow of beauty grow!

(Sources: *The Beauty Food Diet* by M.J. Saffon, 1985; and *Beauty From The Inside Out* by Diana Bihova, M.D., and Connie Schrader, 1987. Adapted from "Nutrition for hair, skin and nails," *Whole Foods*, December 1988.)

CHANGING HIS DIET CHANGED HIS LIFE

According to an article printed in the Baltimore Evening Sun...
Phil Sokolof, a 65 year-old, self-made millionaire from Omaha, Nebraska is spending part of his fortune to fight heart disease and what he calls "the poisoning of America."

After his attack Phil Sokolof brought his cholesterol down within the limits recommeded by the National Heart, Lung and Blood Institute.

He simply stopped eating hamburgers, hot dogs, chili and pastries, all laden with saturated fats. And, he switched to fruits and vegetables, pasta and beans. Fish and chicken are good low-fat alternatives, too.

Commenting on his one-man crusade to save other people's hearts and lives, he said "One man can make a difference. This is a crusade from the heart. When you have enough money for your children and grandchildren, it's time to give something back. How do you compare possible extending someone's life to money?"

Don't Bother Counting the Carotenes

You probably expect this chart to tell you how much beta-carotene is in different foods. It doesn't.

Only in the last year or two have researchers had the technology to analyze the *beta-carotene* content of most fruits and vegetables. The figures below are estimates of *all* carotenes, including beta-, alpha-, and zeta-carotene, as well as beta-cryptoxanthin, lycopene, and others.

So why use old figures, rather than specific numbers for beta-carotene? Because these are the numbers researchers used in the studies that found a link between cancer risk and what many called beta-carotene. Yet, for all anyone knows, it could be some other carotene—or something else in these vegetables—that reduces the risk of cancer.

If you're wondering how many International Units (IU) are enough, don't expect a solid answer. The U.S. Recommended Daily Allowance is 5,000 IU per day, but in various studies, the people in the lowest risk groups (for lung cancer) consumed anywhere from 2,000 to 13,000 IU per day. And the 22,000 doctors participating in the ten-year study of beta-carotene are taking 83,000 IU every two days.

Perhaps the best advice is to forget about IUs and follow this simple rule of thumb from Gladys Block of the National Cancer Institute: "Eat at least five fruits and vegetables a day. At least one should be rich in vitamin A."

Food	Vitamin A (IU)	Food	Vitamin A (IU)
Sweet potato, *cooked (1)*	24,880	Tomaato sauce, *cooked*	1200
Carrot, *raw (1)*	20,250	Broccoli, *cooked*	1100
Carrots, *cooked*	19,150	Tomato juice, *(6 oz.)*	1010
Spinach, *cooked*	7370	Nectarine, *(1)*	1000
Butternut squash, *cooked*	7140	Prunes, *dried (5)*	840
Hubbard squash, *cooked*	6160	Tangerine, *(1)*	770
Dandelion greens, *cooked*	6080	Aspargus, *cooked*	750
Kale, *cooked*	4810	Romaine lettuce, *shredded*	730
Turnip green, *cooked*	3960	Avocado	700
Beet greens, *cooked*	3670	Plantains, *cooked*	700
Mango	3210	Tomato, *(1/2)*	680
Red pepper	2850	Savoy cabbage, *cooked*	650
Papaya	2800	Brussels sprouts, *cooked*	560
Swiss chard, *cooked*	2760	Green peas, *frozen, cooked*	530
Cantaloupe	2580	Endive	510
Apricots, *dried (10)*	2530	Peach, *(1)*	465
Bok choy, *cooked*	2180	Orange, *(1)*	269
Mustard greens, *cooked*	2120	Banana, *(1)*	92
Collards, *cooked*	2110	Apple, *(1)*	74
Spinach, *raw, chopped*	1880		

Serving size is 1/2 cup, unless otherwise noted.

—EDITED FROM *NUTRITION ACTION HEALTHLETTER*
VOL. 15, DECEMBER 1988

How to Add Time to Your Day

The key to saving time is finding your own best work type.

There is no one right way to get organized.

In fact, the system that works well for your office neighbor may actually make you less productive. Ann McGee-Cooper, a Dallas-based management consultant and author, says that the secret to working more efficiently and enjoyably is to develop personalized habits that fit your own way of thinking.

"For years I taught traditional time-management skills, such as 'stick to your to-do list,' 'complete one task before beginning another,' and 'work at a neat desk,'" she explains. "But my own inclination was to work contrary to those rules. Many people I taught didn't operate according to these rules either."

What may actually determine individual work style is *brain dominance*. The right and left hemispheres of the brain are associated with different skills and behavior tendencies. The right side originates artistic images, intuition, fantasy, and emotional responses; the left side is the souce of sequential or rational thinking, and mathematical and verbal processes.

Although we use both hemispheres, most of us develop a greater dependence on one side.

"The point here is not which brain dominance or work method is better," stresses McGee-Cooper. "What really matters is discovering which work style is most comfortable and effective for you."

> **You are LEFT-brain dominant if you:**
> • like to establish priorities • adhere consistently to a plan • work in a sequential, orderly fashion • love structure and predictable routines • set strict deadlines • prefer working alone
>
> **You are RIGHT-brain dominant if you:**
> • crave variety and visual stimuli • stay flexible and take on new challenges • often try to innovate • take time out for fun • need to see work out in the open rather than filed out of sight • enjoy jumping from project to project • work in short spurts

Discovering which side of your brain is dominant is the first step toward creating a personalized system of time management. Are you left-brain dominant? Give yourself large chunks of uninterrupted time. For right-brain types, spread a project out and add other tasks for variety.

—Written by Barbara Lau, based on ideas in the book
and five-tape album entitled
Time Management for Unmanageable People,
by Ann McGee-Cooper, P.O. Box 64784,
Dallas, TX 75206.

Fiber:
How does it work?

Many of our customers are interested in increasing their fiber intake. Like most Americans, they know it is beneficial to their health. But not many of us understand how it works.

The effects of psyllium

A recent study describes the effects of psyllium supplements. The study shows that 3 teaspoons per day can lower blood cholesterol by as much as 15%. Psyllium, used mainly as a stool-bulking laxative, has this effect because it is a water-soluble fiber.

Like certain other types of soluble fiber, psyllium binds bile acids and carries them out of the body. Bile acids are chemical derivatives of cholesterol. Normally, they are secreted into the intestine and then reabsorbed. Through a somewhat complicated chain of cause-and-effect, removing bile acids from the intestine leads to lowered levels of blood cholesterol.

Fibers are not created equal

Not all types of fiber will have this effect, however. Wheat bran, the most familiar form of dietary fiber, does not. This is because it is not soluble, and therefore doesn't interact chemically with bile acids.

How can you increase the soluble fiber in your diet if you do not wish to take psyllium, a laxative? There are a number of whole foods that you can add to your diet that will have this effect.

Whole-food fiber sources

According to James Anderson and his colleagues at the University of Kentucky, authors of the psyllium study, eating adequate amounts of food high in soluble fiber can reduce moderately high blood cholesterol by around 20%.

In contrast, the American Heart Association diet, which is low in fats but not high in fiber, typically reduces cholesterol levels by 3-7%.

Foods rich in soluble fiber include oat bran, flax, corn, legumes such as kidney beans, pinto beans, lentils and peas. They recommend a diet with 20 to 25 grams of total fiber a day, 7 to 12 grams of which consist of soluble fiber.

Fiber from fruits

Other research has shown that high cholesterol levels can be lowered by an average of 11% with a diet high in pectin, another form of soluble fiber. Pectin, found in fruits, is most concentrated in tart apples, citrus, cranberries, and sour plums.

Whole grain products

We use a variety of flours and grains in Natural Ovens bread, muffins and cookies to make them naturally high in fiber. Our Oat Bran Delite bread, Blueberry-Oat and Cherry Almond Oat Bran Muffins are particularly high in the soluble fiber from oat bran and flax seed.

So when you are planning your high fiber diet, include fresh fruits and vegetables, oat bran and flax seed products, and legumes. And don't forget healthful Natural Ovens products to keep your meals interesting and delicious.

Adapted from *Harvard Medical School Health Letter*, 13:12, October, 1988.

Here's a convenient chart to help convert these recommendations to recognizable quantities:

Food	Soluble fiber
	(grams/cup)
Oat bran, dry	6.0
Oatmeal, dry	4.0
Beans, cooked	4.0
Corn, cooked	3.5
Energy Drink Mix *(Oat Bran and Flax Seed)*	4.0g per 2 T.

Winning the fiber game

The recommended daily intake of dietary fiber is at least 25 to 35 grams. Fiber is actually a wide variety of substances with widely different properties. In simple terms, every fruit, vegetable, and whole-grain product contains varying amounts of two basic types: *Insoluble fiber* (found in large quantities in wheat bran and whole grains) tends to move food quickly through the digestive tract, increases stool volume, and may protect against colon cancer. *Soluble fiber* (found primarily in oats, beans, carrots, apples, and oranges) may lower blood cholesterol and helps control blood sugar levels in diabetics. In addition, when you eat high-fiber foods, you leave less room on your plate—and in your stomach—for high-fat foods.

The National Research Council suggests that you eat at least five servings of fruit and vegetables and at least six servings of breads, cereals, and legumes a day (servings are not large: one slice of bread, for instance, is considered a serving). In case you don't always follow this advice, use this chart to make simple trade-offs that will increase your intake of both soluble and insoluble fiber. Remember that each food listed as high in one type of fiber also has some of the other kind. Blackberries, for instance, contain insoluble along with soluble fiber, though they are rich in the latter. Chopping or cooking foods does not have any significant effect on the fiber content.

Note: Despite a much publicized report in the *New England Journal of Medicine* (January 18) suggesting that oat bran by itself may not make a significant dent in blood cholesterol levels, nutritionists still recommend eating a variety of high-fiber foods.

To get more insoluble fiber

INSTEAD OF	CHOOSE	TO GAIN
1 cup corn flakes (.4g*)	1/3 cup whole grain granola (6g*)	5.4g*
1 slice white bread (.5g)	1 slice 100% Whole Grain Bread (5g)	4.5g
10 cherries (1.2g)	1 pear (5g)	3.8g
1/2 cup cooked, sliced squash (.7g)	3/4 cup cooked asparagus (3.1g)	2.4g
1/2 cup cooked spinach (2.0g)	1/2 cup cooked brussels sprouts (3.9g)	1.9g
2.5 tbsp. all-purpose flour (.7g)	2.5 tbsp. whole-wheat flour (1.8g)	1.1g
1/2 cup cooked white rice (.1g)	1/2 cup cooked brown rice (2.4g)	2.3g

To get more soluble fiber

INSTEAD OF	CHOOSE	TO GAIN
1/3 cup Cream of Wheat, dry (.5g*)	1/3 cup oat bran (4g*)	3.5g*
12 grapes (.5g)	1/2 cup blackberries (4.5g)	4.0g
1cup celery (1.3g)	1/2 cooked carrots (2.3g)	1.0g
1/2 cup raw mushrooms (.9g)	3/4 cup cooked lima beans (4.4g)	3.5g
1/2 cup cucumber (.5g)	1/2 cup cooked corn (3.9g)	3.4g
1/2 cup cooked macaroni (.6g)	1/2 cup cooked peas (4.1g)	3.5g
2/3 cup apple juice (1g)	1 apple, with skin (2.8g)	1.8g
1 cup honeydew (1.4g)	1/3 cup canned prunes (5.8g)	4.4g

*All figures are for total dietary fiber and represent average serving sizes.
Source: *Plant Fiber in Foods*, by Dr. James Anderson.

—*UNIVERSITY OF CALIFORNIA, BERKELEY WELLNESS LETTER*

You needn't starve to keep off lost pounds

If you're one of the estimated 65 to 80 million Americans who are currently dieting, we have news for you. Once you've shed those excess pounds, simply adding some exercise to your usual routine appears to be more effective at keeping them off than constantly counting calories and giving up food. Researchers at California's Stanford Center for Research in Disease Prevention found that out when they looked at a group of 90 men who had just spent a year on a weight-loss diet and then took some pains to make sure the pounds didn't creep back on.

Those who tried to maintain their newly trimmed physiques by cutting down on the number of calories they consumed tended to regain more of their lost weight than those who simply increased the amount of time spent walking, jogging, and engaging in other forms of aerobic exercise. Over the course of 12 months, in fact, the calorie watchers regained and average of seven pounds each, while the exercisers' total gain worked out to fewer than two pounds per person. It's true that the exercisers were eating an average of 138 fewer calories each day than they were before trying to lose weight in the first place. But the calorie counters were averaging 335 calories fewer—yet still regaining more weight!

The moral of the story: Once you've gone to the trouble of losing weight, by adding an extra two to three hours to your weekly exercise routine you can keep the weight off.
—*TUFTS UNIVERSITY DIET & NUTRITION LETTER*

...Foods for good health that will take the weight off and keep it off: Lots of fresh fruits and vegetables, whole grain, legumes, seeds, sprouts...the whole foods with good fiber. Add to that: 7-8 glasses of pure water daily coupled with exercise such as brisk walking, and, of course, Natural Ovens breads, muffins, cookies, rolls, granola and Energy Drink...loaded with nutrients and a healthy portion of fiber. ♥

...but personally......

The right way to read in bed...Place several pillows behind your back and neck to prop yourself up as if sitting in a chair...and place a pillow under your knees. *Aim:* Proper back support, so that the neck doesn't bend at too sharp an angle, straining the muscles attached to the back of the skull. *Traps:* Keeping legs *straight* in front puts stress on lower back muscles...lying on your abdomen leads to neck and back strain and stress in the shoulder area.

—*BOTTOM LINE PERSONAL*

• • • • • • •

For strong bones, get a grip on something. Getting a good grip on an old tennis ball can do wonders for thin bones. Doctors found that by squeezing a tennis ball six times a day a group of elderly women not only improved their grips, they also thickened the bones in their forearms.

—*BRITISH MEDICAL JOURNAL*

OVERDOSING ON PROTEIN

The Great Protein Myth has its roots in the last century, and has been perpetuated by well-meaning nutritionists and self-serving industries. According to Joan Gussow, a leading nutrition educator at Columbia Teachers College, "Experimental studies as early as the turn of the century showed protein requirements to be relatively modest—quite close, in fact, to our present Recommended Dietary Allowances (RDAs). But some influential nutritionists insisted that these studies couldn't be relied upon alone."

Instead, researchers like Carl Voit, a famous German physiologist, argued that recommended protein levels ought to reflect what people actually eat. In 1881, Voit analyzed the diets of German men and, on the basis of his findings, suggested a protein intake of 118 grams each day—more than double our present RDAs. Voit's student, Wilbur Olin Atwater, became the first director of research at the United States Department of Agriculture. In the early 1900s, Atwater, following in Voit's footsteps, used the diets of American men to set *his* guideline of 125 grams of protein per day. Subsequently, both Voit and Atwater upped their recommendations even further.

In the 1950s, popular nutrition writers like Adelle Davis were still boosting protein, explaining that, "To obtain too much is...probably impossible; to obtain an adequate amount is to stay young for your years."

Too Much of a Good Thing? Obviously, most Americans eat plenty of protein, and some of us probably eat far too much. Among other things, excess protein may increase the risk of osteoporosis—weak, fracture-prone bones. When people eat more protein, their kidneys excrete more calcium, the mineral that keeps bones strong. If protein intake is doubled, for example, about 50 percent more calcium is lost in the urine. Over time, such heavy losses could lead to osteoporosis.

Epidemiological studies of human populations also suggest a link between high-protein diets and osteoporosis. Among ten groups examined in one study, those that ate the most protein, such as Americans and New Zealanders, had the highest incidence of hip fractures, one measure of osteoporosis. Yet these groups also consumed the most calcium.

People who are losing calcium because they're gorging on protein may be able to keep their bones strong by taking mega-doses of calcium. But by doing so they will load up their urine with calcium. The higher level of calcium in the urine may cause kidney stones in a small number of people.

The Old-Fashioned Kidney. One of the kidney's jobs is to rid the body of nitrogen-containing waste products from protein. But the human body evolved during the eons when humans were hunter-gatherers, and ate large, protein-rich meat meals only rarely. According to Barry Brenner of Harvard Medical School, the kidney probably needs periods of rest. So although people who live in most wealthy countries now regard a continuous high protein intake as "normal," their kidneys may not agree.

Observations of aging laboratory animals suggest that high-protein diets may damage the kidney. "If there were nursing homes for old rats, they'd be full of animals with kidney disease," says kidney researcher Mackenzie Walser of the Johns Hopkins University School of Medicine. "All laboratory rats develop this as they age."

But according to Brenner, kidney disease can be avoided by feeding the animals low-protein diets instead of protein-rich laboratory chow. Similarly, he speculates, if people reduced their protein intake, they might ward off the mild loss of kidney function that typically occurs with aging.

This age-related decline isn't important for most people. But some individuals need all the kidney function they can get. Patients with diabetes and other diseases that impair the kidney are in this category; so, too, may be people who have donated or in some other way lost a kidney. Brenner says protein restriction might help preserve vital kidney function in these individuals.

Low-protein diets (with less than three-quarters of the RDA) are known to decrease weakness, fatigue, and other symptoms in patients with failing kidneys, simply because these diets give the kidneys less work to do. Relieving symptoms with a careful diet is preferable to using a dialysis machine. Furthermore, although damaged kidneys usually grow progressively worse, there's evidence, according to Walser, that low-protein diets (some as low as one-quarter or less of the RDA) can slow this relentless deterioration.

RECOMMENDED DIETARY ALLOWANCES FOR PROTEIN

	AGE (years)	PROTEIN (grams)*
Children	1-3	23
	4-6	30
	7-10	34
Males	11-14	45
	15+	56
Females	11-18	46
	19+	44
Pregnant		30**
Lactating		20**

* One ounce equals 28 grams.
** If you're pregnant, add 30 grams to the figure given for your age group; if you're breastfeeding, add 20 grams.

Source: Recommended Dietary Allowances, National Academy of Sciences-National Research Council, Revised 1980.

FOOD	PROTEIN (% of USRDA)*
Pork chop, trimmed, (4 oz.)	82
Chicken, light, w/o skin (4 oz.)	78
Sirloin steak, trimmed, (4 oz.)	71
White tuna, water pack, drained (3 oz.)	67
Ground beef, lean, (4 oz.)	62
Flounder, (4 oz.)	51
Cheese pizza (1 slice)	33
Low-fat cottage cheese (½ cup)	31
Lentils or split peas, cooked (1 cup)	25
Cheddar cheese (1½ oz.)	24
Milk (1 cup)	18
Peanut butter (2 Tb.)	15
Peas, cooked (1 cup)	14
Egg (1)	13
Hot dog (1)	13
Whole-wheat bread (2 slices)	9
Spaghetti, cooked (1 cup)	9
Brown rice, cooked (1 cup)	8
Corn, cooked (1 cup)	8
White rice, cooked (1 cup)	6
Post 40% Bran Flakes (⅔ cup)	5

* The USRDA for animal protein is 45 grams; for vegetable protein, 65 grams.

Sources: USDA Handbooks 8-1, 8-5, 8-7, 8-13, and USDA Home & Garden Bulletin 72.

Eat more fruit and vegetables, Cancer Institute suggests

CHICAGO, ILLINOIS — Fewer than 10% of Americans - and only 6% of blacks - are eating enough fruits and vegetables, researchers at the National Cancer Institute report.

Nearly a quarter of all Americans do not eat a single daily serving of fruits or vegetables, they say. At least five servings are recommended.

"Twenty-two percent had no servings of fruits and vegetables, not even a slice of onion on a hamburger," said Blossom H. Patterson, a statistician at the institute and principal author of the study. "When you look at the percentage of people who are getting enough, it's less than 10%. That's really appalling."

American distaste for vegetables and fruit contributes to high rates of heart disease and has been linked to some forms of cancer, Patterson said.

Both kinds of diseases occur more frequently among blacks than whites, and poor nutrition could be one reason, she said. The study found that the diets of just 6% of blacks met National Academy of Sciences guidelines for the consumption of fruits and vegetables.

The study is the latest to emerge from data collected by the National center of Vital Statistics in 1980.

The survey findings are consistent with a more recent but less complete 1985 survey, Patterson said.

The study considered one ounce of any fruit or vegetable or two ounces of fruit juice as a serving. Larger portions were counted as two or more servings.

Only 27% of 12,000 adults said they had eaten three or more servings of vegetables in the previous 24 hours. Twenty-nine percent said they had consumed two or more servings of fruit or juice. Only 9% said they had done both.

The figures would have been even worse, Patterson said, if potatoes, which do not have all of the nutritional advantages of green and yellow vegetables, had not been included in the survey. About a quarter of the vegetables consumed were potatoes, she said.

—*MILWAUKEE JOURNAL NOVEMBER 9, 1989*

SIDE NOTE: We felt the information in this news article is so valuable that we decided to reprint it for those who have not read it.

Bodies and brains need nutrients to function at their peak. We at Natural Ovens are doing what we can to supply our customers with the most nutritious, high fibered foods within our ability.

Most Natural Ovens consumers would be aware of the need for fresh whole vegetables, fruits and legumes (brown rice, beans , peas, lentils). We urge you to do all you can to educate and encourage those you know to consume lots of health giving whole foods. Especially the children!

Compound in hot peppers relieves cluster headaches

Capsaicin, a pungent substance found in plants of the hot pepper family, has been found to significantly reduce the frequency of cluster headaches - severe attacks of pain occurring on one side of the head.

In a recent preliminary experiment in Italy, twenty patients applied capsaicin, in liquid suspension into their nostrils as well as massaged it on the outside of their noses. Both treatments were effective in treating cluster headaches. Although the volunteers initially reported painful burning sensations and a heavy flow of nasal secretions, these symptoms subsided by the fifth day of the study.

The majority of the patients - 75 percent - were either pain-free or experienced a reduction in the number of headache attacks after five days of treatment.

It's not yet known whether repeated treatments with capsaicin would offer further help for cluster headache sufferers or if eating capsaicin-containing hot peppers would have a similar effect. But the researchers believe it's a theory worth pursuing.

—*ENVIRONMENTAL NUTRITION SEPT., 1989*

You May Be Salting Away Your Calcium Supply

Salting your food may not only be bad for your heart, it could weaken your bones.

New Zealand researchers restricted nine elderly women to a ten-day diet containing 1.6 grams of sodium a day, and then switched them to a diet that allowed 3.9 grams a day for the next ten-day period. (The average American eats almost 3 grams of sodium a day.) Their calcium intake didn't change, yet urine samples showed that the women excreted almost 30 percent more calcium on the high-salt plan.

British Medical Journal 299 (1989): 834-35

VEGETABLES ARE GOOD FOR YOU

There is no doubt that the widely documented health benefits associated with vegetarian lifestyles, have increased interest in the diet. Current research into the mostly vegetarian diet in China is providing further proof that eating roots, leaves and sprouts is good.

The research, which was a collaborative effort of Cornell University, the Chinese Academies of Preventive Medicine and Medical Sciences and Oxford University in England, found that a diet that is largely vegetarian appears to be protective against the chronic diseases that plague Western nations - heart disease, cancer, obesity and osteoporosis.

"The closer we get to a vegetarian diet, the better off we'll be," says the study's principal American investigator, T. Colin Campbell, Ph.D. Current dietary guidelines, such as those espoused by the American Heart Association or the National Cancer Institute, are easily met with a well-planned vegetarian diet. In fact, in its recent position paper on vegetarian diets, the American Dietetic Association (ADA) states that these guidelines may be more easily met on a vegetarian diet than on a non-vegetarian diet.

Vegetarian Nutrition

One benefit of a vegetarian diet - including fresh or frozen vegetables, fruits, legumes, whole grain breads & cereals, seeds, nuts and sprouts - is that protein intakes are not as likely to be as excessive as in the typical American diet. For years it was believed that plant foods must be eaten in certain combinations to provide proteins as complete as those found in meat. But this is generally no longer thought to be necessary.

Iron deficiency among vegetarians from Western countries is rare. According to George Beaton, Ph.D., professor of Nutrition at the University of Toronto, vegetarians usually have higher iron intakes that non-vegetarians. In his studies of the Chinese, Campbell found that anemia among adults was almost nonexistent, even though most of the iron in their diets came from plant sources.

Anemia among children and pregnant women was not evaluated.

Calcium intakes much lower than the Recommended Dietary Allowance (RDA) of 800 milligrams don't appear to cause health problems in vegetarians. In fact, vegetarians generally have lower rates of osteoporosis than non-vegetarians. Excessive intakes of protein, as in the current American diet, cause increased excretion of calcium, and Campbell notes that most of the calcium in the American diet comes from protein-rich dairy products, while the Chinese get most of theirs from plant foods.

Though experts have expressed concerns that the high fiber intakes of vegetarians might interfere with the absorption of minerals, including calcium, the Chinese study indicates there is no cause for concern.

"Our data did not show any impairment of mineral status at high levels of fiber intake," says Campbell. "In fact, no ill-effects were seen at all, even at fiber intakes as high as 77 grams of fiber per day."

Vitamin B12 is produced by microorganisms and is generally found only in foods of animal origin. Populations that eat strict vegetarian diets do not usually show evidence of deficiency. However, it may be wise for complete vegetarians to take an occasional vitamin B12 supplement.

Child Vegetarians

Well-planned vegetarian diets are adequate for everyone, including infants and children. The position of the ADA is that children who follow vegan or vegan-like diets may need to be given supplements of vitamin D and iron. Care must also be taken that energy needs are met, since vegan diets are bulky and likely to fill small stomachs quickly.

The ADA also states that vegetarian infants who are breast-fed beyond 4 to 6 months of age should be given supplements of vitamin D and iron, just as nonvegetarian infants.

Campbell, however, cites evidence from the Chinese data that growth rates of the children studied, were much slower than the growth rates of American children. In some cases, growth of Chinese children continued up to the age of 21. The average age at which sexual maturity was reached was 17 years, as compared to an average of 12 years in the U.S. The slower rate of growth was associated with decreased risk for the chronic diseases which typically afflict Americans. With later sexual maturity, levels of estrogen were lower in Chinese women and were associated with a decreased rate of breast cancer.

Making the Switch

Changing to a vegetarian way of eating can be easy or difficult. Some people decide to go "cold turkey" and make the switch to vegetarian eating overnight. Most, however, choose to change long-time eating habits gradually.

In sum: Moving toward a vegetarian diet will help to insure that nutritional needs are met without adding the excess dietary baggage that comes with traditional American fare. Research strongly suggests that vegetarian diets greatly reduce the risk of developing such killer diseases as cancer and heart disease. And eating the vegetarian way will contribute to the world's environmental health as well.

-Suzanne Havala, R.D.

—Environmental Nutrition, Inc. April, 1990 2112 Broadway, New York, NY 10023 Subscription Rates: $36/yr.

Orange, Yellow, Dark Green

When you're shopping for food, look for orange, yellow and dark green - the colors of vegetables and fruit rich in beta carotene. If you're like the average American, you should consume two to four times more carotene than you do now, according to Paul Lachance, professor of food science at Rutgers University. He has calculated that people should eat foods supplying 5 to 6 milligrams of beta carotene a day (based on guidelines from the USDA and the National Cancer Institute), while the average American gets less than 1.5 milligrams a day.

A carrot a day will do the trick. Here's another way to make sure you get enough beta carotene - plus other important nutrients. A National Academy of Sciences report in 1989 recommended that Americans eat at least five servings of various fruits and vegetables every day. But one survey showed that on any given day 49% of Americans eat only one vegetable, and 41% eat no fruit at all.

You're better off getting beta carotene from foods than relying on carotene supplements, since the foods will also give you additional nutrients that may play a role in protecting against cancer. Frozen vegetables can retain as much carotene as fresh. Cooking does destroy some carotene (the longer you cook, the more destroyed), but plenty remains. Some research suggests, in fact, that cooking may even allow the body to absorb the remaining carotene more readily.

Note: Don't think it's safe to continue smoking so long as you consume more beta carotene. Your risk of developing lung cancer will remain about 10 times that of a nonsmoker.
— *UNIVERSITY OF CALIFORNIA, BERKELEY WELLNESS LETTER*

Best Sources

Food (3.5 oz)	Beta Carotene (mg)
Dandelion greens (1 cup cooked)	8.4
Carrots (1 large)	6.6
Sweet Potato (1 medium)	5.9
Cress (3/4 cup cooked)	5.6
Kale (3/4 cup cooked)	5.4
Spinach (1/2 cup cooked)	4.9
Mango (1/2 medium)	2.9
Winter squash (3/4 cup cooked)	2.4
Cantalope (1 slice)	2.0
Apricots (3 medium)	1.6
Broccoli (3/4 cup chopped)	1.5
Romaine lettuce (10 leaves)	0.8
Asparagus (7 spears)	0.5
Tomoto (1 medium)	0.5
Peach (1 large)	0.5

Another great source of Beta Carotene is Natural Ovens Energy Drink!

Olive Oil May Lower Blood Pressure

Olive oil has earned the reputation of being heart-healthy. New research from Italy suggests this is especially true for men.

A recent study of 4,903 Italian men and women compared the intake of various dietary fats — butter, olive oil and vegetable oils — with various risk factors for cardiovascular disease.

Consumption of olive oil was significantly associated with lower systolic blood pressure, blood glucose and blood cholesterol levels in both sexes. However, men showed a more significant reduction in diastolic blood pressure than did women.

This is the first large-scale study to suggest that consuming olive oil reduces blood pressure, an important risk factor for heart disease.
— *Journal of the American Medical Association, February 2, 1990, pp. 688-692*

JUST FOR FUN

...ALBERT EINSTEIN'S FIRST WIFE may have been a true genius, too. The original manuscripts for papers that lay the groundwork for the theory of relativity appear to have been submitted under both the physicists' names. *Supporting the theory:* Einstein's divorce settlement stipulated that he pay her the prize money if he won the Nobel Peace Prize. He won. He paid.
— *Bottom Line Personal*

YOUR LIVER-A TRULY VITAL ORGAN!

The liver is one of our most complex and miraculous organs. In ancient Babylon, it was traditional for the priest-physician to study the liver to divine the intent of the gods. To the Chinese, the liver was considered to be the house of the soul. It is no less critical an organ in the modern age.

OVERWORKED DETOXIFIER

The liver is our largest and most important organ for detoxification of the body. With its great store of enzymes, the liver attempts to break the toxins down, convert them to harmless elements and, through the bile, wash them from the body.

But the demands on the liver today are at an all-time high. The liver might easily be considered our most abused organ. It is attacked by the use of alcohol, recreational and prescription drugs, cigarettes, and denatured, preservative-laden foods. Pollution found in the air, water and soil also finds its way into our bodies, and must be filtered out. All of these external toxins overload the liver's capacity to do its job.

TROUBLE

The liver is then forced to act like the harassed office accountant whose increased workload has stacked up to the bursting point. Congestion and backup of the bile can cause the liver to become enlarged, storing unfiltered toxins within its own cells. An overburdened liver is very

often the underlying cause of chronic imbalances in the body, such as PMS, migrains, and hypertension.

This situation of "liver overload" creates both short and long-term problems. the liver is less able to maintain its day-to-day processing of toxins and pollutants. The ensuing hormonal imbances leave us physically drained and emotionally on edge, just not feeling our best.

SERIOUS SYMPTOMS

Symptoms can include dizziness, nausea, chest pains, depression and impairment of appetite. If the process goes unchecked for years it can become the root cause of bodily degeneration and the advent of disease.

The close correlation between physical and emotional well-being is revealed in liver problems. Very often irrational anger, sadness, depression and undue mood swings are the result of liver congestions.

PROTECT YOUR LIVER

One of the most important things you can do to aid your liver is to avoid fats and deep fried foods. This includes concentrated cheeses, fatty meats and oils. Since bile is necessary to digest fats, if the liver is unable to secrete enough bile for digestion, these fats and oils will coat other foods, making them difficult to digest.

Avoid processed or hydrogenated fats, and use cold pressed oils very sparingly. If a salad oil is used, add some

lemon juice to help in its digestion. And avoid the "three whites," salt, sugar and white flour, as well as refined, canned, processed or irradiated foods. It goes without saying that alcohol, tobacco, and drugs should be eliminated or severely limited.

POSITIVE ACTION

In addition to avoiding certain foods, there are some good habits you can cultivate to help keep your liver healthy.

Drink plenty of water. If you don't get enough water, your kidneys can't do their job properly, and can "dump" some of its work on your already-overloaded liver. Keep all the players on your detoxification team healthy and operating.

Eat fresh fruits and vegetables. Some health and nutrition professionals suggest that foods with bitter, hot and sour tastes are especially good for the liver. So adding endive, chicory, dandelion greens, radishes, and lemon juice to a salad would be especially good for your liver.

Increase soluble fiber in your diet. The water-soluble fiber in oat bran, legumes, and fruits help your liver eliminate the toxins from your system.

Adapted from "The Miraculous Organ," Health Shopper, July, 1988.

Be sure to add Natural Ovens products like Oat Bran De-Lite bread, Blueberry-Oat and Cherry-Almond Oat Bran muffins in your diet. Make your liver *and* your taste buds happy!

The A.M. Meal Makes a Difference

The custom of eating a meal at the start of the day is observed in cultures all over the world. Does this make breakfast man's most important meal? Perhaps. Research, for instance, shows that eating breakfast improves intellectual performance and the ability to concentrate and solve problems at the same time as it increases the nutrient content of a person's diet. On the flip side, skipping breakfast has been proven to cause fatigue, decrease the body's metabolic rate, increase snacking during the day and lead to weight gain.

Most of the research on the importance of breakfast has been done with children. Studies show that test scores improve when children are given a morning meal. Not that cereal, milk and juice make kids smarter, but their attention span is increased making it possible for more learning to take place.

Breakfast eaters (both children and adults) consume more essential nutrients like calcium, fiber and vitamins C, B-1, and B-2 than do breakfast skippers. Generally speaking, better nutrition means better resistance to infection.

Stretching that point even further, results of a University of California study showed that breakfast eaters actually lived longer than breakfast skippers. Of course, other factors could be responsible for the findings. For example, people who eat breakfast may also exercise more, and the activity could be the factor responsible for their longevity. Still, the California finding is a provocative one.

Probably the most compelling argument in support of a morning repast is its role in weight management. When a person gets up in the morning with an empty stomach, blood sugar is literally at a "fasting" or very low level. Eating shortly after rising causes the body's furnace to heat up as it burns off the calories of that first meal. Called the "thermic effect of food," it increases after each meal throughout the day. Skipping breakfast, on the other hand, keeps the furnace cold longer and ultimately burns fewer calories.

People who don't eat breakfast have metabolic rates four to five percent below normal, according the Wayne Calloway, M.D. of George Washington University,

Washington, D.C. As a result of this metabolic slump, a breakfast skipper could expect to gain one pound every seven weeks (about 8 pounds per year) - even if his calorie intake remained the same.

Clearly, breakfast is a good idea. To those who say they can't eat in the morning, Dr. Calloway replies, "Nonsense." Eating is an environmental response, he says. And breakfast skippers must condition themselves to eat in the morning by eating lighter and earlier the night before. Even a confirmed breakfast skipper will soon find himself waking up hungry, says Calloway.

But what constitutes a good morning meal? The answer is not as pat as the bacon-and-eggs menu at the local coffee shop would suggest. The choices for breakfast are unlimited.

—*ENVIRONMENTAL NUTRITION*

LOOKING FOR A QUICK & EASY BREAKFAST? Natural Ovens bread makes delicious toast. Or choose from five delectable varieties of muffins. And to drink?...Try our power-packed Energy Drink!

Eat Your Carrots!

You've probably heard about how carotene helps prevent cancer. Carrots are one of the most flavorful, economical, and readily available sources of this important nutrient.

A cup of raw, shredded carrots provides 31,000 international units (I.U.s) of carotene. Because carrots become denser when cooked, cooked carrots have slightly more vitamin A: 38,000 I.U.s per cup.

Carrots are also a good source of potassium; are virtually fat-free; are high in soluble fiber; and are a good source of vitamin C when eaten raw.

PURCHASING CARROTS

Buy smooth, small- to medium-size carrots. They should have a bright orange-red color and a firm texture. Don't buy carrots that are limp, have sprouts, or are decayed at the tips. Greens at the top of carrots are a sign of freshness.

STORING CARROTS

Before storing carrots, remove any tops. Store the carrots in a container in the refrigerator. They should keep for two to three weeks.

Wash carrots thoroughly and peel off the skin before eating them. If you plan to cook the carrots, cut them into small peices and steam them until tender.

DELECTABLE LIME CARROTS

3	large carrots
3/4	tbsp. canola oil
1-1/2	tbsp. lime juice
2	tbsp. water
1	clove garlic
1/2	tsp. honey

Cut the carrots into long, thin sticks. Place in a medium-size saucepan with the oil and cook, stirring over medium heat for two to three minutes. Add the lim juice and water. Push the garlic through a garlic press into the pan. Stir in the honey. Cover and steam over low heat until the carrots are crisp-tender, about 10 to 15 minutes. Makes four servings.

—*Edited from LET'S LIVE Magazine*

All about You & You & You & You...and Me

The human body is an assemblage of more than 100 trillion cells that function as a laboratory, warehouse, pharmacy, farm, electric company, mass-transit system, library, utility company, hospital and sewage-treatment plant. Fascinating facts:

• There is a trace amount of iron in the ethmoid bone (between the eyes) that, like a compass, helps people find direction relative to the earth's magnetic field.

• Eye muscles get the greatest workout of any muscle, moving about 100,000 times in 24 hours. This is equivalent to walking 50 miles.

• One square inch of human skin contains 19 million cells, 625 sweat glands, 90 oil glands, 65 hairs, 19 feet of blood vessels, 19,000 sensory cells and more than 20 million microscopic animals.

• Hair grows in cycles. On the scalp, each hair grows for three to five years, "rests" about three months and is then shed. After another three- to four- month rest, the follicle begins a new growing phase. Eyebrows stay short because their growing phase is only 10 weeks.

• Stomach acid is such a powerful corrosive that it can dissolve a small metal object — a razor blade, etc. — in less than a week. To avoid digesting itself, the stomach produces a new lining every three days.

• The surface area of the lungs is about the size of a tennis court.

—*Edited from BOTTOM LINE PERSONAL*

NOTE: To help all of these parts function best, feed the body fresh whole vegetables, fruits, legumes and whole grains - such as is found in Natural Ovens breads, rolls, muffins, granola & Energy Drink.

Racewalking
STEPPING UP THE PACE

If you're one of the millions now walking a brisk mile or two a day for pleasure and health, you may occasionally be left in the dust by someone speeding along like roadrunner — hips swinging and arms pumping and feet barely skimming the ground. A racewalker, by gosh, and he certainly did look funny (just as joggers caused onlookers to laugh 15 years ago). Walking isn't merely locomotion, but an activity with several potential variations, including walking at the Olympic level. In 1983 the world record for a mile walk was set by American Ray Sharp: 5 minutes, 46 seconds. It takes the average person about three times that long to walk a mile.

Though you may not expect to set an Olympic record, racewalking offers many benefits to the walker who's gotten into good shape and is ready for a challenge. Racewalking can burn as many calories per hour as running, but with much less risk of injury. It's not an expensive sport: all you really need, besides clothing that suits the weather, is an adequate pair of shoes. It's fun to racewalk alone or with a friend, competitively or just for company. And a companion can be very useful for checking your posture and form for you when you're learning to racewalk.

THE "RUSHING CHICKEN" GAIT

The object of racewalking is to move your body ahead as quickly as possible (without running) and to avoid the up/down motions of regular walking. That's the point of the forward-thrusting hip-swivel, which is meant to propel you more efficiently than the normal side-to-side swing of the hips. Here's how to start:

• Think of racewalking as walking a tightrope. In normal walking, your feet make parallel tracks, but in racewalking you must try to put one foot down in front of the other, almost in a straight line. Because of anatomical differences, this form may not be completely achievable for everyone, but come as close to it as you can.

• Swing your hip forward as you step forward — it's the hips and legs that act as the propulsive force.

• Keep your feet close to the ground, with no wasted motion. Each foot should strike the ground solidly on the back of the heel with toes pointed up slightly. Two rules of competitive racewalking are that one foot must always be on the ground, and your legs must be straight at one point in the cycle.

• Use long strides. Your motion should be fluid, efficient, and smooth.

• Keep your torso, shoulders, and neck relaxed, and your head in line with your back. Don't bend from the waist — this can lead to back strain. Some racewalkers angle their whole body slightly forward from the ankles.

• Bend your arms at a 90 degree angle, and keep your wrists straight. With the motion coming from the shoulder, not the elbow, pump your arms rhythmically with your leg motion. When you pump back, your hand should come about 6 inches behind the hip, while on the swing forward the wrist should be near the center of your chest. Keep your hands above your hips. The vigorous arm pumping counterbalances your leg/hip motion, allows for a quick pace, and provides a good workout for your upper body.

GET INTO THE SWING

Since technique is important in racewalking, you will need practice. If there's an experienced racewalker around who can give you pointers, so much the better. Start with leg movement first, build up some speed, and then incorporate the arm motions. See what a difference it makes to have your arms in the proper 90 degree angle position instead of hanging at your sides. Your pace would quicken automatically as you learn to use your arms. Start slowly, walking for 20 to 30 minutes and increasing your pace gradually. Try interval walking — that is, racewalk for a few minutes, then do normal brisk walking. If you're concerned about getting aerobic benefits, pause occasionally to check your heart rate.

AVOIDING INJURY

Racewalking is not as hard on the body as running, but your shin muscles get much the same kind of workout, and most beginning racewalkers experience some shin soreness. To minimize this, try these exercises indoors:

1. To build up the muscles in the shins, walk back and forth across a room on your heels.

2. In a sitting position or standing (balanced on one foot), rotate your raised foot clockwise and counterclockwise in large circles several times. This works shin and calf muscles.

3. For hip flexibility, walk a straight line, practicing hip movement. Exaggerate the movement by walking crisscross over the imaginary line.

4. Warm up and stretch before racewalking; cool down and stretch afterwards.

University of California Berkeley Wellness Letter

TO FEEL GREAT.........

Combine the splendid walking with a highly nutritional diet of fresh whole vegetables, fruit, berries, melons, seeds, nuts, legumes (beans, peas, lentils), brown rice, whole grain breads from Natural Ovens, two tablespoons of Energy Drink daily, and drink 7-8 glasses of pure water. Let us know how you feel after 3-4 weeks.

THE TRUTH ABOUT BREAKFAST CEREALS

Andy Rooney of "Sixty Minutes" reported on a study of all available breakfast cereals. He found the average price to be $3.60 per pound. This sounds pretty high compared to Natural Ovens average bread at $1.20 per pound. The next logical questions — What's inside?...And what'll it do for the body?

Virtually no breakfast cereals are tested to see if they will support life. The questions that if you feed the product to a test animal as a major portion of the diet and add what nutrients are missing, will the animal live a normal life and reproduce? Most all of the boxed breakfast cereals contain so much heat-damaged protein from being burned in the flaking process, that the cereal may actually be toxic. This means that the test animals would live longer on a starvation (no food, just water) diet than they do on the breakfast cereal.

At Natural Ovens, we take an entirely different approach. We do everything possible to prevent heat damage. Secondly, we add the necessary nutrients so the food product is nutritionally balanced. Thirdly, we test our products on three generations of three animal species to make certain our products will support all phases of life — pregnancy, lactation, growth years, middle age and old age. We don't think a mere three week test for toxicity is adequate.

So next time you're in the store and trying decide what to buy for breakfast, remember Natural Ovens bread costs about 1/3 as much as breakfast cereals. You can be sure our breads are made by people who know and care about your long term health and about pleasing your taste buds. ■

SAD Bad For Bones?

In a study at UCLA, Dr. Ron Zernicke and others found that after ten weeks on a diet similar to the Standard American Diet (SAD), young lab animals showed weaker bones and other skeletal defects compared to a group fed a low fat, high complex carbohydrate diet. The SAD group received (in percent of total calories): 21% protein, 39.5% fat, 39.5% sucrose; the control group ate 26% protein, 6% fat, 68% complex carbs. Zernicke believes effect could be due to high fat inhibiting calcium absorption in gut and/or high sucrose diet leading to high insulin levels which may reduce kidney resorption of calcium. Further studies are planned to separate possible fat and sucrose effects.

—*SOURCE UNKNOWN*

Regular Exercise May Prolong Your Life

To Achieve Moderate Fitness

Women:
1) Walk 2 miles under 30 minutes at least 3 days per week
or
2) Walk 2 miles in 30-40 minutes 5-6 days per week

Men:
1) Walk 2 miles under 27 minutes at least 3 days per week
or
2) Walk 2 miles in 30-40 minutes 6-7 days per week

To Acheive High Fitness

Women:
1) Walk 2 miles under 30 minutes 5-6 days per week
or
2) Run 2 miles in 20-24 minutes 4 days per week

Men:
1) Walk 2-1/2 miles under 37-1/2 minutes 6-7 days per week
or
2) Run 2 miles under 20 minutes 4-5 days per week

—MEDICAL JOURNAL BULLETIN

To maximize your fitness, feed your body with whole foods. [i.e.: fresh or frozen whole vegetables; fresh, dried, or frozen fruits; legumes (beans, peas, lentils, etc.); whole grain cereals (brown rice, buckwheat, etc.); whole grain breads; sprouts; pure water; exercise] ■

Fascinating Fact

Many fruit-containing cereals actually have little fruit in them. For a premium price, some of them give you only an ounce or two of fruit in the entire box. Try adding your own dried fruit — or, even better, fresh fruit.

—UNIVERSITY OF CALIFORNIA, BERKELEY
WELLNESS LETTER

338

—from The Office Professional

Why Are Questions Effective Communication Tools?

1. A good question establishes rapport. "What do you think?" "How can we fix it?" Ex-Mayor Koch established rapport with the people of New York City by asking repeatedly wherever he went, "How'm I doing?"

2. Questions enable you to gather information. If you want to turn in work that is flawless, ask, "Can I go over these instructions with you once more to be sure I have understood them?" or "When can I see you if I have any more questions?"

3. Questions can plant ideas that you want to suggest. "What would you think about printing this folder in color rather than in black and white?" "Do you think we should have another meeting before we make the presentation?"

4. Questions can clear up misunderstandings. "What exactly do you want me to say to customers who ask when we will have more price sheets?" "How would you have handled Mr. Dorfmann's complaint?"

5. Questions can organize thinking about problems. "Will starting with a rough draft take too much time?" "If Connie can't do this, whom should I ask?"

6. Questions can help overcome objections. "What are your major concerns about trying flextime?" "What other alternatives do you prefer?" "Why do you think they would work out better?"

7. Questions can encourage people to cooperate with you. "Have you ever made an exception to that rule?"

"Will you go with me if I ask for one more chance?"

8. Questions can reduce risks. "What concerns do you have about our plans for tomorrow? What could go wrong?" "Do you think we have done everything we can? Can you think of anything else we might do to assure the success of the meeting?"

9. Questions can defuse emotional situations. "Is it possible that Sally had good reason for taking that software package home?" "Did you ever say anything and then wish you'd never said it?"

10. Questions can make criticism serve a constructive purpose. "Why do you suppose you feel that way?" "What did you expect me to do?"

Developing the Question Habit

Studies show that it takes between seven and twenty-one conscious efforts to create a new habit. When you make the effort to ask smart questions, however, you will see the benefits so quickly that it will be easy to make the effort habitual.

Make a game of it. Notice how you initiate conversations. The next time you are ready to make a statement, take a keep breath and ask a question instead. By the time you have done this 21 times, you will have acquired a valuable "people" skill that distinguishes exceptional employees from average performers. The habit of asking the right question of the right person at the right time will convert an ordinary conversational skill into a way of improving all of your business relationships. ▨

BABY TALK

Hold the Sugar, Please

Newborns fed water to which sugar has been added appear to have a greater preference for sweets later in infancy. Sugared water as well as sugary beverages should not be given to infants because they contribute calories without providing any of the other vital nutrients that young babies need for proper growth and development. They can also cause gas as well as exacerbate a case of diarrhea.

—Tufts University Diet and Nutrition Letter

CUPBOARD QUERIES

Why Snacking Works

Researchers believe snacking works by controlling the production of certain chemicals in the body.

Insulin, a hormone released by the liver, helps the body produce cholesterol. How much insulin the liver releases into the bloodstream depends on the size of the meals you eat.

Snackers may have lower cholesterol levels because they eat smaller amounts of food, and the liver produces less insulin in response.

Eating more meals throughout the day and adding more fiber to your diet may be keys to keeping your cholesterol levels under control.

Insulin levels dropped. During the study, seven men aged 31 to 51 ate three meals a day for two weeks or 17 snacks a day for two weeks and then switched to the other diet.

The snackers' insulin levels dropped by 28 percent during the study.

Based on the results of this study, researchers believe that nutritious nibbling throughout the day may help you lower cholesterol levels and fight heart disease.

—Natural Healing Newsletter

339

Are you retro active?

Ever wonder why some people run backwards, and why there seem to be more of these "retro runners" than ever? It used to be that if you saw someone running backwards you assumed he was a boxer in training. Today's retro runner is likely to be anyone looking for a change of pace while jogging. But some sports physicians point to the physiological benefits of running, as well as walking, in reverse.

Retro movement helps strengthen the abdominal and back muscles, the quadriceps (the muscles in front of the thigh), and hamstrings (at the back of the thigh). It also stretches the hamstrings and improves overall muscle balance, thus protecting against some running injuries. In addition, if you're recovering from an ankle sprain, back or hamstring injury, or knee surgery, retro running is less stressful and may be undertaken sooner than forward motion.

If you decide to become retro active, however, there are some caveats. Never run backwards on a street or anywhere there's traffic. Choose a smooth surface. You may wish to run with a partner: one of you runs backwards as the other goes forward and acts as guide; then you switch off. When looking over your shoulder, alternate sides to avoid neck cramping. Start slowly to prevent calf soreness; run backwards for only brief periods, adding up to no more than a quarter mile the first week. Don't use retro movement to replace regular running or walking entirely, since it won't give you as good an aerobic workout. Retro running may aggravate heel spurs or arch injuries, so skip it if you're prone to them.

And be prepared for retro spectators.

UNIVERSITY OF CALIFORNIA, BERKELEY WELLNESS LETTER

By Scott Meyer

MAKING EYE CONTACT WITH BETA-CAROTENE

With classes back in session, parents will want to be sure that their kids can see the blackboard clearly. Perhaps they can take a hint from that old kids' favorite, Bugs Bunny. Bugs never had any trouble seeing Elmer Fudd because the beta-carotene in those carrots Bugs was always munching is essential for good vision.

Pro-vitamin A or beta-carotene is a natural pigment in vegetables and fruits that converts to vitamin A once inside the body. Myron A. Winick, M.D., the director of the Columbia University (New York City) Institute of Human Nutrition, says "the primary effect of vitamin A deficiency is damage to the individual's eyes."

The chemical changes that turn electrical impulses into mental pictures require a light-sensitive pigment known as rhodospin, or visual purple. The primary source of rhodospin is vitamin A.

Moreover, xerophthalmia, or abnormal dryness of the eye, is the result of prolonged vitamin A deficiency and is the leading cause of blindness in underdeveloped nations.

"Although severe manifestations are rare in the United States," says Winick, "milder effects are frequently encountered, especially among children."

Beta-carotene supplements can supply much of the 5,000 I.U. of vitamin A that children ages 11 to 18 need each day. You can also ensure that the kids get enough beta-carotene by serving plenty of sweet potatoes, broccoli, spinach, apricots, cantaloupe...and oh yes, Bugs' favorite food.

Watching Your Weight May Keep You Healthier

SOURCES:
Tufts University Diet and Nutrition Letter, Vol. 15, No. 1, March 1987.
Nutrition Action Healthletter, Jan/Feb 1987.
Nutrition Research Newsletter, Vol. VI, No. 1, Jan 1987;
Brownell, Kelly, "A Program for Managing Obesity," Dietetic Currents, Vol. 13, No. 3, 1986.

One out of every five Americans weighs at least 20% more than the desired weight for height in the 1983 Metropolitan Life Tables. These people are considered obese. While many of us watch our weight for personal reasons, scientists are looking at our weight as it relates to disease control. Obese people run a higher risk of dying at younger ages from heart disease, diabetes, and certain types of cancer: colon, rectal and prostate in males; breast, ovarian, uterine, breast and cervical in females. Efforts to achieve a desirable weight--on the scale, by percent fat, or by inches--should focus on healthy eating and exercise habits. Regular physical activity combined with well-balanced, lowfat, high-fiber meals contribute to a trim waistline and reduced risks for many diseases.

VISION OILS

At Oregon Health Sciences University, Martha Neuringer, PhD, assistant professor, and William E. Connor, MD, professor have researched the effects of certain fatty acids on vision. As reported by the University of California, Berkley Wellness Letter, the team focused their studies on the effects of several n-3 and n-6 fatty acids including docosahexanoic acid (DHA). DHA is an n-3 fatty acid which is predominant in the fat of ocean fish.

On this note, Professors Neuringer and Connor studied the depletion of DHA and other n-3 fatty acids in rhesus monkeys. They concluded that deficiencies in n-3 fatty acids (flaxseed, ocean fish) resulted in visual impairment. The discovered deficit in visual acuity may have been due entirely to the effects on the retina, or may also have been mediated by changes in the brain's central nervous system.

Professors Neuringer and Connor found there is evidence that the enzymes for producing DHA and other fatty acids are not yet active in our newborn infants. They point out that human milk contains DHA, however, present-day "formulas" contain none. That means infants raised entirely on "formulas" cannot increase the DHA in the grey matter of their brains. On the other hand, newborns receiving human milk indeed increase the DHA.

Professors Neuringer and Connor summarized that a diet including necessary amounts of n-3 and n-6 fatty acids is important, particularly during pregnancy, lactation and infancy. In general, a diet rich in ocean fish, flaxseed products and primrose oil can ensure proper amounts of essential fatty acids.

Understanding and kindness topped the list of characteristics sought in a mate by both men and women. [Surveyed by the Univ. of Michigan.]

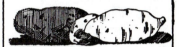

Anybody for Baked Roots?

It used to be if you were trying to diet, you'd stay away from potatoes. But it turns out that that old familiar staple is full of benefits.

Potatoes are a terrific source of carbohydrates, the basic fuel of life. A large baked potato has about 220 calories and 20% of the recommended amounts of potassium, plus 16% of the U.S. RDA for iron and nearly 45% for vitamin C.

Just don't ruin that bounty by pouring on rivers of butter or piles of sour cream.

If you're watching your waistline, try putting a fiber-packed potato onto the center stage on your plate. Top with yogurt, mustard, or a dab of horseradish.

A little low-fat savvy can keep other root vegetables honest too. A half-cup of plain baked sweet potato with the skin provides 40% of the U.S. RDA for vitamin C and *four times* the U.S. RDA for vitamin A. Jerusalem artichokes, or sunchokes as they are sometimes called, have fewer nutrients than sweet potatoes, but only 57 calories for a half-cup's worth of refreshing crunch.

BY MADONNA BEHEN

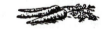 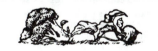 **Best food sources of Vitamin E:**

1 Vegetable oils (but remember to use these moderately, as greater consumption also increases the *need* for Vitamin E)

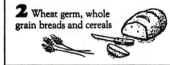

2 Wheat germ, whole grain breads and cereals

3 Dark green leafy vegetables: beet greens, broccoli, chard, chicory, collard greens, dandelion greens, kale, mustard greens, parsley, turnip greens, watercress

4 Some yellow vegetables: carrots, carrot juice, pumpkin, sweet potato, winter squash

Some yellow fruits: apricots, peaches, mangos, papaya, watermelon

5 Legumes (dried beans and peas)

DIETING DOs AND DON'Ts

To beat any challenge, there are basic rules of the game that must be followed. The rules of a high fiber diet are no exception, yet none of them are extreme and most of them will be familiar to you. Here are the rules that promise you success without sacrifice:

DO eat three balanced meals a day. Don't skip breakfast or lunch and then sit down to a huge dinner. Every meal is important because high fiber foods must be distributed throughout the day. In fact, you may find that breakfast is the ideal time to get a really large portion.

DO eat slowly. Chewing promotes a feeling of satisfaction and gives the stomach time to feel full. And fiber needs the juices that chewing stimulates to add bulk.

DON'T eat refined and processed foods wherever possible. White bread and white sugar are both public enemy #1, so avoid them absolutely. If you must use a sweetener, add a bit of honey or real maple syrup.

DO drink plenty of water in addition to other liquids like coffee or tea. At least four 8-ounce glasses a day and more if you can. Fiber needs lots of moisture in order to work.

DON'T consume a lot of meat. Even lean meat has a good percentage of fat. Fish, chicken and many of the high fiber vegetables and legumes will provide you with enough protein. (You may even wish to consider a vegetarian diet.)

DON'T include alcoholic beverages in your diet. There is no room in the high fiber diet for alcoholic drinks because they're loaded with calories that are rapidly converted to sugar. If you must, substitute a small glass of white wine at dinnertime.

DO EXERCISE! No diet in the world will be successful unless it's accompanied by exercise. As you lose weight, you certainly don't want your skin to sag or get flabby. To keep lazy muscles toned up and firm, put aside 15 minutes in the morning before you begin dashing around from chore to chore, or running to catch the train for work. Set up a routine to music and do bend and stretch exercises where you feel the exertion. Within a week you'll notice a difference in how you look and feel.

— HIGH FIBER WEIGHT LOSS DIET
R. Fagen

Nutrition Tip

For a cool and different summer salad that's packed with healthful fiber, turn to whole grains. Cook and cool brown rice, millet or buckwheat and combine with chopped celery, carrots, tomatoes, green pepper and onion for added nutrition. Then season with fresh parsley and lowfat French dressing for a delicious dish than can serve as both starch and vegetable for your lunch or dinner.
—American Institute for Cancer Research Newsletter

YOUR IMMUNE SYSTEM

Germs have gotten a bad rap when it comes to disease. The truth is most people don't get sick from mere germ exposure. Rather, they land in bed because their immune system finally breaks down.

Not too long ago, it seemed that when this happened, people merely took medicine to suppress the offending bug and would be back in commission a few days later.

However, as technology became more complex and sophisticated, so have diseases. Today's incredibly complex immune diseases like AIDS, candidasis, cancer, rhuematoid arthritis and chronic Epstein-Barr virus (CEBV) syndrome have put a damper on that quick fix thinking. These illnesses are caused by something more than a nasty invading organism. They result from a profound breakdown in the immune system.

Although our ancestors struggled with the terrible infectious diseases of their times (i.e. plague and syphilis), ours is the first generation that must fight infectious organisms plus adapt to many thousands of new toxic chemicals in our air, water and food brought on as technology changed.

As a result, we are currently facing terribly complex diseases. Because most of these diseases are seemingly new or at least newly epidemic, scientists and health professionals are, by and large, looking for something novel to combat them. Many believe the solution will be the result of sophisticated drugs and technology. Ironically, hi-tech immune-suppressing drugs are regularly used to treat AIDS and cancer patients.

On the other hand, another group of professionals agree that a hi-tech solution won't be able to control these complex disease. Because the cure is often harder to identify than the cause, these professionals concentrate on prevention.

You may ask, "How have things changed that would affect the immune system?"

Over the years, many people have wondered how it is possible that we could be allergic to "good foods" when it would seem logical that nature would protect us from such problems. Unfortunately, the foods that we are eating today have little resemblance to the foods of 50 or 100 years ago. This is because the use of hormones, antibiotics and other modern chemicals in our farm animals as well as the use of pesticides, hormones and other chemicals in produce. This "modernization" of food production has greatly altered the nutritional value of food and has considerably increased our allergic reactions to certain foods.

Therefore, the target is fortifying the immune system. A diet low in fat and rich in whole foods, vitamins A and C, trace minerals top the list. [Statistics on cancer and chronic illnesses illnesses suggest that a vegetarian version of such a diet is optimal.] Adequate rest and exercise are also necessary to enhance the immune system. Even positive thinking and stress-reducing exercises (i.e. relaxation and meditation) can increase immune cell activity.

It may take a long time to understand the immune system, however we already know the impact of proper diet, exercise and stress management. Now learning how to fortify our immune system can help prevent these complex diseases. Afterall, immune-system maintainance is vital.

Sources: Vegetarian Times and the NOHA newsletter.

Bread for Lightweights

Complex carbohydrates may help us control our weight. They contain very little fat—and they're full of the fiber that bulks food in the GI tract and helps us feel sated. Some scientists also find that calories from carbohydrates are expended faster than calories from fats

Two studies support the "slimming bread" hypothesis. In the '70s Michigan State University nutrition professor Olaf Mickelsen (now emeritus) gave healthy volunteers nine to 12 slices of bread a day for eight to 10 weeks—as part of a low-fat diet. They lost more than a dozen pounds per person on average, and reported no hunger pains. The higher the fiber content of the bread, the greater the loss. "Bread fills the stomach and produces a feeling of satiety," says Dr. Mickelsen.

"Bread is so maligned," says nutritionist Tom Watkins, director of the study. "So many people claim it's fattening, but it's an excellent aid in appetite control and it's completely safe."

American Health

343

The American Dietetic Association, the American Medical Association and three related organizations made headlines recently by alleging that Americans "don't need (vitamin or mineral) supplements to maintain good health."

This statement is clearly refuted by the facts:

In 1980 the U.S. Department of Agriculture completed a nutritional survey of 37,785 Americans. This study covered only 11 of 28 nutrients known to be essential to human health.

Among the findings of the USDA were:

● Only one person in five ingested the Recommended Dietary Allowance (RDA) of vitamin B6.

● Only one person in four got the RDA of magnesium.

● Fifty-one percent of all Americans got **less than 70%** of the RDA of vitamin B6.

● Thirty-one percent got **less than 70%** of the RDA of vitamin A, a nutrient that the National Academy of Sciences, the National Cancer Institute, and the American Cancer Society believe may help prevent cancer.

To summarize, the typical American diet:

● is seriously deficient in several vitamins and minerals;

● is far too high in fat, cholesterol and sugar which tend to crowd out essential vitamins, minerals and dietary fiber;

● may, and almost certainly does, contribute to the high incidence of heart disease, cancer and diabetes as well as to less serious problems such as hemorrhoids, constipation, varicose veins, diverticulitis and tooth decay.

It is true that an ideal diet would provide sufficient vitamins and minerals for most people, without the need to rely upon supplements. However, in view of the fact that the vast majority of Americans consume diets containing less than the RDA of essential nutrients, urging the public not to take vitamin/mineral supplements cannot be justified. Further, it would be very difficult, if not impossible, to induce Americans to improve their diets significantly without massive educational programs. Such programs are not yet on the horizon.

To allege that the obviously substandard typical American diet is sufficiently good so that supplements are unnecessary is a manifestation of gross irresponsibility, or of ulterior finanacial motivation.

A recent USDA study reported that 40% of Americans, largely better-educated Americans, take vitamin/mineral supplements. The percentage increases from year to year, demonstrating that the American public is capable of making intelligent decisions about its health, and ignoring poor advice from organizations which try to impose their outmoded self-serving nutritional ideology upon the public.

NATURAL FOOD & FARMING

Be a Moving Target. Exercise, in particular, can help preserve a youthful body and mind. Reaction time—that is, the time it takes to react to a stimulus (such as a flashing light) with a response (such as pressing a button)—usually slows down with age. The reasons are many: Between the ages of 30 and 80, the number of nerve cells in the spinal cord declines 37 percent, the speed at which nerve impulses travel drops 10 percent, and muscles become less elastic.

NUTRITION ACTION HEALTHLETTER

The Gift Of Health

By Richard P. Huemer, M.D.

What *is* health, anyway? The dictionary seems like a good place to start looking for an answer. My Random House unabridged defines health as vigor, or soundness of body and mind, freedom from disease.

Perhaps the way to "give" health is to nourish ourselves with things of the natural world, to provide a natural harmony in which it can flourish. And so I will take a giant cornucopia, tie a red ribbon around it, and fill it with all the good things of the world: apples, brown rice, spinach, yams, salmon, lentils, spring water, peaches, walnuts, and many others.

It is quite late. Labor Day is over; the heat has abated; the Apple II has survived. My words glow green on a video screen in a dark room. I realize now what the gift of health must be, and where it must come from. It must come from each of us, and be given to each of us, something very ancient: a compelling desire for peace on earth and our expression of good will toward all. We and our ancestors have been talking about that for 20 centuries, maybe longer, and we've meant it every December. Only now, in this winter solstice of our civilization, we must resolve to mean it and work for it all year and all the time to come, forever. □

Tips to Improve That Next Photo

Consider these tips before you take your next photo:

● **Allow more space in front of a moving object than behind it.** If you're dealing with a portrait, leave more space in front of the direction where the subject is looking.

● **Place the subject slightly off center.** This adds visual interest to the photo.

● **Consider using the "rule of threes."** *Here's how:* In your mind's eye, draw two vertical lines. This separates the photo into three identical vertical sections. Then draw two horizonal lines, creating three equal horizontal sections. The points where the four lines intersect are good places to position the main action in the photo.

Healthy Occupations
Work to Walk

Does your job send you striding?

Did you ever notice that certain groups of professions seem to be in better health than others? For many it's because their jobs require them to do a lot of walking.

Scholl, Inc. asked 110 New York workers representing 20 occupations to register their mileage by wearing pedometers at work for one week.

The study showed that nurses topped the list averaging over five miles a day.

Walking between patients adds up the miles for nurses, but not for dentists. They trailed the list with less than a mile. However, those of us with somewhat sedentary professions needn't be discouraged. The survey found the less we walk on the job, the more we like to walk and exercise at other times.

American Health magazine consulted.

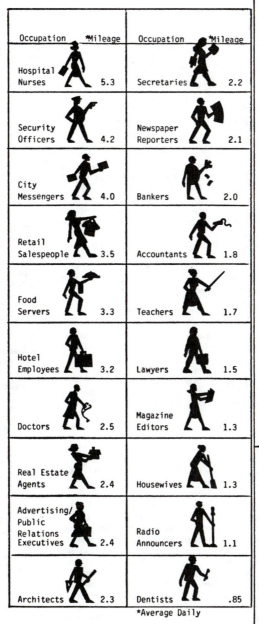

Occupation	*Mileage	Occupation	*Mileage
Hospital Nurses	5.3	Secretaries	2.2
Security Officers	4.2	Newspaper Reporters	2.1
City Messengers	4.0	Bankers	2.0
Retail Salespeople	3.5	Accountants	1.8
Food Servers	3.3	Teachers	1.7
Hotel Employees	3.2	Lawyers	1.5
Doctors	2.5	Magazine Editors	1.3
Real Estate Agents	2.4	Housewives	1.3
Advertising/ Public Relations Executives	2.4	Radio Announcers	1.1
Architects	2.3	Dentists	.85

*Average Daily

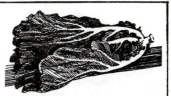

The Rise of the Lowly Collard

Food-writer Waverly Root once described collard greens as "difficult to define except as whatever among edibles causes a Southerner far from home to grow misty-eyed."

They are members of the proud cabbage (*cruciferae*) family, which includes broccoli, Brussels sprouts, cabbage, cauliflower, kale, mustard greens, turnips, radishes, and watercress.

They're rich in many nutrients now being studied as anticancer agents—fiber, beta-carotene, and vitamin C—and contain substances that may help rid the body of toxic chemicals. They're also nearly fat free and sodium free and contain no cholesterol. Low-cal too: One cooked cup of broccoli has only 45 calories, collards only 25. No wonder the National Cancer Institute (NCI) recommends them.

Problem is, collards suffer from the company they keep—for example, high-fat ham hocks and salty seasonings. But collards are delicious in many other incarnations: sautéed in garlic and a little olive oil or combined with wild rice and chicken broth.

BY ALEXIS LIPSITZ

People on a salt-restricted diet (generally less than 2,000 milligrams-a little less than a quarter of a teaspoonful-per day) should determine the salt content of their water supply. Five out of every 100 water supplies contain about 250 milligrams of salt per quart. And home water softeners can increase the sodium content of tap water by as much as 100 milligrams per quart. Solutions: Check with your local water department for information on salt content. If, however, your water comes from a well, have it tested by the local health department or by a private laboratory. If you use a water softener, connect it only to the hot-water lines or leave the kitchen faucet unattached.

Bottom Line PERSONAL

Putting personal idealism before business realism. Providing free breakfast and lunch for employees. Eliminating a flagship product. Doing little advertising. Is this any way to run a business?

Paul Stitt, owner of Natural Ovens of Manitowoc, thinks it is. In a bottom-line-oriented world, he's a proud anomaly.

Natural Ovens makes breads, muffins, rolls, cookies and a high-fibered drink powder used as an energy supplement. The company has expanded from its original Manitowoc base to markets across the Upper Midwest and has gained customers by promoting flaxseed, an ingredient used in all of its products, as health-inducing. And despite Stitt's avowed indifference to financial success, sales of privately held Natural Ovens have increased 130% in the past three years, totaling $5.5 million in 1989.

"I knew from Day One I was going to succeed. I may not make any money, but I was definitely going to succeed." Stitt said. "My definition of success was that I'm going to make food that's good for people and that people are going to willingly buy. They're going to appreciate what I'm doing."

A native of Verona, Ill., 49-year-old Stitt graduated from Beloit College and earned a master's degree in biochemistry from the University of Wisconsin-Madison before becoming a food researcher.

"From what I saw when I was working in the food industry, their whole emphasis is, 'How can we change this food so people will eat more of it?' So they're constantly adding additives to foods to

EDITED FROM

THE MILWAUKEE JOURNAL

Business

Owner's idealism infuses operation of Natural Ovens

stimulate people's appetite to cause people to overeat."

Stitt's goal is to bake products that are healthy for the consumer. All Natural Ovens breads are baked with flax, a grain shown to lower cholesterol levels and to reduce pre-cancerous cells in laboratory tests because it contains a compound known as Omega-3. Fish oils containing forms of this fatty acid also have been highly touted as cholesterol-reducing. Stitt holds a patent on a process to make flax seeds edible.

Natural Ovens' next market niches will be in foods designed to prevent cancer and to enhance athletic performance. These products will use flax, whose action against pre-cancerous cells will be explored in a multimillion-dollar study commissioned by the National Cancer Institute.

Stitt looks out for his employees as well as his customers. Junk food--as well as smoking--is strictly prohibited on Natural Ovens premises. Breakfast and lunch also are provided free to employees; Stitt estimated the cost to the company at 65 to 75 cents per person per meal.

"We want them to experience eating properly prepared natural foods." he said.

Natural Ovens now distributes to the Milwaukee, Green Bay, Chicago and Minneapolis markets.

"We will accept financial success if it's to be," Stitt said. "We're not against wealth, it's just that we don't feel it should

be the one and only priority of a business....I would rather do what's right and fail financially than to do what's wrong and succeed financially."

Such an attitude, however, does not help Natural Ovens fit easily into a financially oriented world. The bakery operates on a slim 1.5% profit margin and is heavily indebted, Stitt says. A big new facility, opened in 1988, operates at only 35% capacity.

Ron Muench, Natural Ovens' corporate controller, maintains that the bakery's loans are proportional to its assets of 1.8 million.

"When you build, you consistently increase your indebtedness to compensate for your expansion." Muench said.

Nevertheless, one of Natural Ovens' short-term goals is to decrease its debt load. Expanding the profit margin through increased volume or price increases also will be explored, Stitt says.

A loaf of Natural Ovens bread retails for $1.79 to $2.98. "Prices are probably too reasonable" considering the quality of the product; said Steve Rayl, assistant vice president of First Interstate Bank of Wisconsin-Manitowoc, Stitt's main lender.

Stitt says, however, that he'll only raise prices to secure the company's financial stability for the time when the company is given over to the employees. Natural Ovens stock is not sold publicly, but given to employees in antici-

pation of a turnover to employee control.

For now at least, Stitt's zeal for nutrition--and his products--is finding more acceptability all the time.

He's also burying some hatchets. Stitt says that since his departure from Quaker Oats and the publication of his book, "Fighting the Food Giants," Quaker has become one of the more nutritionally conscious food companies.

Ron Bottrell, senior manager of corporate communications at Quaker Oats, explains that Americans in general have become more health-conscious, and Quaker is responding to the demand with products such as oat bran, while not overhyping its dietary and nutritional benefits.

"We have a major commitment to wholesome and nutritional foods," he said. "We have tried to be responsible in the marketing."

Stitt and Manitowoc are getting along better, too. Stitt now includes a Manitowoc promotional blurb on every bread label. With the sponsorship of First Interstate-Manitowoc and the Manitowoc-Two Rivers Chamber of Commerce, Stitt and his wife, Barbara, co-owner of Natural Ovens, received the 1988 Small Business Persons of the Year award from the US Small Business Administration's Northeast Wisconsin Advisory Council.

"The amount of free publicity they've provided for this area through their marketing is incalculable," said Martin Owens, Chamber of Commerce president.

Stitt also seems happy with his Manitowoc location:

"We intend to maintain production in the state of Wisconsin. This may be the only food company in the United States that's not for sale."

From the desk of Paul Stitt...

Thoughts in March, 1990

DEAR FRIEND:

You may think that all of the newsletters about Energy Drink and Roy Pirrung is so much hype about a "health fad," but let me assure you that this product is for real. Just telling the plain unvarnished truth sounds to many people like a lot of wild exaggerated claims, but they are not. The plain truth simply sounds too good to be true. For example:

1). The first male athlete to test this product set 17 new national and international personal bests in one year.

2). The first female athlete to test this product set 28 new course records in Wisconsin in nine months.

3). A highly respected cancer researcher from Canada found a 50% reduction in colon and mammary precancerous lesions in 4 weeks with a diet that contained just 5% flax compared to the same diet that contained no flax seed.

But what's more important to you than the above data, is what Energy Drink can do for you. That's what counts in my book.

After three weeks of using Energy Drink according to directions, virtually every person we talk with say they like the added energy and stamina. People who are watching their weight also tell us that it helps them lose unwanted pounds.

The National Cancer Institute is interested in flax. For over two years I have presented all available information that has been published in the last 100 years on the consumption of flax. As a result, the NCI has flax in their $20.5 Million study on the five top health enhancing foods.

The National Cancer Institute recently appointed me as a consultant to review some of the research grant applications that they have received from over forty universities to study ways to develop effective "Designer Foods." The foods that nutritional researchers will be studying for their health enhancing properties are: flaxseed, garlic, the parsley vegetable family (carrots, broccoli, cauliflower, and dark leaf green vegetables), citrus foods and licorice root (not licorice candy).

Because we have been adding fortified flaxseed to our products, Natural Ovens was the only food company mentioned in a February 7th article in the New York Times regarding the National Cancer Insititute research program to develop "Designer Foods." I guess that definitely identifies, our breads, rolls, muffins, cookies and Energy Drink to be in the health enhancing Designer Foods category.

Energy Drink, containing flax, oats and barley is sold in most stores with the Natural Ovens breads. And in some cases it may be found in the cereal or weight-loss section. If you can't find it, you may ask the manager or customer service for its location. Energy Drink may be just the best new product you've ever purchased.

Feeling Good Losing Pounds

Slow and steady is the best way to burn fat. You added fat slowly to your body, and slowly is the only way you'll lose it. Fast weight loss in mostly water and muscle. If you're a scale watcher, one-half to one pound per week is a healthy reduction rate. (Very heavy folks may lose weight a little faster.)

Develop reasonable goals and good habits. A good program tailors your individual caloric needs to your activity level: The more active you are, the more food you can eat and still shed fat. If you eat far too little, you risk a slowdown in metabolism, loss of muscle tissue and an eventual weight rebound. Instead, look for guidelines that ease you into health one step at a time, through wiser food choices, better cooking techniques and increased physical activity. A good plan will focus more on the source of your excess body fat than on the fat itself, which is only a symptom.

Enjoy real foods high in carbohydrates and fiber and low in fat. Low-cal is out, high fiber and carbohydrates are in. Choose up to 60% of your calories from whole-grain bread, cereal and pasta, starches like dried beans, corn and potatoes, and lots of fruits and veggies. These foods will fill you up without adding to your padding. On the other hand, research says fat calories are more fattening, so trim food fats to 20% to 30% of your calories.

—*AMERICAN HEALTH MAGAZINE*

347

WHAT ABOUT
SOLUBLE FIBER

No doubt, there is more to come on the subject of soluble fiber and foods that lower cholesterol. For those who don't want to wait, however, the old dietary advice is still the best: Eat a variety of foods in season every day, including 4 to 6 servings of fruits and vegetables, 6 to 8 servings of whole grain breads and cereals and protein alternatives (dried beans, peas and legumes) and a healthy dose of soluble fiber is guaranteed.

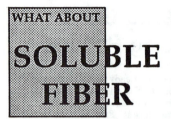

Soluble Fiber Content of Foods		
	Serving	Soluble Fiber (g)
Black-eyed peas, cooked	1/2 cup	5.5
Kidney beans, cooked	1/2 cup	2.5
Oat bran, dry	1/3 cup	2.0
Natural Ovens Great Granola	2 oz	2.0
Figs, dried	2	1.7
Brussels sprouts, cooked	1/2 cup	1.6
Kale, cooked	1/2 cup	1.4
Oat, quick, dry	1/3 cup	1.4
Natural Ovens 100% Whole Grain Bread	1 slice	.8
Apple, raw, with skin	1	.8
Sweet potato, cooked	1/2 large	.8
Plums, raw	3	.7
Brown rice, cooked	1/2 cup	.2
Lettuce	1/2 cup	.1

—EDITED FROM
ENVIRONMENTAL NUTRITION
To subscribe write:
2112 BROADWAY, SUITE 200
NEW YORK, NEW YORK 10023
or call 212-362-0424.

AS WE HEARD IT...

October 23, 1989

DEAR PAUL,

I spoke with you briefly at the Road America Run last weekend, but I wanted to drop you a line and get my "testimonial" in writing. First a little bit about my background. I am 31 years old and have been running, biking, and swimming for 4 1/2 years. I have competed in races, and still do, at least twice a month for the last 4 years. During the last 3 years I've been past the stage of rapid improvement that usually occurs in the first year a new activity is started. PRs (Personal Records) becoming a rarity, and I was satisfied with coming within 5% of them.

After you spoke at our Shoreline Striders meeting early this year, I began using Natural Ovens products. Within a few weeks I was having one to two slices of bread, one tablespoon of Energy Drink mixed with my orange juice, one Natural Ovens cookie and muffin almost every day. I was a little concerned about my training at that time because I had to cut it nearly in half for four months (January thru April) because of another endeavor. After I had been using your products for several months and resumed my regular training in May, I had some pleasant surprises. Below is a list of races I have done both last and this year on the same courses. I've also indicated the time improvements.

Bellin 10K Run...Green Bay
June '88   44:25
June '89   43:54   29 sec.

Spirit's Here Race Festival (biathlon)...Manitowoc
June '88   69:34
June '89   65:55   3 min. 39 sec.

Secura Triathlon...Kimberly
July '88   1:59:13
June '89   1:54:20   4 min. 53 sec.

Kewaskum Kettle 20K Race
Aug. '88   1:41:32
Aug. '89   1:35:11   6 min. 21 sec.

Al's Run...Milwaukee
Sept. '88   34:30
Sept. '89   33:55   35 seconds

In addition to the above, this year I have set PRs in the two-mile, four-mile, eight-mile and, most recently, the marathon. Two weeks ago in the Twin Cities Marathon I beat the Boston Marathon qualifying standard by almost fourteen minutes! Since my training has not significantly changed in the past year and I've had no other changes in my diet (in fact I've averaged five pounds heavier this year), I can only attribute my improvement to your wonderful products. I recommend them to my family and friends. ...My thanks to you and Barbara.

Sincerely,
C.M.,
Sheboygan Falls, WI

Organic Farming and Cost-Consciousness

Stacked near the check-out counter of my local food co-operative are gallons of apple juice. There are two stacks: one of commercial apple juice sells for $3.50, the organic juice for $6.50. Each week when I step up to the counter, my hand hovers between the two stacks. Invariably, my fingers come to rest on the neck of the commercial juice, and I feel that I am being cost-conscious. "The organic juice is simply too expensive," I tell myself.

It is not just juice that brings on this hesitancy. I behave in this fashion whenever a price difference appears between an organically-produced item and its organic equivalent. And I imagine that there are many such "cost-conscious" shoppers, each with their hands wavering.

Are we really cost-conscious shoppers when we behave in this way? Are we "getting a good deal" when we choose the commercial product? The higher price of organic foods partly reflects the small numbers of organic farmers. However, it also reflects other factors which we might refer to as stewardship costs. To illustrate this, let us ask the reverse question. Why are the prices of commercial products so low? There are some significant production costs absent from the prices of commercial items. These include the costs of soil degradation and soil erosion, the water pollution costs of fertilizer runoff, the costs of ground-water depletion, the national-security costs of over-reliance on imported fossil fuels, the health and despeciation costs of herbicide and pesticide use, the agricultural-security costs of reduced plant-species diversity, and the cultural costs of factory farming. Economists have a term for these costs. They are known as "externalities." These costs are not borne by the commercial farmer as part of the production process. They are borne by other individuals or groups, or even by future farmers. They are thus *external* to commercial-farm production and are not reflected in the prices of commercial-farm products. This, in part, explains why commercial food items are so inexpensive relative their organic counterparts.

In contrast to commercial-farm production, organic-farm production *internalizes* many of these costs. Natural soil maintenance (composting), a greater amount of hand care and labor-intensive techniques, integrated pest-and-disease control, and culturally-rich small farms all involve costs the become incorporated into the prices of organic products. When we purchase these goods, we are being "cost conscious" in a very true sense. We are paying for what others would pay in external costs if we had purchased the commercial equivalent.

The recognition of these stewardship costs is quite profound. As it stands, the agricultural system of the United States is guilty of an error of conception that was identified by E.F. Schumacher in his well-known essay "Buddhist Economics." Simply put, the U.S. agricultural system mistakes capital for income. It treats the environmental and natural-resource capital of the United States, which includes the soil, species diversity, ground water, and fossil fuels, as income available on an annual basis into eternity. Organic farming corrects this misconception, treating our environment and natural resources as what they are: capital. The higher prices of organic foods reflect capital-maintenance or stewardship costs. Paying these higher prices, we exercise true cost consciousness.

—by Kenneth Reinert
BUILDING ECONOMIC ALTERNATIVES
SPECIAL THANKS to Kris Olsen,
Minneapolis, MN for sending this article to us.

Caffeine Causes Infertility

Women who drink more than the caffeine equivalent of one cup of coffee per day are half as likely to become pregnant as women who drink less caffeine, a new study finds.

Because of their anti-estrogenic effects, cigarettes have long been known to reduce fertility, but researchers have only speculated on caffeine's impact on fertility.

A group of North Carolina investigators asked 104 healthy women who had been trying to get pregnant for three months about their consumption of caffeinated drinks, alcohol and cigarettes. Coffee was the source of three-fifths of the caffeine the women consumed.

After 13 months, only six percent of the women in the lower caffeine group had failed to conceive, compared with 28 percent in the higher caffeine group. Women consuming high levels of caffeine ahd 4.7 times the risk of infertility of women consuming low levels of caffeine.

—MEDICAL NUTRITION MAGAZINE

(Dis)counting Calories

The more calories you eat, the fatter you'll be, right? Maybe not. A new study from the Stanford Center for Research in Disease Prevention indicates the the *fattier* your diet, the fatter you'll be.

Darlene Dreon and her colleagues reviewed the diets of 155 sedentary, obese, middle-aged men. Each had been weighed under water to determine what percent of his weight was fat.

As it turned out, the fattest men had the fattiest diets; a higher percentage of their calories came from fat, and a lower percentage from carbohydrates. But there was no link at all between the number of calories eaten and body fat.

"Our data suggests that dietary fat can be a contributor to obesity, independent of its calories," says Dreon.

Researchers at Harvard Medical School reached a similar conclusion in a study of 141 middle-aged nurses.

—NUTRITION ACTION HEALTHLETTER,
VOL. 15, NO. 10

Is all wheat bread high in fiber?

The answer is "no." Some wheat breads are made of predominantly white flour. While "wheat flour," "enriched wheat flour," and "unbleached wheat flour" may sound fibrous, all are basically white flour.

Just because a bread looks brown doesn't mean it's high fiber either. Some breads have caramel coloring added, giving them the look of whole wheat bread but not the fiber. And don't be fooled by bread in brown-colored wrappers.

People seeking whole grain nutrition should read ingredient labels and buy bread with one of the following ingredients listed first: "whole wheat flour," "stone-ground whole wheat flour," or "100% whole wheat flour."

—ENVIRONMENTAL NUTRITION
Vol. 12, No. 8

EDITOR'S NOTE: You can be sure that all Natural Ovens foods are made with only the finest whole ingredients available—making them truly the very best.

349

The POWER OF FLAX

Flax is endowed with power that no other food has. According to published scientific papers, small amounts of substances found in flax (at high levels) can help lower blood pressure, prevent and remove cholesterol plaques from the arteries, prevent selenium toxicity and increase learning ability. All of these powers can be demonstrated even with low levels of flax in the diet.

How can it do all of this? Why wasn't it discovered long before this? How much flax does it take? I'll answer the last question first. One to two tablespoons of flax per day contains plenty of the necessary compounds to accomplish the aforementioned feats, according to qualified scientific reports.

History of Flax

Flax has been used for thousands of years; as long as wheat and barley. But until a few years ago, no one realized that flax contained high levels of many beneficial compounds. At the office of Natural Ovens and Essential Nutrient Research Corporation, we have pieced together this amazing story from hundreds of published scientific research articles. On our demonstration farm we have demonstrated how beneficial flax is for the healthy growth of pigs, chickens, and horses. To our knowledge no other research organization has ever before put the whole story together and proven it in a practical way with animals.

Flax Components

Whole ground flaxseed contains many compounds that are readily available to the human digestive system. These compounds are:

Alpha-linolenic acid	20%
Soluble and insoluble fiber	39%
Lignans	80mg/g

Alpha-linolenic acid (ALENA) has a long and well kept secret of the many different actions it can have in the human body. Each action is

By Paul Stitt, M.S.
Biochemistry
President, Natural Ovens of Manitowoc

separate from each and every other action, yet it adds up to being a very powerful substance. In brief, ALENA has been shown to improve learning ability in rats and monkeys, prevent agglutination of platelets in humans, remove cholesterol from arteries and prevent dry, scaly skin.

ALENA Performs Hundreds of Functions

First of all, ALENA, or its direct derivations, comprise 65% of some parts of the brain. It is directly involved in the interconnectedness of the brain which makes the brain such a powerful organ. Japanese researchers have found that rats fed a diet enriched in ALENA had a superior learning ability.[1] The same compounds, which are extremely sensitive to light, are involved in the retina of the eye which enable it to be such an amazing organ, converting light energy into electrical energy.

ALENA also becomes an important part of platelets to keep them from sticking together when they shouldn't.[3] This is important to prevent unwanted blood clots. Yet, ALENA does not cause the other extreme either — it does not cause excessive bleeding or thinning of the blood like fish oils.[4]

Derivatives of ALENA are found at high levels in cold water fish. Eskimos, on their native diet of cold water fish, scarcely ever develop heart trouble, arthritis and other degenerative diseases even though their diet contains over 60% fat.[5]

Flax is a Super Energy Source

ALENA is also an excellent source of energy because it can easily be converted, via Beta oxidation, to acetyl co-A which produces ATP. Runners have found that when they use flax during training, and just before races, they set new personal records because of the sustained energy released from flax.

ALENA has been proven to be an Essential Fatty Acid by its' ability to heal skin lesions, nerve damage and other skin disorders.[8] ALENA has revealed itself to be an excellent promoter of healing of the skin.

Flax: An Excellent Source of Fiber

ALENA is not the only substance of importance in flax. More is known about ALENA than the rest of the substances in flax, but it may not be the most important. It also contains high levels of dietary fiber — 39% according to Dr. David Jenkins at the University of Toronto. Two thirds of it is soluble fiber and one third is insoluble. Soluble fiber is known to attach to cholesterol and bile acids in the intestinal tract and thus be removed from the body. Bile acids are made from cholesterol and so, the more they are removed, the more one's cholesterol levels are lowered. Insoluble fiber is known to remove other toxins from the body. Together, the two types of fiber keep the intestinal track moving.

Lignans

A special compound, called lignan, in flax is converted by bacterial enzymes in the intestinal tract to anti-estrogen compounds. These compounds help prevent excess levels of estrogen from causing estrogen related tumors.[6,10] Dr. Lillian Thompson at the University of Toronto, and others, are actively working in this exciting area of research.

350

Choose your Foods!

The foods you choose can make a big difference in how you feel, how much energy you have for sports or schoolwork, and even how you look! To be your best, you must choose a variety of foods.

Today, many foods that Americans eat every day can be bad for your health if you eat too much of them. These foods are usually high in sugar, fat, salt, or chemical additives. They are sometimes called "junk" foods. These foods can cause you to be overweight, have poor skin, get tooth decay, or develop heart disease when you get older.

If you want to be at your best, find ways to avoid these types of food and replace them with fresh whole foods. Here's a way for you to find out what you have been eating, and try to find ways to make more healthy food choices.

ACTIVITY

1. Carry a notebook with you throughout an ordinary school day. Make a list of all the foods you eat for breakfast, lunch, dinner and snacks.

2. Look at the Food Guide on this label. On your list, mark a large "X" next to the foods that are under Foods To Avoid.

3. Make another list of all your foods marked with an X. Beside each of these foods write a food from the "Eat More" column that you might eat instead. Try to make these good food choices whenever you can. You'll not only look and feel better, but will discover the great taste of fresh foods.

Adapted from *Ladybugs and Lettuce Leaves,* written, illustrated and produced by Project Outside/Inside, Somerville Public Schools, Somerville, MA. A publication of the Center for Science in the Public Interest, Washington, D.C.

Snack Food Guide

Eat less of these...	Because they are...	Eat more of these...
Soda pop, fruit drinks, milkshakes	High in added sugar	Unsweetened fruit juices, unsalted club soda, fruit juice mixed with club soda, water, lowfat milk, milk-banana-fruit shake
Candy bars, doughnuts, cakes, pies, cookies, pastries	High in added sugar and fat	Fresh fruits (bananas, apples, berries, melons), Natural Ovens muffins (Blueberry Oat, Raisin Bran, Cherry Almond Oat Bran, Banananut), Natural Ovens breads (Kidz Bread, Nutty Wheat, Happiness, English Muffin, Sunny Millet and all the other good Natural Ovens breads), Natural Ovens Cookies (Scotch Oaties, Sunnypower, Happy, Goodbites, Choco Chip)
Bacon , hot dogs, cold cuts, processed cheese	High in fat, salt, and additives	Baked or broiled fish, chicken or lean meats, yogurt, cottage cheese
Potato chips, corn chips, cheese puffs, french fries	High in fat, salt	Unsalted popcorn, pretzels, nuts & seeds, roasted soybeans

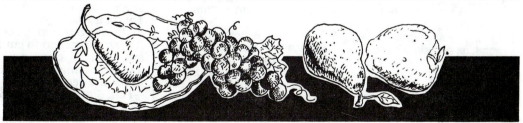

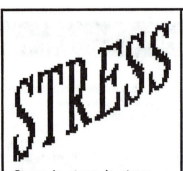

Stress is stress is stress — whether it's from physical or emotional causes.

HOW TO REDUCE STRESS

First address your diet — the foods and beverages you consume.

Go for the best for your health and vitality: lots of fresh grown and colorful vegetables, fruits, melons, berries, beans, lentils, seeds, nuts, sprouts, whole grain breads and cereals, pasta, fish, organically grown chicken or turkey.

Be on the alert for food or chemical sensitivities. If you especially love a food, avoid it for five days, then eat it first thing in your day, and pay attention to how you feel. If a food or drink makes you feel depressed, irritable or tired, avoid it.

Your body needs and loves 6 to 8 glasses of pure water daily between, before and after meals. Excellent bottled water is available in most areas.

WALK IT OFF

Exercise reduces stress faster and better than any drugs. Brisk walking 25 minutes daily can do wonders, especially if you walk near trees and/or water. Fifteen to 20 minutes of yoga exercises can help you start the day with a feeling of being in balance.

LISTEN TO SOOTHING MUSIC

Breathe from your stomach like a baby. Force the air *out* of your lungs; the air will then come in naturally.

If you feel yourself becoming upset, walk away, concentrate on deep breathing. In a couple of minutes you'll feel the stress easing.
—*Barbara Stitt*

Saga of Natural Ovens May 1988

May was an exciting month at Natural Ovens. The horses were put on fresh grass, which they dearly love. We had finished seeding oats with the horses and we were looking forward to a good crop.

The bakery was operating much better. We installed circulating fans in the oven, which improved the baking tremendously. We've increased muffin production, and have stared looking for a muffin making machine that would make muffins more uniformly. When they are formed by hand, some muffins are too large and don't bake all the way through. And who likes raw muffins! When the muffins are baked properly, we don't seem to have much competition.

May was a very exciting month for me, since I attended the American Oil Chemists meeting in Phoenix. These people study the extraction of fats and the effects of various kinds of fat on people's health — a very exciting topic.

I was especially interested in what was new about alpha-linolenic acid (alena), which is found so abundantly in flax, and in our breads, muffins and cookies.

Dr. Ed Emker from the USDA Northern Regional Reseach Center reported that alena is efficiently and rapidly utilized by some people. This is the first conclusive scientific report of this finding. He reported that the type of other fats in the diet had a strong effect on the utilization of alena. For example, polyunsaturates inhibit the metabolism of alena, while a low fat diet seems to speed up its use. This is another good reason to follow Surgeon General Koop's suggestion to cut fat and protein consumption, and eat more whole grains, fruits and vegetables.
—*Paul Stitt*

Breakfast

The poetry of breakfast starts with its meaning: breaking the fast of a night's sleep.

BRAIN FOOD

The classic Iowa Breakfast Studies, conducted from 1949 to 1961, set a precendent for the importance of breakfast. Researchers studied 121 people of all ages: When they didn't eat breakfast, the subjects worked less efficiently in the late morning hours. All did significantly more work when they ate an adequate breakfast than when they didn't. The no-breakfast kids also had a poorer attitude toward school work.

Eating a mid-morning snack *in addition* to breakfast provided no benefit, however. Nor was omitting breakfast any help in weight control. Indeed those who didn't eat breakfast had more trouble controlling hunger.

A recent study confirms earlier findings that breakfast boosts performance in children. Professor of Pediatrics Alan Meyers and colleagues at the Boston University School of Medicine studied low-income children who participated for the first time in a federal school breakfast program. Stardardized achievement tests given before and after the breakfast program showed that it brought a significant improvement in academic performance. Absenteeism was also slightly lower, and tardiness significantly lower, after kids were put on the breakfast program.

STAYING TRIM

Since Iowa, both animal and human studies have proved the benefits of eating three or more meals a day. When people eat fewer meals, they are likely to have more body fat, gain more weight (or lose less), and have high blood cholesterol levels. They are also likely to consume more fat and dietary cholesterol, fewer essential vitamins and minerals, and less dietary fiber.

Those who eat fewer than three meals a day tend to eat less during the morning and early after noon and more in the late after noon and night. That's not optimal. A good rule of thumb is to consume about two-thirds of the day's foods by late afternoon, leaving about a third for dinner and snacks.

Clincial experience in weight control confirms the improtance of breakfast in regulating hunger throughout the day. So finds endocrinologist C. Wayne Callaway of George Washington University in Washington, DC. His research reveals that people who skip breakfast have metabolic rates 4% to 5% below normal.

Each meal we eat sparks a little increase in the rate at which we burn calories. It's called the "thermic effect of food." Eat just one big meal a day and you'll burn fewer calories than someone who eats the same amount of food spread out over breakfast, lunch and dinner.

Dr. Callaway finds many overweight people tend to skip breakfast, eat hardly any lunch, then eat too much for dinner and late at night, so they're not hungry for breakfast the next day. If they *do* eat breakfast, they report, it makes them *hungrier* for the next meal — which can lead to binging. That's not a result of eating breakfast, however, but of the pattern of daily deprivation they bring to the morning meal.

The key is to eat three meals (each having at least 25% to 30% of the day's calories) spaced throughout the day so that hunger never becomes a problem to control. If you retrain yourself to eat a good breakfast, then within about two weeks you'll start waking up hungry for breakfast — and less hungry later in the day.

—American Health Magazine
Harlan, IA 51537-3015
(10 issues – $14.95)

Some suggestions for an excellent breakfast: freash fruit, melon or berries plus oatmeal, cold baked potato, minestrone soup, corn or oat bran muffins, brown rice and lentils. Also delicious day starters are Natural Ovens Oat Bran DeLite toast, Great Granola and any one of our four varieties of muffuns .

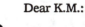 FROM OUR MAILBOX

 Q. Dear Paul and Barbara:

We love your breads but we are a little confused. You show Omega-3 on the label however no fish oil is shown in the ingredient list. Would you please explain the source of the Omega-3?

K.M.,
Minneapolis, MN

A. Dear K.M.:

We use ground fortified flaxseed in our breads. The flaxseed is high in alpha-linolenic acid which the body uses as Omega-3. Omega-3 is an essential fatty acid that has been found to help reduce cholesterol, help lower blood pressure and also contribute to the increase in learning ability.

In some of our high-fibered breads, no oil is added, with the only oil being that which naturally occurs in the flaxseed. When it is necessary to add a small amount of oil. We use canola oil which also contains Omega-3.

Thank you for writing. We are always happy to hear from our wonderful customers.

Sincerely,
Paul & Barbara Stitt

```
Did you know that...
```
happily married women gain an average of 18.4 pounds in the first 13 years of marriage, while *unhappily* married women gain an average of 42.6 pounds? On their wedding days the average weight difference between these women is only five pounds.

--Bottom Line Personal

The New York Times

SATURDAY, AUGUST 19, 1989

Patents | Edmund L. Andrews

Using Flax To Get Benefit Of Fish Oils

WASHINGTON

PAUL A. STITT, a Wisconsin biochemist-turned-baker, this week patented what he said is a way to put the health benefits of cod-liver oil — without its notoriously foul taste — into bread, cookies, salad dressings and even fruit drinks.

In recent years, some medical researchers have suggested that a particular ingredient in fish oils, a fatty acid known as omega-3, may have numerous health benefits, although others dispute the claims. The Heart, Lung and Blood Institute, a part of the National Institutes of Health, has found that consuming large volumes of fish oil may alleviate some heart symptoms, like angina. Researchers at the National Cancer Institute, meanwhile, say that animal studies indicate that omega-3 may also have some ability to prevent cancer.

Nevertheless, the oils are too unpalatable for use as food supplements.

Mr. Stitt, the founder of Natural Ovens of Manitowoc Inc., in Manitowoc, Wis., believes he has a solution. He won patent approval this week for a method of incorporating flax into foods. Flax is the source of linseed oil and is also rich in omega-3.

Mr. Stitt said linseed oil has many of the same ingredients as fish oils, but typically becomes rancid quickly and as a result is just as foul-tasting as its chemical cousins. The new patent covers a method for stabilizing the flax, even after it has been ground into meal.

"What we discovered is that if you do not extract the oil from the seed, and treat the flax with zinc and vitamin B-6, you end up with a stable product that tastes good," he said.

Mr. Stitt said he was now selling flax-filled breads, cookies, muffins and drink supplements through about 800 supermarkets in the Midwest. The new products now account for 65 percent of his concern's $5.5 million sales, he said.

Mr. Stitt received patent 4,857,326.

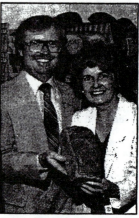

Paul A. Stitt has patented what he says is a way to put the health benefits of cod-liver oil into baked goods and other foods without the oil's notoriously foul taste. Mr. Stitt is shown here with Barbara Reed Stitt, his wife and co-president of the company he founded, Natural Ovens of Manitowoc Inc.

MAGNESIUM ALERT
Curb the Cola

Before you reach for your next can of soda, consider this: Too much cola could lead to deficiency of the vital mineral magnesium, setting the stage for heart disease and other disorders.

Kenneth Weaver, M.D., associate clinical professor of obstetrics and gynecology at East Tennessee State University in Johnson City, Tennessee, found that many of his pregnant patients who suffered from high blood pressure and magnesium levels well below the normal level (1.7 mg per deciliter). Examining their

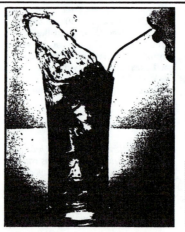

diets, he found they downed can after can of cola.

Cola is high in phosphoric acid, a form of the mineral phosphorous, which binds with magnesium and pulls both minerals out of the body. Weaver says that one 12-ounce can of cola contains 36mg of phosphoric acid — which extracts 36mg of magnesium.

—*NUTRITION DYNAMICS*

Bad exercises for bad backs
are those done with *unbent* knees — toe touches, straight-leg raises, straight-leg sit-ups, straight-leg push-ups, etc.
—BOTTOM LINE PERSONAL

Dietary Fiber Recommended In New Government Cancer-Prevention Pamphlet

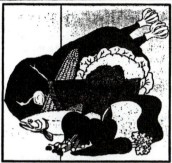

A pamphlet recently released and offered free by the U.S. Department of Health and Human Services underscores the importance of dietary fiber in preventing many types of cancer.

"Diet, Nutrition & Cancer Prevention: The Good News," prepared by the National Cancer Institute Office of Cancer Communications, deals with a variety of nutritional factors that may help prevent cancer. The booklet explains what dietary fiber is and what it does:

"Dietary fiber is material from plant cells that humans cannot digest or can only partially digest. It helps move food through the intestines and out of the body, promoting a healthy digestive tract. A diet high in fiber and low in fat may reduce the risk of cancers of the colon and rectum," the booklet says.

The publication also says that the National Cancer Institute recommends that Americans eat between 20 and 30 grams of fiber per day. The current intake in this country is about 11 grams daily, it said.

Several food groups were specified as having a high fiber content. These include breads, rolls, pastas and cereals made with whole grains or whole-grain flours from wheat, corn, rye, oats and their brans; fresh and frozen fruits and vegetables, including apples, peaches, pears and potatoes with their skins; and cooked dry peas and beans.

The booklet includes a chart of high-fiber foods that shows grams of fiber and calories per serving for a variety of foods. It is available free by writing to: The Consumer Information Center, Department 517T, Pueblo, Colo. 81009.

FIBER FACTS

On the average, a slice of Natural Ovens bread contains 2g of fiber.

TIPS FOR THE HOLIDAYS

Scrumptious dressing
Combine:
1 loaf of Sunny Millet with 4 slices of Happiness Bread. Toast by laying the slices on a wire rack in a 350° oven. Turn over when tops are lightly toasted. When toasted on both sides, collect the slices in a large bowl or pan. Holding 3 slices at one time, run medium hot water over them soaking well. Lightly squeeze some of the water out and crumble into a large steel bowl.

Saute in a saucepan:
¼ c. extra virgin olive oil or Canola oil
1 med. to lge. onion-chopped or diced
3 stalks fresh celery-chopped or diced

Pour mixture into bowl of crumbled toast. Add:
Sage to taste-1 or so teaspoons
Vegesal or salt to taste [approx. ½ tsp.]
2 or 3 eggs
¼ c. chopped walnuts [optional]
Mix well with wooden spoon. Stuff the cavity of the bird and turn the remaining into a baking dish. Bake 25 minutes. Serves 6-8 hungry people.
Note: Any of Natural Ovens breads work beautifully as dressing. This happens to be the favorite of Paul and Barbara.
Delicious served with cornish hen, chicken, turkey, ham[or as is for vegetarians]. Round out your meal with raw vegetables and apples baked with cinnamon and maple syrup.

Summer's Freshest Flavors

Summer brings the freshest of fruits and vegetables — the tastiest, most colorful and most nutritious foods we see all year. Season this newly-picked produce with equally fresh herbs. Summer's bounty includes the distinctive flavors and fragrances of fresh parsley, basil, thyme, rosemary, chervil and other delights.

Herbs are among the easiest plants to grow and are increasingly available fresh in local markets. Here are a few rules of thumb for using fresh herbs to perk up your summer cooking:

- Use two or three times the quantity of fresh herbs when substituting for dried, since their flavor is much more subtle.

- Most cooking calls for herb leaves, but stems usually have the strongest flavor.

- Robust herbs, including sage, sorrel, marjoram and oregano, retain their flavor even if cooked for a long time.

- Fine herbs, such as basil, chervil, tarragon and dill, have a more delicate flavor that should be added to dishes just before serving. □

Summer Herbs

Here are a few suggestions on how to use summer's luscious herbs.

	Flavor	Try with
Basil	mildly peppery with a trace of mint and clove	tomato sauces, salad dressings, poultry, fish
Chervil	warm, part-anise, part-parsley flavor	omelets, green beans
Chives	mild, sweet onion taste	salads, omelets, potatoes
Coriander*	strong sage flavor with a sharp citrus bite	chicken, beets, onions, chilies, curries
Dill	slightly sweet with sharp tang	fish, eggs, carrots, cauliflower, spinach, apples, potatoes, cucumbers, dips or sauces
Fennel	soft, nutty anise/celery flavor	fish, cabbage, soups, salads, breads
Marjoram	mild oregano taste with hint of balsam	stuffing, eggplant, squash
Mint	cool, refreshing, sweet	tea, fruit, carrots, peas
Oregano	pungent, peppery, slightly bitter	tomatoes, mushrooms, poultry, lentils
Parsley	gentle, green flavor	chicken, shellfish, pasta pasta
Sage	pleasantly bitter, lemony zest	breads, stuffing, potatoes
Summer Savory	light, sweet with a peppery tang	beans, lentils, vegetable juices
Sorrel	lemon-like or vinegary sour taste	spinach, cabbage, lettuce, fish, mixed salads, coleslaw
Tarragon	anise-like	chicken, fish, young vegetables, vinaigrettes
Thyme	pleasant, fresh taste with faint clove aftertaste	poultry, salad dressing, dried beans

*Also known as cilantro or Chinese parsley

American Institute for Cancer Research NEWSLETTER

SUMMER PICKINS

BROCCOLI FLORETS contain eight times as much beta carotene (a vitamin A-like compound) as the stalks. However, the stalks are still a good source of vitamin A. And, like the florets, the stalks contain B vitamins, vitamin C, calcium, iron and fiber.

LETTUCE RATED *Most nutritious* (in descending order): Swiss chard ... bok choy ... chicory ... watercress ... romaine. *Least nutritious:* Endive ... iceberg ... butterhead (Boston, bibb, limestone).

WHEN GROCERIES SIT IN THE CAR...keep perishables cold by using a picnic cooler. The cooler slows the thawing process — allowing time to take care of other errands.

These tips come from BOTTOM LINE PERSONAL. *We think it's a most informative and interesting publication.* To subscribe write: BOTTOM LINE PERSONAL, P.O. Box 58446, Boulder, CO 80322.

Banishing Brittle Bones With Boron?

Boron, an element long known for softening water, may play an important role in hardening bones, Agricultural Research Service scientists report.

A 6-month study indicates that boron, not even considered an essential nutrient for people and animals, may be a key to preventing osteoporosis, say nutritionist Forrest H. Nielsen and anatomist Curtiss D. Hunt at ARS' Grand Forks, North Dakota, Human Nutrition Research Center.

They believe the results of the study--the first to look at the nutritional effects of boron in humans--"will generate a lot of interest in the element."

In the study, 12 postmenopausal women consumed a very low boron diet (0.25 milligrams per day) for 17 weeks then were given a daily 3-mg supplement--representing the boron intake from a well-balanced diet--for 7 more weeks.

Within 8 days after the supplement was introduced, they lost 40 percent less calcium, one-third less magnesium, and slightly less phosphorus through the urine. In fact, their calcium and magnesium losses were lower than prestudy levels, when they were on their normal diets.

"These elements are important in maintaining the integrity of bone," says Nielsen, who is director of the Center.

Each day the women took the 3-mg boron supplement they retained an average of 52 mg more calcium. "That's a gram of calcium every 20 days. The body contains roughly 1,100 grams of calcium, so over a period of several years, that's a significant savings in calcium," Nielsen says.

"Boron has a remarkable effect on indicators that the body is conserving calcium or preventing bone demineralization," he says.

Since boron isn't considered essential for people, there is no recommended intake and no boron supplement on the market. Nielsen says the supplement of sodium borate used in the study was specially prepared based on the amount of boron a person would get from a well-balanced diet containing fruits and vegetables. He says the average boron intake is about 1.5 mg--or half the experimental dose--"but average means a lot of people get less and a lot get more."

Hunt cautioned that large doses of boron can be toxic, even lethal. The lowest reported lethal dose of boric acid is about 45 grams (1.6 ounces) for an adult and only 2 grams (0.07 ounce) for an infant.

People can get ample boron--up to 4 or 5 mg per day--by eating plenty of fruit--especially apples, pears, and grapes--nuts, leafy vegetables, and legumes. These foods have the highest levels of the element as well as many essential vitamins and minerals, Hunt says.

Nielsen points out that "Seventh Day Adventists, who are vegetarians, have a much lower occurrence of osteoporosis than Americans as a whole; but Eskimos, who eat almost no fruits or vegetables, have a very high incidence of bone demineralization."

Osteoporosis affects as many as 15 to 20 million older Americans, predominantly women, according to a 1984 conference sponsored by the National Institutes of Health. Each year, osteoporosis contributes to about 1.3 million fractures (primarily in the hip, sprine, and wrist) in people 45 years old and over. This costs an estimated $3.8 billion annually.

Calcium supplement sales are at an all-time high as women try to prevent bone loss, but little evididence exists to support the claim that adequate calcium alone prevents the loss of bone. According to Mark Hegsted, professor emeritus of nutrition at Harvard University, "osteoporosis looks like a dietary problem but not a calcium problem."

Nielsen says, "We've only scratched the surface with our research. If boron is involved in adding the hydrogen-oxygen group that steroid hormones need to be biologically active, it may be important in preventing a lot of other diseases of unknown cause--including some forms of arthritis."

Edited from AGRICULTURAL RESEARCH/November/December 1987

HOW COFFEE CAN MAKE YOU SLEEPY. If you drink a lot of coffee or caffeinated soft drinks, can the caffeine make you sleepy on the job? It sure can, says Dr. Richard Coleman, Ph.D., former codirector of the Stanford University Medical School Sleep Clinic.

"People use coffee to try to make themselves feel alert," says Coleman. "They feel that if they use coffee, they will function better on the job.

"But actually, if you drink coffee in large amounts—say ten cups per day—it may make you sleepier," he warns. Consequently, people will be less productive and more prone to accidents. Here's why:

Coffee has paradoxical effects. First, after each cup of coffee, the drinker suffers a depression or "crash" within a few hours. Many coffee drinkers drink more coffee to boost themselves out of this depression. By doing so, they create more "crashes" and want more coffee.

Second, the brain gets used to high levels of caffeine, and it then needs more to stay alert. Before they know it, coffee drinkers are drinking endless cups of coffee but are unable to get enough caffeine to stay alert. It's a vicious circle.

"People become dependent on coffee," Coleman says. "We find that shift workers who are heavy coffee drinkers often are excessively sleepy and risk not operating their machines safely." Soft drinks are not always a safe alternative, since many—especially colas—contain more caffeine than coffee does.

Eat, Sniff and Be Wary

Although for most people, flowers make a tasty and colorful addition to a meal, some allergy and hay fever sufferers get nothing but a runny nose and blotchy skin from them. So before you indulge, test a flower to see if you're allergic to it. Denise Diamond, in her book *Living with the Flowers*, suggests rubbing an herb or a flower on your wrist; if your skin reacts to the plant, don't eat it.

Whether you pick your flowers from your own garden, gather them from an open field or buy them from an organic nursery, make sure you positively identify them before you nibble. Unwary or untrained florivores have come down with rashes, stomachaches or more severe illnesses because they weren't eating what they thought they were. Also, because of varying soil conditions, flowers that are perfectly safe in one region may cause illness in another.

Don't purchase blooms from a florist. The blossoms found in floral shops may contain dangerous levels of chemicals. The government does not regulate the amount of pesticides that can be used on flowers because they are considered ornamental rather than edible plants. Also, don't eat flowers you find by the roadside—they could contain lead and other poisonous residues from auto fumes. Finally, some flowers—like sweet pea and autumn crocus—are definitely poisonous and should never be eaten. Here are some of the flowers considered edible by both Diamond and Robert Kourik, author of *Designing and Maintaining Your Edible Landscape Naturally.*—*Drew DeSilver*

Apple blossom (*Malus* species)	Lemon blossom (*Citrus limon*)
Carnation or pink (*Dianthus* species)	Lilac (*Syringa vulgaris*)
Chamomile (*Matricaria recutita*)	Marigold (*Calendula officinalis*)
Daisy (*Bellis perennis*)	Nasturtium (*Tropaeolum majuis*)
Dandelion (*Taraxacum officinale*)	Orange blossom (*Citrus sinensis*)
Day lily (*Hemerocallis fulva*)	Pansy (*Viola wittrockiana*)
Geranium (*Geranium* species)	Petunia (*Petunia hybrida*)
Gladiolus (*Gladiolus* species)	Primrose (*Primula vulgaris*)
Hibiscus (*Hibiscus rosa-sinensis*)	Rose (*Rosa* species)
Hollyhock (*Althea rosea*)	Tulip (*Tulipa* species)
Honeysuckle (*Lonicera japonica*)	Violet (*Viola odorata*)

Sweet Rice-Stuffed Hibiscus

Large, showy, trumpet-shaped flowers reveal hibiscus' tropical origins. The sweet, mild flavor of hibiscus blossoms makes the flowers ideal for use in teas, as well as this recipe. Begin preparation of this dish one day before you plan to serve it.

    1 cup raw brown rice
    1 tsp. herbal salt replacer
    ½ clove garlic, minced
    2 cups boiling water
    ¼ cup virgin olive oil
      Dash nutmeg
    1 Tbs. honey
    1 cup sliced almonds
    1 cup almond butter (optional)
    15 hibiscus flowers
    ⅛ cup green peas, cooked,
      for garnish

The day before serving, combine all ingredients except almond butter, hibiscus flowers and peas in a large saucepan or pot. Bring to a boil, cover and simmer about 40 minutes. Mix in almond butter, if desired, to thicken mixture. Place in refrigerator overnight.

Before serving, gather and wash flowers. Gently cut off green stems but leave enough of the base to hold the flower together. Fill with cold mixture and top with one or two green peas. Makes 15 servings. ▼

Per serving: 133 calories; 3g protein; 8g fat; 13g carbohydrates; 8mg cholesterol; 8mg sodium

A Peek Into The Natural Ovens 1988 Scrapbook

We're proud of the fact that we work hard to make excellent products for our customers, and we're very pleased that you respond by buying our products and allowing us to continue to serve you. But we must admit that it's very gratifying to be recognized for our work by our peers in the business world.

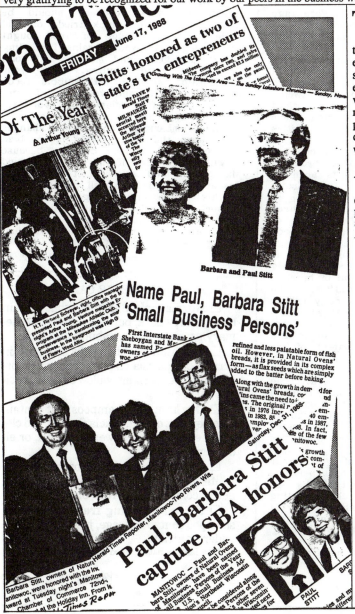

Barbara and Paul Stitt

Thanks to You

Thanks to our skilled employees and the continuing support of our customers, Natural Ovens has grown from a small-scale bakery to a regional bakery. We are very proud of the fact that we can offer delicious breads, rolls, muffins and cookies to health-conscious people throughout Wisconsin, in Chicago and Minneapolis-St. Paul areas as well as across the nation via UPS.

A Year For Awards

During 1988, Natural Ovens owners Paul and Barbara Stitt have been presented a number of honors by local and state business organizations. Awards include:

- Industry of the Year Award from Manitowoc-Two Rivers Area Chamber of Commerce
- Entrepreneur of the Year Milestone Award, given by Arthur Young and *Venture* Magazine
- Small Business Persons of the Year, awarded by First Interstate Bank of Wisconsin-Sheboygan and Manitowoc counties
- Small Business Persons of the Year, awarded by the U.S. Small Business Administration's Northeast Wisconsin Advisory Council

Our Pledge To You

The most important reason we have been chosen for recognition by our peers is because more and more of you are choosing our products—and recommending them to your friends. You can trust us to deliver the best products made with the highest quality ingredients. And our pledge to you is that we will continue to offer that excellence, and serve you in whatever way we can. That's the promise Natural Ovens is built upon, and that's what will help us to continue to grow.

359

Nutrition & Your Child

Basically the standards of good nutrition hold true for both children and adults. However, the effects of violating these standards during the growing years are profound and decisive for life. Inadequate nutrition before age five can cause a brilliant and attractive child to become physically and mentally dull.

A child's growth rate is extremely rapid between birth and two years and during two other growth spurts from ages five to seven and twelve to sixteen. It is imperative that a child receive maximum nutrition during these times; however the in-between times are equally important.

We advocate the conversion of children from a diet featuring refined products to a diet rich in whole foods such as grains, seeds, nuts, honey, fresh fruits and vegetables.

Recently there has been a flurry of articles applauding the merits of junk foods. It is true that these foods can contain a significant percentage of the daily protein requirement. It is also true that they are extremely high in calories for the amount of nutrients supplied. A fast food meal can easily supply half the total daily calorie needs for a sedentary teenager, most of those calories from fat. That is not to mention the calories from sugar and the extremely high salt content of fast foods.

The cold cereal you may serve at breakfast is another fast food. The real villain here is sugar-some favorite cereals are more than half sugar-and the victim is the young child who in time becomes accustomed to it's taste. These children lose their appetites for other foods.

The easiest way to deal with sugar is not to allow your child to experience it in the first place, but if it's too late you must alter your child's eating habits try substituting fruits and root vegetables [such as beets and yams] for concentrated sweets, and by making your own desserts, using ever decreasing amounts of honey, maple sugar and/or barley malt and rice syrup as sweeteners.

Encourage and develop a respect for whole foods in your family. Supplements can never replace fresh, whole foods. Learn to eat what comes naturally with as little done to it as possible. Vegetables, when cooked, should be lightly steamed or quick fried, oriental style. The remainder of food ought to be legumes, whole grains [including rice, buckwheat, and millet], and some eggs, fish and poultry. Keep your refrigerator stocked with nibble foods like fresh fruits and vegetables [carrot sticks and stuffed celery are favorites]. raw nuts and chunked white cheese.

When embarking on these changes make sure the whole family is involved and committed to the change, because it will never work if the child is served six grapes and a piece of cheese for dessert while dad is still putting sugar in his coffee and eating pie for his dessert. Also help your children to understand the necessities of a healthful diet, and that means more then just telling them "It's good for you".

Harvest Day Newsletter

HERBAL HAIR CARE*

☐ **Normal hair.** Shampoos that contain black cherry bark, burdock, cloves or rosemary promote manageability and gloss.

☐ **Oily hair.** Use shampoos that contain orris root, quassia chips, lemon grass, orange leaf, peppermint, willow bark or hazelnut bark.

☐ **Dry hair.** Use shampoos that contain comfrey root or leaf, acacia flowers, red clover, meliot, orange flowers and peel, or elderberry flowers.

☐ **Dandruff.** Use shampoos that contain white willow bark, birch bark, peppermint, nettle, comfrey leaf or root, or quassia chips.

☐ **For a refreshing fragrance.** Use a shampoo containing sage, juniper, pine, lavender or arnica. ∎

*Available in natural-food stores.

Bottom Line
PERSONAL

Ask the expert
Q: Will hot drinks keep you warm in cold weather?

A: Hot liquids have undoubted psychological benefits in the cold, but they don't do much for your body temperature, according to Dr. Murray Hamlet, director of the Cold Research Division of the U.S. Army Research Institute of Environmental Medicine at Natick, Massachusetts. You would have to drink a quart of hot liquid (130° F.) at one time to generate some extra body heat, but it would be hard to keep down that much hot fluid. Hot liquids may dilate skin blood vessels and make you feel warmer. However, that actually causes a small amount of heat loss—nothing to worry about, but you won't be ahead of the game.

If the temperature of a liquid doesn't matter, what does? The real problem, in cold as in heat, is getting enough to drink. A study at the Natick labs showed that people who were severely dehydrated in the cold were almost 20% colder (as measured by skin temperature of the fingers) than others. As you lose fluids, your body begins to lose the ability to regulate its temperature. Fluid can be lost by sweating in activity and—particularly in winter—during breathing. The dry winter air is warmed and moistened by the respiratory system. As you breathe out, you lose water. It's the water droplets that allow you to "see" your breath. And, of course, you lose water through urine production, which is stimulated by the cold as well as by coffee, tea, and alcohol.

By causing the blood vessels near the skin surface to open, alcohol also increases heat loss. The notion that alcohol is warming, or that it ought to be given to a person suffering from cold, is a myth. It makes you colder, not warmer.

It's true that if you drink very cold liquids in winter, your body needs a few more calories to warm them up as they go into your digestive system. But this is not significant. Many people find that cold liquids quench thirst better than hot ones, in winter and summer. The important thing is to drink plenty of nonalcoholic, non-caffeinated liquids, whatever their temperature may be.

UNIVERSITY OF CALIFORNIA, BERKELEY WELLNESS LETTER

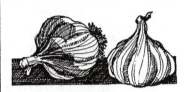

Garlic's Strength

Few foods are as Old World as garlic. Biting when raw, gentler as it cooks, it's the essential ingredient in many Italian, French, Greek, and Spanish dishes—as well as in the cuisine of China, Thailand, and other parts of the Far East.

If you like garlic's pungent punch, it can help give personality to dishes cooked with little salt. But it's more than flavor; garlic is a boon to the entire cardiovascular system.

The same chemical that causes garlic's odor—*ajoene*—reduces the tendency of blood to form artery-damaging clots. It's as effective as aspirin, studies show.

Other clinical studies find that garlic—in amounts normally eaten—lowers high levels of blood cholesterol, another heart-disease risk factor.

Garlic is also a good source of selenium, a trace mineral that, in the tiny amounts found in food, may help protect the body from cancer. Scientists are now busily exploring the cancer-protection possibility. But garlic's benefits have been known for centuries. Sir John Harrington wrote in *The Englishman's Doctor*, published in 1609: "Garlic then have power to save from death/Bear with it though it maketh unsavory breath."

BY ROBERT BARNETT

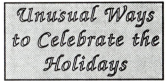

Unusual Ways to Celebrate the Holidays

☺ **Reminisce with close friends** about how they've celebrated past holidays. Incorporate some of their most successful ideas into your own celebration.

❄ **Have a healthful holiday** with a skinless turkey, baked potatoes, steamed vegetables, sugarless cranberry sauce, etc. Invite dieting friends.

☺ **Cheer up the holidays** for someone who has to work. Take a basket of seasonal goodies to the local police station, fire department, etc.

❄ **Rent a sleigh** or a horse and buggy and take your family for an old-fashioned ride in the country.

☺**Visit the neighborhood** where you grew up.

❄ **Pick up the telephone** to personally thank everyone who sends you a Christmas card.

☺**Visit a cathedral** on Christmas Eve for Midnight Mass.

❄ **Organize a stocking-stuffer party** to which the guests all bring tiny gifts for each other. *Set a theme:* travel, sports, personal development, etc.

Thoughts in December, 1989

The Rise and Fall of Ancient Greece

Since returning from our trip to Greece with Roy Pirrung, and having been a part of his heroic feat of running 155 miles in 27 hours and visiting the ruins of the ancient cities of Greece, I have become very interested with the ancient Greek civilization...how it came about... what it was like...why it collapsed.

Since returning, I have been studying the effect of Greek diets during the rise and fall of the Greek civilization. I noticed that the ancient Greeks ate what I consider the perfect diet — lots of fresh vegetables and fruits, olive oil, bread made with flax, beverages of barley and flax, some fish and sparse amounts of meat. I believe they adopted this diet more by accident than by design. It worked. The diet helped develop the finest athletes the world has ever known. No athlete today has ever repeated the feat of Pheidippides (the messanger who ran 300 miles in three days) or the feat of many other Greek athletes. The athletes of ancient Greece had such beautiful bodies of which copies of copies of copies of statues are still being sold to this day.

You might ask, "If the diet was so great, why did their civilization fall?" The answer is simple. Their diets changed. Why? I believe it was because they didn't know that it was the *Spartan diet* that made them so strong. Instead, they began thinking that it was because of their genes, their culture, their climate, and because they were chosen by God to be the best in the world. So they started doing a lot of celebrating. Instead of having feast days every couple of months, they began having them every month, then every fortnight, and eventually every day. They over-indulged in the "King's Dainties". They didn't even pay lip service to the Spartan diet which had made them strong.

With over-indulgence came debauchery. This, in turn, produced such weak bodies that they couldn't even run around the block. Not to mention they declined marching for hundreds of miles each week, like the original Greeks did. History clearly records this is the scenario for the fall of Alexander the Great. He became so fat that he couldn't even mount his horse. Then he became so weak he couldn't stay on his horse. Some leader he made!

Remember that the more you embellish the diet with excess animal fat, protein and sugared products, the weaker you become and the fatter you can get.

Reading health books, talking about nutritional foods, even lecturing others on the subject will not make you healthy, wealthy and wise. You must experience the benefits of nutritional foods.

362

Dear Paul and Barbara:

Just a few words to describe an anecdotal experience that I had recently at the Olympic Ice Rink in Milwaukee...

The day was December 21, 1989, with a record-low temperature of 15° below zero, combined with a powerful northwest wind. That day I wondered if I could "survive" the wind-chill factor of 58° below zero while skating twenty-five laps or six and one-half miles.

Although I am not a competitor or someone who is training for anything...and certainly far from being young—I am 59. I had no dificulty in handling the tissue-freezing temperatures.

In fact, I skated a total of fifty laps nonstop, attributable, I believe, to using your ENERGY DRINK and eating eight to ten slices of your OAT BRAN DELITE BREAD and 100% WHOLE GRAIN BREAD daily. (I had fourteen slices yesterday.)

All possible, continued success.
Respectfully,

J.K.,
Brookfield, WI

The Staff of Life, Improved

*Flax is the secret
ingredient in Paul
Stitt's healthy bread.*

BY TIMOTHY WALSH

More and more these days, Paul Stitt finds himself having to tell smooth-talking financiers that his bakery is not for sale. It's not surprising, given the national publicity his Natural Ovens of Manitowoc has received recently, especially by way of the National Cancer Institute, for championing of flax, a grain whose many benefits are just beginning to be appreciated. In the wake of an article about him in Forbes late last year, for instance, Stitt says he received about five buyout offers a day. But his business is definitely, emphatically, not for sale.

The soaring demand has been fueled in part by a growing interest in a basic ingredient used in most Natural Ovens products: flax. Recently, the National Cancer Institute announced $20.5 million program to study the anti-cancer properties of some select food substances, including flax. (The new NCI study marks a significant shift in cancer research. In the past, the focus has been on identifying foods that my cause cancer. The emphasis is now on finding foods that restore vital compounds to the body and therefore may fortify the body against carcinogens.)

Stitt holds the patent for stabilizing flaxseed for use in food. He expects to sign a cooperative research and development agreement with the NCI under which Natural Ovens will be a major supplier of foods for the study. The patent gives Stitt considerable control over the market for flax used in food, and he has recently sold stabilized flaxseed to food giants Kellogg's and General Mills.

He began using flax, a once-popular grain that had virtually disappeared from the American diet, when he was searching for a seed with a high oil content to replace processed oil in his breads. When Stitt—who holds a master's in biochemistry from the UW-Madison—tested flax, he couldn't believe what he saw. Here was a grain rich in fiber, vitamins and minerals, and with extremely high concentrations of Omega-3, the essential oil also found in fish and known to lower cholesterol and blood pressure levels.

Stitt's radical approach to nutrition carries over into his equally unconventional facilities in northeastern Wisconsin. On a 55-acre tract nestled amid the sprawling farmland just west of Manitowoc, the cathedral-like bakery rises up amid fields of oats, hay and wheat. A magnificent, three-story stained-glass window illuminates the building's reception area where Natural Ovens products are displayed and sold. Stacks of nutrition articles and the newsletters Stitt encloses with every loaf of bread are available for the taking, and free samples of whatever's coming out of the oven are offered.

Stitt himself can often be found in the reception area—which also doubles as an art gallery—talking to the legions of curious who drop in for one of the bakery's free tours. Indeed, the Manitowoc-Two Rivers Chamber of Commerce reports that Natural Ovens tours alone draw as many as 50 people to the area per day at the height of tourist season. Many of the visitors drive up from Milwaukee or Chicago to have a look at the bakery.

Natural Ovens employees are treated to free breakfasts and lunches, in keeping with Stitt's belief that a healthy diet is life's most essential factor. Looking ahead, Stitt sees the future of Natural Ovens closely tied to another product, Energy Drink, which also contains large amounts of flax along with oat bran and barley and a host of other nutrients.

One person who agrees with Stitt's view is ultramarathon champion Roy Pirrung of Sheboygan. Last September Pirrung, who is 42, finished fourth in the grueling 155-mile Spartathlon in Greece, consuming only Energy Drink, Natural Ovens bread and water along the way. "I set 18 personal bests in 1989," the year he began using Natural Ovens products, says Pirrung, "and I hadn't seen personal bests for four or five years before that."

Pirrung will be sponsored in next month's [September] Sparthathlon by Natural Ovens. He's gearing up for the race now by runnning an average 15 miles per day and consuming Energy Drink, Natural Ovens breads every day.

Stitt claims that Energy Drink promotes a "speeded-up recovery time" in athletes. "The body heals so much faster that athletes can go out and have a good workout the day after a tough meet or a tough game, and they're not sore," he says.

Other professional athletes are interested in the supposed healing powers of Energy Drink, too. Recently Stitt was invited to give a presentation to the Buffalo Bills football team. And four members of the Green Bay Packers organization, including Greg Blache, the defensive line coach, have been using Energy Drink, with what one calls "excellent results."

For the present, Stitt's immediate concern is simply keeping up with demand for his bread in Milwaukee, Minneapolis-St. Paul, Madison and Chicago his primary markets. Since no preservatives are used, Natural Ovens breads have a shelf life of just four days, which poses considerable distribution problems. "We spend more money delivering bread than we do making it," says Stitt.

Tours at Natural Ovens are given on Monday, Wednesday, Thursday and Friday at 9, 10, and 11am. Large groups should call 414/758-2500 for reservations. ∎

The following is an article from the Fond du Lac, Wisconsin weekly Action Sunday, July 22, 1990 edition. We thought many of you would be interested in another local athlete who has discovered the benefits of Energy Drink:

ATHLETE OF THE WEEK

With an eye on Olympic trials

Penny Braatz alters running pace

Much celebrated Fond du Lac runner Penny Braatz is shifting gears—both downward and upward, at the same time.

Braatz, the winner of nearly 200 trophies for a variety of short and middle distance event first place finishes where bursts of speed were in demand, is slowing her running pace.

Penny is becoming a marathon runner. Instead of the quick pace of 2- and 3-mile and 5- and 10-kilometer runs, Penny is eyeing the demanding 26.2 mile marathon where a steady pace and stamina are at a premium.

And with good reason. She feels that the marathon offers her the best opportunity to participate in the Olympics. But to even qualify for the Olympic trials, Penny has realized she must step up and intensify her training.

Preparations for a fall marathon are already in high gear. Penny trains nearly four hours each day including 4 a.m. workouts on a treadmill, biking and swimming. Then, after an 8-hour day at Prestige-Pak, Penny puts in another two hours of weight lifting and running.

"My goal is to get to the Olympic trials and to do that is going to require a lot of work," said the 26-year-old runner. "I've been successful in racing. But to be successful, you have to work at it. That's what keeps me going."

The marathon is a new challenge for Penny. She ran her first marathon in 1987 in Lake County, IL, and raised a few eyebrows with her performance. She not only won her age division, but she was the overall women's winner, quite a fete for a first attempt. Her finish in three hours and 50 seconds is still the fastest time for any female Fond du Lac runner.

"After that first marathon—and with winning it—I felt I realistically could make the trials," said Penny who admits she was just hoping for a top 10 finish in the race. "I really hadn't taken the time or trained as much as I could have, either. I feel I have the potential, as long as my knee holds up."

Because of bow legs, Penny has had some problems with a knee. But a recent readjusting of shoe supports seems to have corrected the problem. Before that, Penny had been limited to the amount of running and training she could complete.

"I'm getting results. The knee feels better than ever. And the adjustments I've made are working out, too, so I'm pretty confident that I'll be able to run and train the way I want."

Although she did not finish her second attempt at a marathon, she found out that she has the capability of making the qualifying time of two hours and 45 minutes that is needed to make the Olympic trials.

The last marathon was in Las Vegas and "I hit the wall at 21 miles," said Penny. "I was on the pace and would have done it, but it was just not my day."

Penny will try again this October in the Lakefront Marathon which is one of a select few races in which runners can qualify for the Olympic trials which will be held in Long Beach, CA, next year.

Only the top three runners at the trials qualify for the Olympics. Joan Benoit won the trials in 1987 after claiming a gold medal for the United States in the 1984 Summer Olympics.

For now, Penny is concentrating on this fall's marathon. She runs in the shorter races nearly every weekend, but, is not out just to finish first and add to a big trophy collection.

"I use the races as a speed workout," she explained. "And then I add to that with the longer runs." Her weekly regiment includes at least one run of between 15 and 20 miles, she noted. That is usually to her parents' home in Eden and back.

"To me, the time in a race or in training is more important," explained Penny. "It is the quality that I get out of a run that is important to me right now."

The results, though, as far as her supporters are concerned, have been the same. At a recent run, Penny left the field far behind and in the process, saved a whopping 59 seconds off her old record in the 5-K event.

It's been a long time since Penny was not the first female finisher in a race. Since May of last year, she has set 46 course records in 5-K and 2-mile races.

Penny credits her recent success—better times—with a diet that includes Energy Drink, a flax and oat bran mix that can be taken with a liquid or blended with a favorite fruit. It is made by Natural Ovens of Manitowoc and used by many other local athletes as an energy snack which aids recovery after prolonged exercise.

Penny also includes a lot of carbohydrates in her diet. Meals of pastas and breads supply energy. And since beginning to train for marathons, she has been experimenting with drinks that quickly replenish liquids and nutrients.

Penny quickly adds that she could not have accomplished what she has without help. And she knows she won't be able to go it alone from here on out, either. ■

Congratulations on your successes, Penny!

Fibers

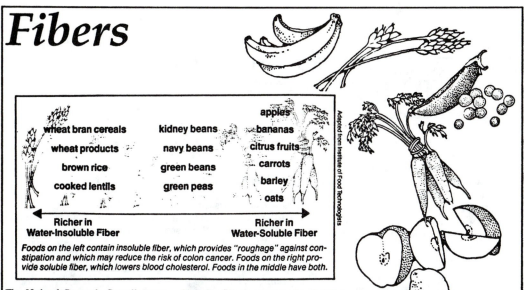

wheat bran cereals	kidney beans	apples
wheat products	navy beans	bananas
brown rice	green beans	citrus fruits
cooked lentils	green peas	carrots
		barley
		oats
Richer in Water-Insoluble Fiber		**Richer in Water-Soluble Fiber**

Adapted from Institute of Food Technologists

Foods on the left contain insoluble fiber, which provides "roughage" against constipation and which may reduce the risk of colon cancer. Foods on the right provide soluble fiber, which lowers blood cholesterol. Foods in the middle have both.

The National Research Council recommends that adults eat five or more daily servings of fruits and vegetables and six or more servings of breads, cereals and legumes—a diet that provides a good mixture of soluble and insoluble fiber. "Don't stick to one type of fiber," they advise. "The combination of fibers is very important."

Basically, fiber is any part of a plant that mammals can't digest. But just as the term "vegetable" includes foods as diverse as bell peppers, rhubarbs and bok choy, "fiber" encompasses a variety of substances with widely different properties. Its forms range from the rigid, insoluble cellulose that puts the snap in a stalk of celery to the gummy, soluble fiber of oat bran.

FROM SCIENCE NEWS, VOL. 136, Published every Saturday by SCIENCE SERVICE, Inc., 1719 N St., N.W., Washington, D.C. 20036; Phone 1-800-247-2160; Subscription rate: 1 yr., $34.50

Not just any green...broccoli

Broccoli is a superstar. Higher in nutrients than almost any other plant food, one cup of this leafy green vegetable, cooked, has 165 percent of the recommended dietary allowance for vitamin C, nearly half the daily vitamin A allowance (in the form of beta carotene), more than 20 percent of the RDA for calcium, 10 percent for iron, and some B vitamins, potassium, and other minerals. All this for only 45 calories—with negligible fat or sodium.

Few vegtables can top broccoli in fiber content as well. Cup for cup, it has more fiber than cauliflower, spinach, cabbage, or string beans.

As one of the brassica or cruciferous family of vegetables, broccoli also scores extra points because of evidence that these vegetables may be linked to the prevention of cancer, particularly of the lung, bladder and digestive tract. The Surgeon General specifically recommends cruciferous vegetables, which include, along with broccoli, cauliflower, bok choy, Brussels sprouts, cabbage, kohlrabi, mustard greens, rutabaga, collards, kale, and turnips.

Fresh broccoli, available year-round and often less expensive than frozen, is one of the better green vegetable buys. And as growing consumption figures attest (we now eat more than five times the broccoli we ate in 1972), this versatile vegetable fits easily into countless popular dishes. It is delicious on its own, raw or lightly steamed, in salads, as a companion to rice and other grains, chopped or puréed in soups, baked in casseroles, in sauces over pasta, and minced into omelettes or frittatas.*

—TUFTS UNIVERSITY DIET & NUTRITION LETTER

*A plate of vegetables with 1 or 2 slices of Natural Ovens Hunger Filler, 100% Whole Grain, Light Wheat or Sunny Millet Bread makes a deliciously satisfying meal.

WITH INTENSE EXERCISE

The most important thing is to drink, period—even if you don't feel thirsty. Thirst is satisfied long before you have replenished lost fluids. Research shows that cool water (40° to 50°) is absorbed more quickly than lukewarm water. In hot weather drink at least 16 to 20 ounces of water two hours before exercising and another 8 ounces 15 to 30 minutes before. While you exercise drink 3 to 7 ounces every 10 to 20 minutes. After exercising, drink enough to replace the fluid you've sweated off (weigh yourself before and after you workout; drink one pint for each pound lost) and eat whole foods.

UNIVERSITY OF CALIFORNIA, BERKELEY
WELLNESS LETTER
TO SUBSCRIBE:
P.O. BOX 420148
PALM COAST, FLORIDA
32142

A BIT ABOUT
BARLEY
BY PAUL A. STITT, M.S. BIOCHEMISTRY

Barley has been used for food for over 8000 years. It was one of the first domesticated plants along with wheat and several varieties of flax. According to ancient history the Spartans used a drink of barley and flax to keep them going for months at a time during battle.

● ● ● ● ● ● ● ● ● ● ● ● ● ● ● ● ● ● ●

Barley has been found to help ward off heart disease, constipation, other digestive ails and, possibly, tumors.

Experiments at the University of Wisconsin Medical School and Nutrition Science Department proved that capsules of barley oil could lower blood cholesterol up to 18% in patients who had bypass surgery. Barley, like rice, contains tocotrienol, which slows down the HMG reductase enzyme. This, in turn, produces the bad kind of cholesterol, the LDL type. Limonene, from lemon oil, also acts to reduce HMG reductase activity. Together, the two are more effective than either one separately.

Barley also contains protease inhibitors, like other grains, which suppresses tumor causing agents in the intestinal tract and may act as an antidote to over-growing cells.

Barley comes in various forms. Pearled barley has some of the bran removed and is excellent in almost any soup. Malted barley is barley that has been sprouted and some of the starch has been broken down to maltose. This is the variety that tastes sweet. Barley flour can also be used in bread baking, but it tastes somewhat bitter and is not preferred by most people. One place you won't find much barley is in beer. Before the beer is made, most of the good part in the barley is removed and used for animal feed.

Natural Ovens uses barley in our breads in the malted form to help bring out the sweetness in other grains as well as adding the health promoting properties in this very nutritional grain.

Fun things that don't cause cancer

RELAXATION — Some people go fishing. However you relax, it's important. Laboratory studies have indicated a link between chronic stress and cancer risk.

FRESH AIR — So fill up your lungs with it every chance you get. And don't smoke. Research shows that more than 20% of all cancers are caused by smoking. Whether it's your own or breathing someone else's.

HIGH FIBER FOODS — Like popcorn, whole grain breads, fruits and vegetables are just plain good.

A PINEAPPLE, AN ORANGE OR A PEAR— Fruit is a natural source of vitamins you need to stay healthy. And a healthy person has a better chance of staying that way.

BROCCOLI, LEAF LETTUCE OR CARROTS — When your mother told you to eat all your vegetables, she was right. Without them you dont' have a balanced diet. And that's critical.

EXERCISE — It helps to relax you, energize you, *and* keep your weight down. As that goes down so does your cancer risk. Brisk walking near trees and/or water is especially refreshing.

A GOOD DAY'S PAY — Earning money doesn't cause cancer, but where you earn it can. Strive for a clean-air work environment.

Author Unknown

Fun Fact...

● It's the release of a sulfur-containing substance in a newly cut onion that irritates your eyes and the lining of your nose. To help minimize the effect, refrigerate onions before you slice or chop them.

—UNIVERSITY OF TEXAS LIFETIME HEALTH LETTER

AND THEN CAME
NATURAL OVENS

In 1976, Paul Stitt [M.S. Biochemist, University of Wisconsin] began Natural Ovens because he saw a need — a need for fresh, preservative-free, whole-grain food in the Midwest. He saw that as scientists discovered more and more about the dangers of chemical additives and preservatives of synthetic sweetners and artificial flavorings, of white bread and white sugar, consumers became more concerned about their family's health.

As a biochemist, Paul knew the value of whole grains. He knew that they provided plenty of complex carbohydrates, protein, vitamins and minerals, as well as important dietary fiber.

So Paul started Natural Ovens, developing his own recipes and baking techniques to insure maximum nutrition.

Together with his wife, Barbara, their beautiful 28,000 square-foot bakery now stands as proof that delicious, nutritious, preservative free breads, cookies, muffins and rolls can be produced and successfully marketed.

Today Natural Ovens products are offered in over five hundred supermarkets in Wisconsin, Illinois and Minnesota.

NATURAL OVENS BREAD IS
WORTH THE FULL PRICE

The creation of bakery foods that truly promote healthful eating and the well-being of their customers is uppermost in the minds of Natural Ovens bakers.

At Natural Ovens, bakers embrace the lengthy and labor intensive sponge-and-dough bread production method. This procedure requires that the doughs ferment for more than three hours. It is this lengthy fermentation period that is responsible for the distinctive and robust flavors of Natural Ovens breads and rolls.

After the sponge has fermented, it is re-mixed with additional whole grain flours, flax-seed and fourteen vitamins and minerals to produce the dough.

Bakers then allow the bread to rise in an atmospherically-controlled chamber that further allows them to develop their natural bread flavors.

After the loaves have risen, bakers load them into a custom-designed hearth oven. The hearth oven's special design imparts the characteristic crusts that Natural Ovens customers desire.

Once the loaves cool, bakers slice and package Natural Ovens bakery foods into two packages. The inner package is a heavily constructed, airtight barrier bag. Just before the loaves are sealed in the airtight package they flush out the air and replace it with carbon dioxide. This expensive, controlled-atmosphere packaging process is used extensively in Europe to promote the freshness of bakery foods instead of using preservatives. Natural Ovens is the only domestic baker that packages its breads using this advanced, controlled atmosphere packaging technology.

From the very first step of the baking process to the last step of product packaging, Natural Ovens bakers have but one goal in mind. That is to produce only the finest nutritionally-dense bakery foods available anywhere. At any price.

WHAT'S COOKIN?

1988 marked the beginning of a new year in our new bakery. In January, Natural Ovens picked up and moved to our spacious, countryside location just south of Manitowoc along I-43.

Needless to say, it was quite a welcomed change. The new bakery is four times the size of our previous facility, stretching across a 55-acre countryside setting on County Trunk CR, 1½ miles south of Manitowoc.

You can witness the wonders of Natural Ovens whole-grain baking at our bakery located just south of Manitowoc off I-43. Tours are given on the hour Mondays, Wednesdays, Thursdays, and Fridays 9am—2pm and Sundays noon—2pm. Stop in and visit! [For large group reservations, call 414-758-2500.]

The first half of 1988 has been most exciting for Natural Ovens and Paul and Barbara Stitt. In January they moved into the newly constructed, 28,000 square foot bakery. In March, Natural Ovens was name, "The Industry of the Year," by the Manitowoc / Two Rivers Chamber of Commerce and on June 16th, Paul and Barbara Stitt received one of the four 1988 Arthur Young Entrepreneur of the Year awards for the state of Wisconsin. Presented with the Milerstone Award, Paul and Barbara were recognized for their perserverance in transforming a small-scale bakery into a successful, growing bakery that is now serving thousands of people in three states.

Natural Ovens beautiful Belgian parade horses have completed another summer making appearances in parades and state fairs from Minneapolis to Milwaukee. Their grandest display was as the traditional introduction team for the Great Circus Parade in Milwaukee. Watch for Buck, Bingo, Dick and Walker around your town next summer.

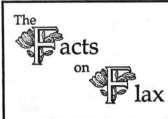

The Facts on Flax

Flax, *Linum Usitatissimum*, has a long and useful history as food and fiber. Linen cloth is spun from the plant's fibers, and flaxseed supplies oil and food protein, and lots of both.

History, ancient and modern

Archeologists say flax was being cultivated in Babylon at least as far back as 5000 B.C. Egyptian tombs contain bolts of finely woven linen, and even chairs with seats made of linen cord. In the 5th century B.C., the physician Hippocrates used flax to relieve abdominal pain and inflammation. Flax seeds have been found embedded in clay pots from many ancient cultures, indicating that flax has long been used as food.

Flax was a popular export product in this country, finding both food and industrial uses in Britain, Europe and Scandinavia, where it remained a major food oil until after WWII.

Buried treasure

Flaxseed and the oil it contains are rich sources of the "essential" Omega-3 fat called alpha-linolenic acid. Once consumed, it can be transformed by enzymes in the body to the ultrapolyunsturated fats, EPA and DHA, commonly found in fish. These fats form vital structural parts of every cell in the body, especially brain cells.

This was not widely known when Natural Ovens started experimenting with the use of flaxseed in bread several years ago.

Until 1985, Natural Ovens breads had been made with polyunsaturated oil to keep them soft and moist. At that time Paul Stitt received a phone call from a concerned doctor in Aurora, Illinois. He pointed out that all refined oils presented significant aflatoxin and rancidity problems.

When Paul asked what the doctor suggested he use instead, the reply was, "I don't know. You're the biochemist; you figure it out."

"Figuring it out"

There followed a period of experimentation. What kind of oil could be used that was not refined? Soybean presented rancidity problems. Olive oil had an inappropriate flavor. Could whole oil seed be used?

This led to the decision to try flaxseed. A test batch showed it worked; texture and taste were fine. Grinding techniques took a while to work out, but the problems of working with the small, hard, slippery seeds were not insurmountable.

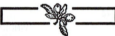

Meanwhile, Paul Stitt was finding out everything there was to know about flaxseed. At that time the data was pretty thin. A trip to the Flax Institute in Fargo, North Dakota yielded little information; searching through several libraries yielded less. But perseverance paid off, and the information trickled in. Little by little, an interesting picture was taking shape.

In 1985, articles appeared about the benefits of the essential fatty acids in fish oil, and controversy began about alpha-linolenic acid (nicknamed ALENA), found in flaxseed. Could enzymes in the human body transform ALENA into the same Omega-3 fats in fish oils? Controversy abounded.

Trying it out

It was time for more research. Through Essential Nutrient Research Corporation (ENRECO), Paul Stitt developed a product called Fortified Flax, made of ground flaxseed with added zinc, since flaxseed is low in that nutrient, and vitamin B6, since flaxseed contains a B6 antagonist.

He gave Fortified Flax away to thousands of volunteers in the community, and collected comments in an informal study. By the hundreds, people reported lowered blood cholesterol and blood pressure, less arthritic discomfort, better skin, and relief from constipation. (If you would like a copy of the study results, send a stamped, self-addressed envelope to Natural Ovens.)

Animals receiving flaxmeal showed similar benefits. Horses had shinier coats and stronger hooves. Chicks showed higher tissue levels of Omega-3 and stronger bones. Mink, fox—even tigers, bears and buffalo—given the meal ate their rations better, grew faster, had shinier coats and better dispositions.

The good news

Today, research continues on the benefits of flaxseed and Omega-3. The Flax Council of Canada has recently committed half a million dollars toward research on the effect of flaxseed on humans. A NATO-sponsored workshop held in Italy last June focused on Omega-3 fatty acids, with ALENA, the Omega-3 fatty acid found in flaxseed, getting the lion's share of attention.

New information is being compiled, and new products are being designed. High Energy Diet Food (see article on back of label) is a new product featuring human grade flaxseed.

As we find out more good news, we'll continue to share it with you. To your good health!

❀❅❀❅❀❅❀❅❀❅❀❅❀❅❀❅❀❅❀

The best all-around exercise

Cross-country skiing has lagged behind the downhill variety in popularity in the U.S., but in terms of all-around aerobic benefits it's the front runner. Using muscles in the shoulders, back, chest, abdomen, buttocks, and legs, cross-country skiers can burn as many as 600 to 900 calories per hour. Champion cross-country skiers expend upwards of 1000 calories per hour and have set records for the highest levels of oxygen consumption ever, indicating excellent aerobic fitness. The kick-and-glide technique, combined with the poling motion that propels you along, can provide a more complete workout than running or cycling, which emphasize lower-body muscles. It can also help develop coordination.

Another advantage of cross-country skiing is that it has a lower risk of serious injury than skiing on the slopes. Also, you can rent (or buy) skis, poles, and boots for a fraction of what you would pay for downhill gear. You don't need to make any reservations at high-priced ski resorts, because you can cross-country ski in a nearby park or even your own backyard. Most people don't need a lesson before starting out, yet a good instructor can help with advanced technique.

Burning so many calories generates a lot of heat even on the coldest days, so it's best to dress in layers that your can peel off. You can start off in loose fitting jeans or knickers (which are good for mobility), long cotton underwear, a couple of shirts, and a wool sweater. And don't forget a wool hat and lightweight insulated mittens or gloves.

-edited from the **University of California, Berkeley Wellness Letter**

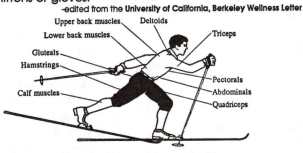

Upper back muscles — Deltoids
Lower back muscles — Triceps
Gluteals
Hamstrings — Pectorals
Calf muscles — Abdominals — Quadriceps

Major muscles and muscle groups conditioned by cross-country skiing.

Manitowoc County has some excellent cross-country trails to offer. Fox Hills Resort in Mishicot has a rental service and trail excellent for beginners. Point Beach State Forest has beautiful trails that wind through this lakeside site. For more information on Manitowoc County's cross-country ski trails and lodging call the Manitowoc Lakeshore Development Bureau, 414/684-3678 or write them at 1515 Memorial Drive, Manitowoc, Wisconsin 54220.

❄

Baking Soda

A Simple Solution to Many Everyday Troubles

𝕋he solution to dozens of your most nagging problems is probably sitting on a shelf in your kitchen. Sodium bicarbonate, commonly called baking soda, has unique physical and chemical characteristics that allow it to...

Eliminate odors. In the refrigerator, litter box, dishwasher, etc. Place open one-pound boxes in the refrigerator and freezer. Cover the bottom of the cat litter box with baking soda and add the usual amount of litter. Sprinkle a quarter cup in the bottom of the disherwasher between loads.

Treat acid indigestion. Dissolve a level half teaspoon in half a glass of water and drink.

Relieve poison ivy and bee stings. Make a paste of baking soda and water and apply it to the affected areas.

Eliminate acid build-up on car battery terminals. Apply a baking soda paste to the terminals and wipe clean.

Help disinfect your swimming pool. Baking soda can provide reserve alkalinity to help prevent pH swings. Ask your pool supply dealer about the appropriate amount for your pool.

Improve the efficiency of your septic tank. The bacteria that break down waste in septic tanks produce acid...but they function better in a neutral environment. One cup of baking soda per week (just flush it down the toilet) neutralizes the acids.

Put out *small* kitchen and electrical fires. Baking soda contains carbon dioxide, which smothers fire. *Warning:* Do not use it on deep-fat fires--the fire could spread.

Brush your teeth. Baking soda will leave your mouth feeling cleaner than comerical toothpaste and it removes plaque without abrasion.

Make skin feel softer. Add about half a cup to your bath water.

Make your dish detergent more effective. Add one tablespoon to dishwater when you wash dishes.

Get your laundry cleaner, for less money. Use only half the regular amount of liquid bleach and add half a cup of baking soda to top loaders, a quarter cup to front loaders. The bleach will work more effectively...and it won't leave a strong smell on your clothes.

-Bottom Line Personal
to subscribe write:
Bottom Line/Personal
Subscription Service Department,
P. O. Box 58446
Boulder CO 80322
bi-monthly, $49/yr.

Children and nutrition:

Behavior problems…or symptoms of inadequate diet?

Are your children getting adequate nutrition—not just enough to eat, but the right kinds of food?

You may be surprised to learn that 1 in 5 American children are not receiving the Recommended Daily Allowance (RDA) of major nutrients, including iron, thiamin, riboflavin, niacin, vitamin B6, magnesium and zinc, as well as about 17 other nutrients.

Eleanor Whitney, R.D., Ph.D., is the author of three leading college nutrition textbooks, and co-owner of the Nutrition Co. of Tallahasse, Florida, a resource and eduction center for nutrition professionals. Dr. Whitney has compiled a list of behaviors and symptoms that could signal nutrient deficiencies.

Nutrition deficiency symptom checklist

Iron—fatigue, weakness, headaches, pallor, listlessness, irritability, learning disorders, anorexia, apathy, a tendency to develop lead toxicity.

Thiamin—confusion, poor coordination, depressed appetite, irritability, sleep disturbances, fatigue, general misery.

Riboflavin—depression, hysteria, psychopathic behavior, lethargy, hypochondria.

Niacin—irritability, agitated depression, headaches, sleeplessness, memory loss, emotional instability.

Vitamin B6—irritability, insomnia, weakness, mental depression, fatigue, headaches.

Vitamin C—hysteria, depression, listlessness, lassitude, weakness, aversion to work, hypochondria, social introversion, fatigue.

Magnesium—apathy, personality changes, hyperirritability.

Zinc—poor appetite, failure to grow, irritability, emotional disorders, mental lethargy.

The care and feeding of your family

Children and adults alike need good food, but we cannot always control what our kids eat.

However, we can keep good foods on hand. Fresh fruits should be kept on hand and in sight. Fresh vegetables cleaned and cut up in the refrigerator are convenient and accessible. A bowl of popcorn can tempt a hungry teenager to forget about sweets. Fruit juice will do, if there is no soda.

Natural Ovens products are tasty and nutritious. Branana Nut, Blueberry-Oat or Cherry-Almond Oat Bran Muffins can fill a child up with good nutrition.

If your child is exhibiting serious symptoms, check with your family doctor. You may need to use nutritional supplements. But try adding wholesome, whole foods to your child's diet—and your own. Find out how good you can feel!

Nutrition Mistakes Moms Make

Though your intentions are good, your way of getting your kids to eat better may be bad for them.

By Rosalind Charney, Ph.D.

Edited from REDBOOK Magazine, October 1989

"You have to eat, even if you're not hungry."
Parents need to realize that all children, even finicky eaters, will eat when they're hungry. Never force a child to eat against his will. Reprimands such as "Clean your plate," or "Drink all your milk," only undermine a child's natural ability to determine whether or not he or she needs to eat. Instead, ask your children questions like, "Are you hungry?" or What would you like to eat?"

"No snacking between meals!"
Just as a parent should never force a child to eat when the child isn't hungry, neither should a parent forbid a child to eat. There is nothing wrong, of course, with enforcing a rule of "no snacks right before dinner" if a parent feels that snacks will spoil a child's appetite. Parents can further reinforce a child's healthy eating habits by making sure that all the food in the house is nutritious, even the snacks.

"If you're good, you'll get a treat."
The connection between food and love runs very deep in many of us. But it is important that children see food for what it is: good-tasting fuel for the body, *not* a form of love. Parents should give affection and approval through direct words and actions, not through food. Children who are constantly told, "You can have a snack because you were a good girl," or "If you're nice to the babysitter, she will bake you some cookies," may begin to associate food with approval and may then feel loved only when rewarded with a special treat. Later in life, when they're feeling sad or lonely, they may again turn to food as a source of comfort, which can then lead to problems such as overeating.

Food also should never be used as a punishment. A child should not be deprived of food as a way of pressuring him to behave; nor should he be forced to eat a food he dislikes because he has misbehaved. Such tactics can lead to severe eating disorders later on.

"It's important to be thin."
Americans are victims of a cruel paradox. We are continually being encouraged to eat, while also being reminded of how important it is to be thin. Teach your child that each individual has a weight and shape that is appropriate for that person, and that not everyone can, or should, be "model" thin. Children who are taught that thinness doesn't make a person smarter, nicer or more desirable, will grow up to be more accepting of themselves and others.

"I hate my body."
The best way to teach your children healthy attitudes toward food and eating, of course, is to set a good example yourself. Ideally, this means that you respect your body no matter what its size, eat nutritious foods* and do so only when you're hungry. Always reinforce your child's healthy attitudes and behavior. Remember, the younger the child, the better your chance of helping establish good eating habits. ▫

*Nutritious foods are: whole fresh vegetables, fruits, grains, whole grain breads, beans, lentils, brown rice, seeds, nuts, sprouts, etc.

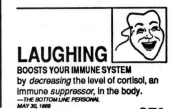

LAUGHING
BOOSTS YOUR IMMUNE SYSTEM
by *decreasing* the level of cortisol, an immune *suppressor,* in the body.
—*THE BOTTOM LINE PERSONAL*
MAY 30, 1989

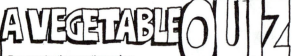

A VEGETABLE QUIZ

Try answering these questions and see how many you know. Then ask the rest of your family to try them, maybe sometime when you're all eating together.

1. What is the most ancient vegetable still grown today?

2. What's the biggest selling vegetable in the U. S. today?

3. What vegetable do you eat that is related to the morning glory? (Hint: It's often eaten at Thanksgiving.)

4. What vegetable is usually used to make pickles?

5. Name a vegetable that you can eat both the leaves and the roots of.

6. Name all the vegetables that you can think of that are reddish in color, inside or outside or both.

7. What vegetable is a member of the cabbage family and looks like miniature cabbages?

8. When this vegetable was first grown in the U. S., you'd have to take a train to Kalamazoo, Michigan, to get some. What is it?

9. There is a vegetable that is related to the lily. What is it?

10. About how many kernels are on a corncob about eight inches long?

11. How come people sometimes say that someone is "cool as a cucumber"?

12. What kind of vegetable is an "aubergine"?

13. What vegetable is very dangerous to pick wild and eat?

14. Which state in the U. S. grows the most spinach?

15. Which vegetable is sold mostly in October?

A VEGETABLE QUIZ ANSWERS

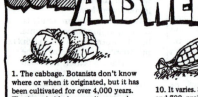

1. The cabbage. Botanists don't know where or when it originated, but it has been cultivated for over 4,000 years. That's probably because it grows almost anywhere.

2. The potato is first, followed by lettuce and tomatoes.

3. It's the sweet potato.

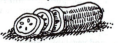

4. Cucumber, usually, though people have been known to pickle all sorts of things, including the rind of watermelons.

5. You can eat the greens and the roots of the beet and turnip. Do you know any others?

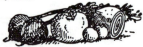

6. Some reddish vegetables: beets, red cabbage, red onions, tomatoes, radishes.

7. Brussel sprouts.

8. It's celery.

9. The onion is related to the lily.

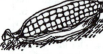

10. It varies. Somewhere between 600 and 700, probably.

11. That's because a cucumber really is cool inside, about 20 degrees cooler than the air outside on a warm day.

12. "Aubergine" is the French name for the eggplant. It's used in Great Britain too.

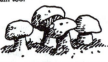

13. Mushrooms. Some mushrooms are highly poisonous and can cause death.

14. Texas.

15. Pumpkins, of course. About 80 percent of all the pumpkins sold each year are sold in October.

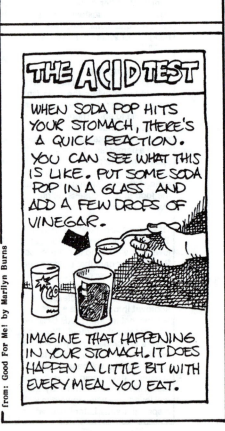

from: Good For Me! by Marilyn Burns

THE ACID TEST

WHEN SODA POP HITS YOUR STOMACH, THERE'S A QUICK REACTION. YOU CAN SEE WHAT THIS IS LIKE. PUT SOME SODA POP IN A GLASS AND ADD A FEW DROPS OF VINEGAR.

IMAGINE THAT HAPPENING IN YOUR STOMACH. IT DOES HAPPEN A LITTLE BIT WITH EVERY MEAL YOU EAT.

A SUGAR TEST

HERE'S SOMETHING FOR YOU TO TRY THAT GIVES YOU A CHANCE TO ACTUALLY FEEL WHAT SUGAR DOES.

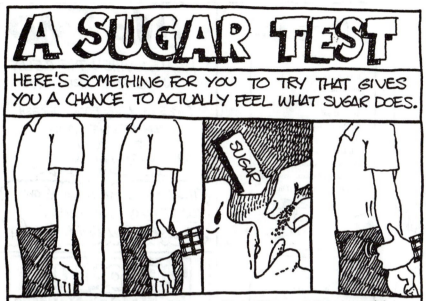

You need a friend or one of your parents or a sister or brother to help out. What you do is stand, arms at your sides, with the palms of your hands facing out and the backs of your hands against your leg.

Have the other person hold your wrist and try to pull your arm away from your body while you do your best to resist. It may or may not be possible for the person to pull your arm up. That's not as important as you feeling how your are able to tighten up your arm muscles and resist the pull. Try this now to get that feeling.

Now the other person will do the same thing again. But first, take a small pinch of sugar, about the amount that you can hold in between your thumb and forefinger. Put that teeny pinch on your tongue and swallow it. Now have the other person pull on your arm again.

What will happen is that you won't be able to resist this second time. Remember, it's not a tug-of-war between the two of you. It's an experiment to help you judge your own ability to use those upper arm muscles with and without the influence of sugar. Right after putting the sugar on your tongue, your arm muscles just won't work for you in the same way.

What's happening here? It's the sugar. Your body is reacting against the sugar in a very special way — you lose strength in your arms — and instantaneously. It's a startling experiment, and it gives you a clue to how your body really feels about sugar.

You might want to try this with someone who is stronger than you are, someone whose arm you couldn't possibly pull away. See if you can do it when they've put that pinch of sugar on their tongue.

from: *Good For Me!* by Marilyn Burns

What kind of fish can you put on bread?   A Jellyfish!

HIGH JUMP

If you exercised every day, could you jump as high as a house? You sure could—because a house can't jump!

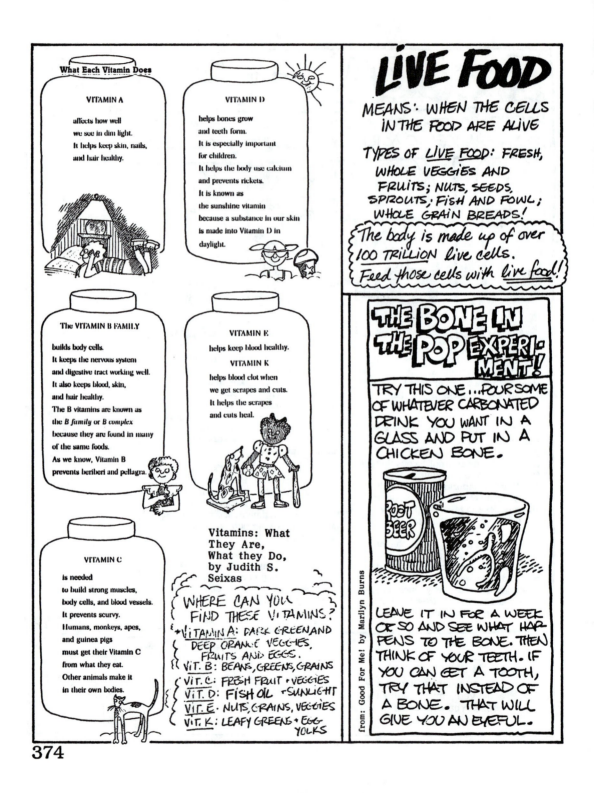

What Each Vitamin Does

VITAMIN A

affects how well
we see in dim light.
It helps keep skin, nails,
and hair healthy.

VITAMIN D

helps bones grow
and teeth form.
It is especially important
for children.
It helps the body use calcium
and prevents rickets.
It is known as
the sunshine vitamin
because a substance in our skin
is made into Vitamin D in
daylight.

The VITAMIN B FAMILY

builds body cells.
It keeps the nervous system
and digestive tract working well.
It also keeps blood, skin,
and hair healthy.
The B vitamins are known as
the B family or B complex
because they are found in many
of the same foods.
As we know, Vitamin B
prevents beriberi and pellagra.

VITAMIN E

helps keep blood healthy.

VITAMIN K

helps blood clot when
we get scrapes and cuts.
It helps the scrapes
and cuts heal.

VITAMIN C

is needed
to build strong muscles,
body cells, and blood vessels.
It prevents scurvy.
Humans, monkeys, apes,
and guinea pigs
must get their Vitamin C
from what they eat.
Other animals make it
in their own bodies.

Vitamins: What
They Are,
What they Do,
by Judith S.
Seixas

WHERE CAN YOU FIND THESE VITAMINS?
+ VITAMIN A: DARK GREEN AND DEEP ORANGE VEGGIES, FRUITS AND EGGS.
VIT. B: BEANS, GREENS, GRAINS
VIT. C: FRESH FRUIT + VEGGIES
VIT. D: FISH OIL + SUNLIGHT
VIT. E: NUTS, GRAINS, VEGGIES
VIT. K: LEAFY GREENS + EGG YOLKS

LIVE FOOD

MEANS: WHEN THE CELLS IN THE FOOD ARE ALIVE

TYPES OF LIVE FOOD: FRESH, WHOLE VEGGIES AND FRUITS; NUTS, SEEDS, SPROUTS; FISH AND FOWL; WHOLE GRAIN BREADS!

The body is made up of over 100 TRILLION live cells. Feed those cells with live food!

THE BONE IN THE POP EXPERI-MENT!

TRY THIS ONE...POUR SOME OF WHATEVER CARBONATED DRINK YOU WANT IN A GLASS AND PUT IN A CHICKEN BONE.

ROOT BEER

LEAVE IT IN FOR A WEEK OR SO AND SEE WHAT HAPPENS TO THE BONE. THEN THINK OF YOUR TEETH. IF YOU CAN GET A TOOTH, TRY THAT INSTEAD OF A BONE. THAT WILL GIVE YOU AN EYEFUL.

from: Good For Me! by Marilyn Burns

374

Nutrition • You Are What You Eat

In olden times, farmers grew plants not only to eat, but also for their ability to cure certain diseases. Plants were given names such as Heart's Ease, Heal-All, Boneset, and Eyebright. The plants were named this way because the farmers felt that these plants helped their bodies to remain healthy. The health-giving properties of plants were discovered over hundreds of years of experimentation.

What early farmers didn't know about (at least in the way we do today) was the science of nutrition. **Nutrition** is the study of food and how it affects our health. To remain healthy, our bodies need a daily supply of **vitamins, minerals, proteins, fats, and carbohydrates.** These are called **nutrients.** The vegetables and even the flowers in your garden contain these nutrients. Without them you would become sick, and if you don't eat enough of them, perhaps you are not as healthy as you might be.

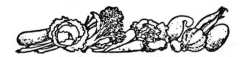

LADYBUGS & LETTUCE LEAVES
The Center for Science in
the Public Interest

Vegetable and Fruit Nutrition Chart
— Serious vitamin deficiencies are rare in the United States and Canada —

VITAMIN	BEST SOURCES	WHAT IT DOES FOR YOU
A	Pumpkins Winter squash Sweet potatoes Collard greens Carrots Kale Broccoli Spinach Red peppers Watermelon Tomatoes	Keeps eyes healthy and capable of seeing well at night (prevents night blindness)
B	Broccoli Peanuts Peas Turnip greens Lima beans Brussels sprouts Collard greens Dried beans and peas	Keeps skin, eyes, and hair healthy. Helps nerves function properly. Helps the body make blood. Enables you to use the energy found in carbohydrates (bread, potatoes, pasta).
C	Green peppers Collard greens Brussels sprouts Oranges Strawberries Tomatoes Grapefruit Canteloupe	Helps heal wounds. Helps make cementing materials that hold body cells together. Keeps gums healthy Fights infection.
D	Not found in vegetables, but if you work in the garden you'll get plenty of it from sunshine. It's called the sunshine vitamin; eggs and milk also contain this vitamin.	Helps calcium make strong bones and teeth.
E	Vegetable oils Green leafy vegetables	Helps keep membranes surrounding cells strong and healthy.

MINERALS

Calcium	Collard greens Broccoli Kale Swiss chard Dried beans	Works with Vitamin D to build bones and teeth.
Iron	Broccoli Peas Beans Leafy green vegetables	Helps blood carry oxygen.

CHICKEN WITH BASMATI RICE, CASHEW NUTS, AND ORANGES

A one-dish meal.
1 tbsp. extra virgin olive oil
3 to 3½ lb. whole frying chicken (with or without skin), quartered
1½ c. chicken broth
1 c. water
1½ c. uncooked brown basmati rice
1 large red or green bell pepper, cut into one-inch strips
2 ribs celery, with leaves, thinly sliced
1 medium size onion, diced
1 to 2 cloves garlic, minced
Sea salt, black pepper and/or cayenne, to taste (optional)
¼ c. orange honey
2 tbsp. grated orange rind
2 scallions, thinly sliced
2 tbsp. finely chopped fresh parsley (save half for garnish)
1 c. lightly toasted, unsalted cashew nuts or equal amount whole or sliced almonds or pignolia (pine) nuts
Paprika, for garnish
1 to 2 medium-size oranges, sliced or cut into attractive garnish

In large skillet (preferably cast iron), heat oil over high heat until very hot. Place chicken in pan, skin-side down. Cover and braise until slightly browned. Turn and continue to braise until slightly browned on other side. Remove from skillet and set aside. Pour off excess oil from skillet, return to heat, and pour in chicken broth and water. Stir vigorously to deglaze pan. Add rice and bring to boil. Cover, reduce heat to low simmer, and cook 30 minutes. Uncover, add next five ingredients, and stir into rice. Drizzle one-eighth of the honey over rice and sprinkle in one tablespoon of the orange rind. (Add one-half cup water, if necessary.) Place chicken on top of rice. Drizzle remaining honey over chicken along with a sprinkle of remaining orange rind, salt, and a little paprika, if desired. Cover and cook over medium-low heat for 30 minutes. Uncover, remove chicken, and set aside. Add scallions, parsley, and nuts, and quickly stir into rice. Cook another three minutes. Place rice on large heated platter and arrange chicken over mixture. Garnish with paprika and parsley, and place orange slices around chicken in an attractive manner. Serve immediately. Yields four abundant servings. □

Fascinating facts

• By her thirteenth wedding anniversary, the average married American woman has gained 23 pounds, while her husband has put on 18 pounds, according to the American Dietetic Association.

• You must brush your teeth for at least five minutes to remove plaque effectively, according to a study done at the University of Iowa. The typical American brushes her teeth for only 30 seconds, long enough to remove only 10% of accumulated plaque.

UNIVERSITY OF CALIFORNIA, BERKELEY WELLNESS LETTER

The Mind/Body Connection

People have always known that the mind can affect the body, but that knowledge was forgotten, or at least ignored, during a good part of the 1900s. *Reason:* It is only in this century that we've developed specific treatments for illnesses—antibiotics for bacterial infections, etc. These new treatments, which often mean the difference between life and death, are so potent that we forgot the mind/body connection. Now the pendulum is swinging back.

BREAKING THE STRESS CONNECTION

People under stress have an increase in common ailments—stomachaches, headaches, indigestion, back pain and the common cold. *What to do:*

• *Improve your lifestyle.* People who live on fast foods and cigarettes need to pay attention to what they are putting into their bodies and start getting some exercise.

• *Understand your symptoms.* Illness is a feedback system. In order to get well, you have to understand why and how a particular symptom hits you.

• *Regulate your autonomic nervous system* via psychophysiological self-regulation—using your mind to help regulate your body. This begins with learning how to breathe, followed by relaxation exercises.

AVOIDING MIND TRAPS

Because your body is completely connected with your thoughts, it's easy to feel that whatever is on your mind at any given moment is all there is. When you're worried about something, your whole body is worried.

It's important to learn to identify less with the thoughts that fill your mind and to become a detached, objective observer of those thoughts. Then you can begin to develop discrimination—to decide when you need to take further action on a problem and when you should simply let it go.

We found this article interesting and thought you may also. These tips came from: Bottom Line/Personal, Box 1027, Millburn, N.J. 07041 (24 issues for $39). We think it's a great magazine.

THE BUGS BUNNY DIET

"Are carrots really good for your eyes?" asks the straight man in the old joke. Answer: "Did you ever see a rabbit wearing glasses?" Carrots are definitely good for your eyes, since they are the world's richest source of beta carotene, which the body converts to vitamin A, a crucial nutrient for the health of the retina. Besides that, beta carotene, an antioxidant, is now also believed to be a protector against cancer. And carrots may also help lower blood cholesterol.

Carrots are a smart way to get your beta carotene and vitamin A. Just one three-ounce carrot has enough beta carotene to supply your body with five times the vitamin A it needs daily. A carrot also contains one to two grams of dietary fiber--and it's the kind of fiber that helps lower cholesterol. Carrots are among the sweetest-tasting vegetables, yet that three-ounce specimen has only 35 calories.

A word of caution about the rabbits-and-glasses issue: vitamin A won't cure nearsightedness or farsightedness and can improve vision only if vision problems result from a vitamin A deficiency, which is a rare condition in this country.

Source: University of California, Berkeley
Wellness Letter

☐ Note: Natural Ovens newest loaf, KIDZ Bread is supplemented with beta-carotene. As a matter of fact, the beta-carotene is what gives KIDZ Bread its "already-buttered" look. Two slices of KIDZ Bread provides 1/3 of the Recommended Daily Allowance.

ZINC TABLETS EASE COLD DISTRESS

Sucking--not swallowing--tablets of zinc gluconurate can ease cold symptoms, according to Dr. David Tyrell of the British Medical Council's Common Cold Unit. He did a study of zinc gluconurate to follow up an accidental finding by an American, George Eby, whose younger daughter said her cold got better when she sucked the tablets she was taking for a zinc deficiency.

Dr. Tyrell's study found fewer sneezes and sniffles in cold patients who got the zinc tablets than in those who got a placebo.

Reason: Zinc may work by preventing cold virus reproduction, say the researchers. They found no evidence that zinc tablets can prevent colds or stop their spread . . . but symptoms are eased and this mineral may be preferable to drugs!   THE NUTRITION & DIETARY CONSULTANT

Young Americans Getting High

Behavior Today magazine reports that American adolescents use illicit drugs more widely than their peers in any other industrialized nation. They stated that fifty-eight percent use unlawful drugs before finishing high school. Moreover, one in twenty uses alcohol or marijuana **daily**.

Solution: Change food selections to provide the youngster with lots of fresh vegetables, fresh fruit, whole grains (brown rice, whole wheat, etc.), seeds, legumes (lentils, beans, etc.), 6-8 glasses of pure water, and exercise. Eliminate refined and processed foods, soft drinks and other sugared or caffeine products.

Results: Better health, better grades, and much better self image. Happy, healthy children grow up to be healthy, happy adults. Addictive foods, starting with the sugared cereals, candy, soft drinks and colored sweet drinks set up a pattern for addiction. Avoiding these addictions can lead to another high--getting high on life.

Kristina's Potato Salad

Scrub 6 medium potatoes and boil them in their skins until they're tender, but not mushy. (You might want to save the water you boiled them in for soup stock.) Drain and cool.

Combine:
The potatoes, skins & all, diced
2 chopped, hard-cooked eggs
2 diced, medium tomatoes
a chopped red or green pepper
2 minced scallions
a chopped cucumber
chopped, fresh parsley
alfalfa sprouts
½ cup toasted cashews
¼ cup, mixed, toasted sunflower and sesame seeds
3/4 - 1 cup mayonnaise
1 - 2 tsp. Vegesal
fresh black pepper
dash of tamari
½ cup cider vinegar
½ tsp. dry mustard
½ tsp. tarragon
1 tsp. prepared horseradish

Chill well. Serve on fresh spinach with olives and lemon wedges.

From Moosewood Cookbook by Mollie Katzen

Making choices

Can certain foods cause or prevent cancer? The answer, so far, is maybe. This chart outlines the smart choices.

SUBSTANCE	MAJOR DIETARY SOURCES	SUSPECTED ROLE IN CANCER	COMMENT
POSSIBLE PROTECTORS			
Beta carotene (transformed into vitamin A by the body)	Yellow, orange, and green leafy vegetables and fruit, such as carrots, cantaloupe, broccoli, yams, spinach	Deficiency may increase risk of lung, stomach, cervical, bladder, and other cancers.	This antioxidant is thought to be more anticarcinogenic than dietary vitamin A. Extra carotene is stored in most tissue for future use. Not toxic.
Vitamin A	Liver, egg yolk, fish oil	Deficiency may cause abnormal cell growth, possibly leading to cancerous tumors.	Much of its protectiveness is due to beta carotene (above).
Vitamin C	Citrus fruits, tomatoes, broccoli, strawberries, potatoes, peppers, kale (C is destroyed by improper storage or long cooking)	Deficiency of this antioxidant may increase risk of cancer of stomach and esophagus. May block conversion of nitrites and nitrates to cancer-causing agents.	Adult RDA is 60 milligrams, supplied by 4 ounces of fresh orange juice. Unused C is excreted. Megadoses (over 1 gram daily) can cause diarrhea
Vitamin E	Nuts, liver, whole grains, wheat germ, dried beans	An antioxidant. Shown to protect lab animals against some cancers.	Enjoy dark green vegetables, eggs and wheat germ.
Selenium	Seafood, liver, meats, grains, egg yolks, tomatoes	An antioxidant. Shown to protect lab animals against some cancers.	No RDA. Plentiful in most diets. Supplements can be extremely dangerous.
Fiber	Found only in plant foods, such as fruits, vegetables, whole grains	Promotes healthy bowel function. May lower risk of colon and rectal cancer.	Choose whole-grain breads and cereals. Eat fruit and vegetables with skins when possible.
Cruciferous vegetables	Vegetables of the cabbage family, e.g., broccoli, kale, Brussels sprouts, cauliflower	Contain antioxidants that may block production of potential cancer-causing agents in lab animals.	Eat at least 2-3 servings each week. Excellent sources of fiber, minerals, and vitamins.
POSSIBLE VILLAINS			
Fats	Meats, poultry skin, whole milk and milk products, vegetable oils	Excess consumption of fats may contribute to cancers of the digestive and reproductive systems and to obesity, another risk factor for cancer.	Choose lean meats; trim all visible fat and discard poultry skin; don't fry meats. Eat fish. Avoid high-fat processed foods.
Alcohol	Beer, wine, liquor	Heavy drinking, especially combined with smoking, contributes to cancers of the mouth, throat, liver, and bladder. May also be a factor in breast cancer.	Drink only in moderation, if at all: no more than 2 drinks a day.
Nitrites	Used to preserve cured meats, such as bacon, hot dogs, sausages, ham	Promotes cancers of stomach and esophagus in lab animals.	Avoid eating cured meats habitually. Use low-temperature cooking methods.
Aflatoxins	Poisons formed in moldy peanuts, peanut butter, seeds, corn, and other crops	If eaten in large amounts, can cause liver cancer, a rare disease in this country.	Discard moldy, shriveled, discolored peanuts. Refrigerate freshly ground peanut butter; discard entire jar if moldy.
Browned foods	Meats grilled, barbecued, or fried at high temperatures	These cooking methods create cancer-causing agents. Most dangerous when cooking fatty meat over a heat source.	As often as possible, choose other cooking methods—steam, bake, roast.

UNIVERSITY OF CALIFORNIA, BERKELEY WELLNESS LETTER

A papaya a day keeps the doctor away. Papayas have 48 times more vitamin A, 14 times more vitamin C, four times the calcium, triple the potassium and more than double the vitamin B of apples--and fewer calories.

Appendicitis prevention: Eat plenty of peas, beans, brussels sprouts and cabbage. Theory: These foods subdue bacteria that inflame the appendix.

Bottom Line
PERSONAL

Sprouting Seeds to Eat

Seeds of certain plants can be sprouted easily and eaten as nutritious, low-calorie vegetables. Alfalfa seeds, mung beans, chick peas, lentils, and wheat grains are among the most commonly sprouted seeds. Sprouts are crisp and delicious in sandwiches, soups, salads, and just plain. To sprout seeds, follow these directions. (Be careful not to sprout too many seeds at once. Because seeds increase greatly in size after sprouting, use about ¼ cup of seeds for every quart jar you would like to fill.)

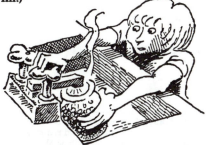

1. Rinse seeds in a jar and soak them in warm water overnight.

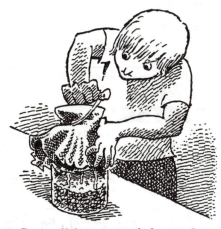

2. Drain off the water and place seeds in a large jar. Secure several layers of cheesecloth or fine plastic mesh over the mouth of the jar with a rubber band.
3. Keep the jar in a warm (68° to 74°), dark place.

4. Rinse the seeds 2 to 3 times each day with warm water, leaving the cheesecloth or wire mesh in place.
5. After rinsing, leave the container inverted so the excess water will run off.

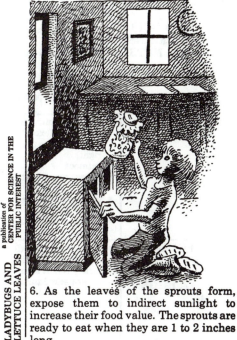

LADYBUGS AND LETTUCE LEAVES a publication of CENTER FOR SCIENCE IN THE PUBLIC INTEREST

6. As the leaves of the sprouts form, expose them to indirect sunlight to increase their food value. The sprouts are ready to eat when they are 1 to 2 inches long.

SPROUTZA

Here's a fun, easy, and delicious way to combine sprouts with a favorite food: pizza. The recipe is adapted from Jane Brody's "Pizza Patty," in Jane Brody's *Nutrition Book*, W.W. Norton and Company, Inc. 1981.

Makes two servings

Equipment
Broiler
Knife
Spoon

Ingredients
2 slices English Muffin or Kidz bread
2 tablespoons tomato sauce
2 slices tomato
Bean sprouts
Oregano

Directions
Top each slice of bread with tomato sauce, one tomato slice, a sprinkling of oregano, and enough sprouts to cover.
Broil until bread is toasty.

Do you have to give up all your favorite foods just because they're not the healthiest foods? No! Just eat them <u>less</u> often, and eat the more healthful ones <u>more</u> often. This list can help you know how.

YOUR EATING GUIDE

	ANYTIME	IN MODERATION	NOW & THEN
BEANS GRAINS & NUTS	• wholegrain breads & rolls • dried beans & peas • brown rice • plain popcorn • whole grain cereal • whole wheat pasta	• white bread or rolls • pizza • pasta (except whole wheat) • peanut butter • nuts • granola • white rice	• presweetened breakfast cereals • doughnuts & sticky buns
FRUITS & VEGETABLES	• all fresh fruits and vegetables (except those listed to the right) • potatoes • unsweetened fruit juices • unsweetened frozen and canned fruits • unsalted vegetable juices	• avocado • dried fruit • fruits canned in syrup • cole slaw • french fries • vegetables canned in salted water	• coconut • pickles
POULTRY FISH MEAT & EGGS	• most fish (not fried) • chicken (w/out skin) • turkey (w/out skin) • water-packed tuna	• pork loin or shoulder* • oil-packed tuna • lamb leg or loin* • veal* • steaks: flank, round or lean sirloin* • roasts: rump, arm-bone, or round* • chicken/turkey with skin *Trim all outside fat	• eggs (about 3/week) • untrimmed red meats • roasts: rib or blade • spareribs • fried chicken and fish

EAT, THINK, AND BE HEALTHY! by Paula Klevan Zeller and Michael F. Jacobson, Ph.D.

HEALTH HELPERS
AND HEALTH HURTERS

Which of these are "health helpers?" Which of these are "health hurters?" Cross out the squares below that are "health hurters," and circle all which are "health helpers."

Good nutrition and being good to your body will help you stay healthy. Knowing what can harm your body and what will help it is the key to good health.

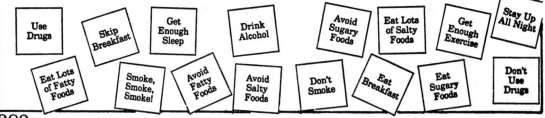

Use Drugs — Skip Breakfast — Get Enough Sleep — Drink Alcohol — Avoid Sugary Foods — Eat Lots of Salty Foods — Get Enough Exercise — Stay Up All Night — Eat Lots of Fatty Foods — Smoke, Smoke, Smoke! — Avoid Fatty Foods — Avoid Salty Foods — Don't Smoke — Eat Breakfast — Eat Sugary Foods — Don't Use Drugs

CARBOHYDRATES

Carbohydrates play a very important role. They provide the human body with energy.

Carbohydrates come in three major forms:
<u>simple sugars</u> which are sweet to taste
<u>complex carbohydrates</u> or starches which are found in cereal grains and legumes and
<u>fiber</u> which is very important to digestion.

Carbohydrate snacks containing sugars and starches provide the body with almost instant energy because they cause a sudden rise in the blood sugar level. However, the blood sugar level drops again rapidly, creating a craving for more sweet food and even fatigue, dizziness, nervousness and headache.

Overindulgence in sweet foods may crowd out other essential food and result in tooth decay and obesity.

On the other hand, it's important to eat necessary amounts of carbohydrates for your body or you may experience a loss of energy or depression.

What kind of carbohydrates are right for your body? Include fruits, whole grains (like whole grain breads and cereals) and legumes (like beans and lentils) in your diet. These foods are healthful for you and taste good too.

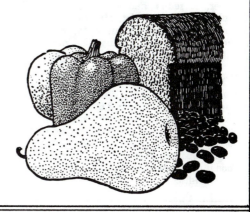

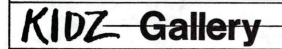

KIDZ Gallery

A peaceful moment is....

A piece of wheat dancing with the wind, just then the sun faintly spots a kind hand, picking the wheat so gently, appreciating every piece; putting them into another state of being a beautiful loaf of bread where everybody can share a beautiful moment.

Heather Lassa, age 13
Muskego, Wi.

My tooth is loose,
see it wiggle
I can make it
jiggle, jiggle
And back and forth
and round about
What shall I do
when it comes out
Will I grow one
to take its place
Or will I leave
a whistling space

by Mark Mattek,
age 6
[submitted by his grandparents,
Mr. & Mrs. Karl Kluenker, Manitowoc]

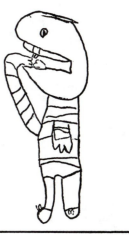

Leaves • Food Factories

For many years, people were bothered by the question, "How does a plant get the food it needs for growth?" People knew that they themselves needed to eat to survive. "But," they asked, "does a plant eat or does it make its own food?"

After a lot of hard thinking and investigating, the mystery was finally solved. It was discovered that the leaves of every vegetable, tree, and blade of grass contain a kind of 'food factory'. Although a leaf may appear as thin as paper, it really has an inside which makes food from **light, air, water, and soil**! The leaf is like a sandwich, with all the equipment for making food packed between its upper and lower surfaces.

One scientist found that a large tree working for 10 hours a day from May to September could create 3,600 pounds of food. A garden vegetable such as a watermelon makes about 20 pounds of food, while a carrot plant makes about 4 ounces of food. Just imagine how much food is made each year by all the plants in the world!

Carrot-Orange Salad (Israel)

Equipment
Grater
Measuring cups
Measuring spoons
Knife
Cutting board

Ingredients
1 pound carrots,
   washed and grated
1/2 cup orange or
   pineapple juice
2 tablespoons sesame
   seeds (optional)
1/2 cup raisins
2-3 oranges, tangerines,
   or tangelos--peeled
   and sectioned

Directions
   Combine all ingredients
in a bowl.
   Serve plain or on fresh
salad greens.

How the 'Food Factory' Makes Food

The 'food factory' goes into operation as soon as sunlight strikes and penetrates the surface of a leaf. Once inside the leaf sandwich, the sunlight is trapped. The trapped **sunlight** then combines with **air** and **water** to make **sugar**.

This combining of sunlight, air, and water to make sugar is called **photosynthesis**. Photosynthesis is the first step in the making of all food on earth. It happens everywhere that sunlight falls upon green plants.

LADYBUGS AND LETTUCE LEAVES

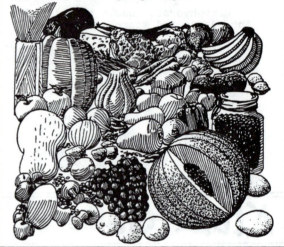

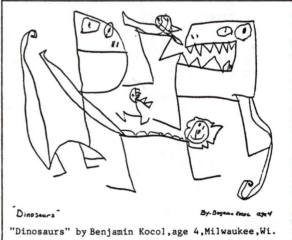

"Dinosaurs"   By-Benjamin Kocol age 4

"Dinosaurs" by Benjamin Kocol, age 4, Milwaukee, Wi.

How can mental imagery benefit recreational athletes?

Step by Step

1. Set the goal you want to achieve in the visualization. For example, if you want to improve your tennis service, decide   what specific improvement is needed. You may be able to define this yourself, or you may need the help of an instructor.

2. Detail each of the concrete steps necessary to achieve your   performance goal.

3. Achieve a relaxed state through any relaxation technique you prefer.

4. Visualize yourself performing the desired set of movements or actions in a competition or practice scene. Notice how your body moves and feels as you correctly perform the tennis serve or other movement.

5. Practice, both in the quiet of your room and in practice matches, and then integrate the mental skills into actual play.

—Richard Suinn, Ph.D., is professor and head of the Department of Psychology at Colorado State University in Fort Collins.

Weight Loss and Endurance

You don't have to be a big-league star to use mental preparation to help you in sports. If you are out of shape, you can motivate yourself to get fit by imagining how you'll look and feel 20 pounds lighter. When you're running up a steep hill, don't think about how tired you are; instead, project a mental image of how good you'll feel when you reach the top.

—From the Athlete Within by Harvey B. Simon, M.D., and Steven R. Levisohn, M.D.

We know many of you are athletes and/or weight conscious. By combining a healthful diet including whole fresh vegetables, fruits, seeds, legumes and whole grains plus exercise, good pure water, and imagery you may enjoy the most success in both worlds.

When Your Back Hurts...

First, rest it so it can heal.

Then an exercise regimen can strengthen back muscles and help prevent a relapse.

Keeping Your Back Healthy
If your back is pain-free, you can help keep it that way by adhering to the following guidelines:

- Exercise regularly to keep your back muscles strong.

- Maintain good posture, with your abdomen and chin held in and the curve in your lower back kept as straight as you can.

- Lose weight if you're overweight; excess pounds add to your back's burden and can distort posture.

- When seated, don't slouch; and rest your feet securely on the floor.

- Don't bend over from the waist; squat down to pick up items from the floor.

- When lifting, bend your knees and keep your back straight. Carry objects as close to your body as possible.

We subject our backs to a lot of abuse each day — from carrying around extra weight to picking up items we have no business lifting by ourselves. And it's easy to take a healthy back for granted. But if you'll give your back the care and attention it deserves, you can avoid painful and debilitating back injuries.

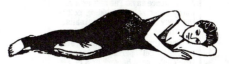

Rest is best, when your back is sore. One comfortable position: On floor or very firm bed, on your side, knees bent, pillow between knees.

—UT lifetime Health Letter
P.O. Box 53817
Boulder, CO 80322-3817

The "heat" from eating a chili pepper triggers perspiration, which may be one reason spicy foods are popular in hot climates.

Hero may be beta-carotene

By Patricia Tennison
Chicago Tribune

Beta-carotene is not exactly a household word yet, but scientists and nutritionists are enthusiastic about this misunderstood nutrient.

Paul A. Lachance, professor of food science and nutrition at Rutgers University, is one of its

SMART EATING

promoters.

"We, as scientists, were fooled by previous studies that worked with vitamin A," Lachance says.

About 30 studies done since 1950 that link diet to lower cancer incidence in humans state that the difference was vitamin A. But scientists who did the studies may have credited the wrong nutrient, Lachance says. The real hero may be beta-carotene.

The two are closely related. Beta-carotene is a nutrient found naturally in plants, algae and bacteria. Animals, including humans, don't produce beta-carotene. We get the nutrient by eating certain fruits and vegetables — particularly carrots — and from drinking milk or eating meat from animals, such as chicken or lobster, that have eaten plants or algae.

One of the important values of beta-carotene is that it creates vitamin A. When a molecule of beta-carotene splits it becomes two molecules of vitamin A.

However, only about 25 percent of beta-carotene turns into vitamin A, Lachance says. The rest of it has many other roles, including coloring body fat and, perhaps, inhibiting cancer.

"Sometimes there is damage to a healthy cell, perhaps an oxygen (molecule) goes berserk or a cell is ruptured," Lachance says. "The (beta-carotene) sitting in the membrane of the cell traps the oxygen or radical that went berserk. . . . It turns on the defense system and naturally prevents many cancers of the lung, intestinal tract, cervix and skin."

Eating an orange gives you up to 60% more vitamin C than drinking the juice.

"It's easy to get enough vitamin A, yet not get enough beta-carotene," Lachance says. That happens when consumers eat mostly animal products and shun fruits and vegetables rich in beta-carotene.

Americans need 5 to 6 milligrams of the nutrient a day, but they typically get only one-fourth that amount, Lachance says. The best sources of beta-carotene include the yellow and some of the orange fruits and vegetables, as well as dark green vegetables. ●

★

In Brief

Cholesterol Level Is Affected By Stress

Stress may affect blood cholesterol levels, according to Redford B. Williams, Jr. M.D., Director of Behavioral Medicine Research Center at Duke University. What happens is that hormones produced in response to stress stimulate the release into the blood of cholesterol from fat tissue. The stress-induced hormones may also increase cholesterol synthesis by the liver. Both reactions result in higher blood cholesterol levels. Dr. Williams also says that hostility and stress can interfere with the effectiveness of cholesterol-lowering drugs.

ENVIRONMENTAL NUTRITION

★

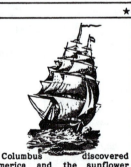

Columbus discovered America and the sunflower seed. He took the seeds back to Europe. Today, they are eaten mostly abroad. The Russians discovered that a pectin in the sunflower seeds is a "detoxifying" substance: a substance that helps you get rid of contaminants.

The Body's Need For Water

By Sandi Mitchell, Ph.D.

There's no substitute for water. Even though it undergoes no change in our body, it's absolutely essential to the performance of vital functions so that life is maintained.

A decade ago, a British mountain climbing expedition reached the summit of Mt. Everest, the roof of the world. For a number of years, Swiss climbers, considered among the best in the world, had failed in a series of assaults on the peak. When Dr. Hunt, the physician of the British expedition studied the accounts of the Swiss failures, he found that the climbers drank only two to three glasses of water daily, concentrating instead upon energy-giving foods.

Dr. Hunt ordered the British climbers to drink 12 glasses of water a day: the expedition was a success.

HARVARD UNIVERSITY TESTS

Critics stated that too much emphasis is placed upon drinking water so Harvard University conducted these tests:

A group of athletes was placed on a treadmill running at a speed of 3½ mph with 5 minute rest breaks. The first group was allowed no water. They ran for only 3½ hours before giving out. The second group was allowed to drink as much water as they wanted. They ran for 6 hours. The third group was forced to drink as much water as their bodies lost. They went for 7 hours and were going strong when the tests ended.

Conclusion: thirst is no criterion in determining the body's need for water... it needs to maintain its balance by replacing its losses continually for maximum performance.

++++++++++++++++++

The Human Body
- Requires 30 pounds of air daily
- Can survive 10 minutes without air
- Takes in 3 pounds of food daily
- Can go 5 weeks without food
- Consumes 4 pounds of water daily
- Can go without water for 5 days
- The kidneys use 5 glasses of water daily
- Loses 10 glasses of water daily

384

Dr. Donald B. Ardell, *Ardell Wellness Report*

The Problem With Modern Medicine

is that we expect too much from it ...and too little from ourselves

Americans spend a lot of money treating diseases that they could have prevented for free — through their own wellness-focused lifestyles.

Wellness is much more than the absence of illness or injury...and it is not the same as *holistic health*, which focuses on curing illness.

Wellness involves paying close attention to your health, your lifestyle and your environment. It's not very hard work, yet it can drastically reduce your risk of illness and premature death. Wellness can bring you much greater satisfaction in life.

PRINCIPLES OF WELLNESS

•**Avoid known disease-causing behaviors.** There is no miracle cure for a disease that was caused by years of high-risk behavior—smoking, drinking alcohol, eating high-fat foods, etc.

•**Examine your doctor before he examines you.** Doctors who ignore their own nutrition, fitness and overall well-being are not likely to promote healthy lifestyles in others.

•**Take resonsibility for your own well-being.** Others can give advice, but in the end *you* are responsible for you.

Example: When you visit a doctor, don't consider yourself a ;atient, which implies submission. *Better:* Consider yourself a *client* who is resonsible for his/her own actions.

•**Let nature take its course.** Americans are pill freaks. Although there are occasions when medicine is warranted, natural remedies, time, determination and a positive lifestyle are sufficient treatments for many, many ailments.

•**Don't change your lifestyle until you're ready.** Reform initiatied by guilt or pressure from others won't last. When you understand why you are doing something and anticipate its benefits, you will welcome the changes.

DIMENSIONS OF WELLNESS

•**Stress control.** Long-term stress is a major factor in most illnesses—major and minor. *Key:* Learn to cope with stress-causing events and stop worrying. *Also important:* Express your emotions and creativity instead of stifling them. That generates stress.

•**Self-responsibility.** Take an active, *positive* role in your life. *Progressive benefit:* The more things you do *for* yourself, the fewer things you'll do *against* yourself. *Important:*

•*Experience your physical and emotional feelings.* This will make you more aware of the mind-body connection. *Helpful:* Keep a journal observation, insights, emotional responses, experiences, etc., and review it periodically to see how you act and react.

•*Go after what you want.* It's the only way you'll get it. *Helpful:* Visualizing what you want will help you get it.

•*Get paid to do something that you love.* There is little happiness—or wellness—in doing something you hate...especially when it's your job.

•**Nutritional awareness.** Five of the 10 leading causes of death are diet-related—heart disease, cerebrovascular disease, cirrhosis, diabetes mellitus and arteriosclerosis. *Nutrition basics:* Eat a *balanced* diet...limit sugar and fat...increase intake of fiber, raw vegetables, fresh fruits and whole grains...avoid processed foods, caffeine and alcohol.

•**Physical fitness.** Unlike machines, our bodies wear faster from *disuse* than from use. *Helpful:* Set a fitness goal and work towards achieving it. Any goal, whether it's walking a mile or running a marathon, is fine as long as it challenges *you.*

—Bottom Line/Personal

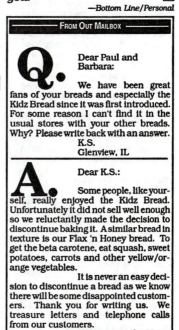

A Balanced Diet May Be Best Defense Against Disease

A person's health depends in large part on how well the immune system works. The intricate workings of the immune system enable the body to fight off diseases and infections, and destroy abnormal cells that may cause cancer. To perform at its peak, the immune system requires several nutrients. The latest research shows that certain vitamins and minerals — such as vitamins C, E, D and zinc — are especially important in helping to ward off disease.

A Carrot A Day

Beta carotene and other carotenoids — pigments that give carrots, cantaloupe and spinach their bright orange or dark green colors — are touted for their potential to protect against cancer. Studies have indicated that, on average, people who often eat carotenoid-containing foods have fewer cases of lung cancer than those who don't. Researchers say carotenoids appear to spark immune system activity with macrophages — blood cells that surround and destroy bacteria, abnormal cells and other invaders.

Recently, Dr. Joel Schwartz of Harvard School of Dental Medicine found that mouth tumors in experimental animals could be shrunk or even prevented with injections of beta-carotene.

Antioxidant Immune Protectors

Vitamin C is one of several antioxidants that protect the lungs and other organs from damage done by cigarettes, smog and pollution. Research has proven that smokers need more vitamin C than non-smokers to protect their cells from the harmful effects of cigarette smoke.

Dr. Raymond Bridges of the University of Kentucky, compared an equal number of smokers and non-smokers and looked for differences in their vitamin C status. He found that smokers had less vitamin C in their blood, fewer immunoglobulins (antibodies) in their blood streams and more inflammation — a sign of infection. Part of his findings occurred because the smokers consumed less vitamin C in their diets, but Dr. Bridges also determined that the more cigarettes a person smoked, the less he could find in their white blood cells.

Some of the most exciting research in nutrition and immunity involves the protective powers of the antioxidant, vitamin E. One of that vitamin's most important roles is to protect cells from free radicals (unstable oxygen molecules that damage cells). Vitamin E's protective powers lie in its ability to become part of the membrane, or "skin," of cells.

At Colorado State University, researchers found that a large dose of vitamin E (six times the amount in a normal diet) helped protect animals from bacterial infections. And at the U.S.D.A. Human Nutrition Research Center on Aging at Tufts University, Simin Meydani, Ph.D. boosted the immune activity of white blood cells in elderly subjects by giving them 400 I.U. of vitamin E — a dose well above the Recommended Dietary Allowance of 8 to 10 I.U.

A Sunny Forecast

Exciting research at the Texas A&M College of Medicine suggests that vitamin D is a crucial ingredient of resistance to certain diseases. David N. McMurray, Ph.D., of A&M fed guinea pigs a diet lacking vitamin D and found that the deficient diet weakened their immune systems and worsened the animals' ability to fight off tuberculosis. McMurray believes this is because two types of blood cells important to the immune system — macrophages and lymphocytes (white blood cells) — need vitamin D to function properly. "Most interesting," explains McMurray, "is the fact that in the early 1900's people were sent to Arizona or sunny mountain resorts to recover from tuberculosis. Now we know why."

Zeroing in on Zinc

Of all the minerals in our diet, zinc is the best known for its effects on the immune system. One of zinc's primary roles is to activate thymic hormone (manufactured by the thymus gland) which is responsible for the development of T lymphocytes (white blood cells that fight disease-causing invaders). Because the thymus gland is most active in young children, dietary zinc deficiency early in life can permanently damage the body's ability to produce T lymphocytes.

Zinc deficiency is common in people with Acquired Immune Deficiency Disease or AIDS, a disease that seriously compromises the body's ability to ward off life-threatening infections. According to Susanna Cunningham-Rundles, Ph.D. at the New York Hospital-Cornell University Medical College, zinc deficiency can be found in people even before they're diagnosed as having AIDS and regardless of whether or not they are taking zinc supplements. "We are looking for ways to use nutrition to improve immunity, and zinc is one of the key nutrients," says Dr. Cunningham-Rundles.

But zinc is not the only important nutrient. For example, McMurray found that zinc-deficient animals can still fight off tuberculosis, as long as there is enough vitamin D. in their diets. He concluded that the body can compensate for certain deficiencies if other parts of the immune system are adequately nourished.

Breast Feeding May Be Best

Researchers at the University of Texas Medical Branch at Galveston have found that several nutrients in human milk boost the immune system's infection-fighting abilities. Most important, perhaps, is that breast feeding can enhance an infant's ability to fight infection without inflammation.

Inflammation is one of the body's natural defenses against infection, but in an infant it has the potential to damage the delicate gastrointestinal and respiratory tracts. Human milk also contains several antioxidants crucial to the immune system.

The Bottom Line

Other nutrients — including iron, selenium, folic acid and vitamin B-6 — are an integral part of the immune system. Paradoxically, though, the same vitamins and minerals, when given in large amounts, weaken immunity and increase the risk of infection. In addition, polyunsaturated fats which are promoted for their cholesterol-lowering abilities can decrease the immune system's ability to fight infection if consumed to the exclusion of other types of fats. For this reason, most experts agree that the best defense is a good offense — eating a well-balanced diet. Too much or too little of some nutrients can compromise the immune system.

—Mindy G. Hermann Zaidins, M.B.A., R.D.
from ENVIRONMENTAL NUTRITION

386

Grains—back to the future

A square meal isn't what it used to be: at many tables vegetables, pasta, and other foods high in complex carbohydrates have begun to edge out meat as the center of interest. Of course, potatoes, pasta, and rice can all be turned into excellent meat substitutes when combined with beans or cheese, for instance. Whole grains, though, such as cracked wheat and barley, are too often overlooked as potential main or side dishes. While grains have been used as main dishes since Biblical times, many American cooks are unaccustomed to handling them, except in the form of flour or breakfast cereal. Such foods as kasha or bulgur may sound a little too mysterious. And often only health food stores stock special grains.

Yet whole grains are rich in protein and fiber, as well as some B vitamins. Many are also fairly good sources of calcium and iron. The average cup of cooked whole grains contains only about 200 calories and is as easy to prepare as rice or dried pasta.

Kasha is simply a term for roasted buckwheat kernels that are cooked like rice; bulgur is precooked whole-wheat berries, which can also be handled much like rice. Mediterranean and Middle Eastern cuisines feature many famous whole-grain dishes: couscous, a delicious combination of cracked whole-wheat berries (millet can be used, but the packaged product is usually ground semolina) with meat, vegetables, or even fruits; tabbouleh, a cold salad made of cracked wheat or bulgur, chopped tomatoes, mint, and parsley; and pilafs, cooked combinations of grains with meats or vegetables. There are endless adaptations of these dishes using everyday ingredients. Other whole grains, such as rye and oats, while not ready substitutes for rice or pasta on the dinner plate, can be incorporated in bread, meat loaf, and other baked dishes. And one grain can, of course, be mixed with another.

Three unusual names on the chart below are amaranth (from the Greek, meaning "immortal grain"), triticale (the term combines *triticum* and *secale*, Latin words for "wheat" and "rye") and quinoa (pronounced KEEN-wa, an Andean word meaning "the mother grain"). Amaranth and quinoa are native to South America. Both are high in protein, minerals, and vitamins; supermarkets and health food stores carry them. Triticale, another high-protein "miracle" grain, is a hybrid created about a century ago.

Remember that many whole grains, especially wheat, keep best in the refrigerator. The natural oils in the bran and the germ (the outer parts, which are removed in refining) tend to spoil quickly, especially in warm environments. This is why whole grains tend to be relatively costly, and one reason why most grains are refined in the first place—to increase their shelf life in grocery stores and home pantries.

Comparing grains (3.5 ounces dry, about 1 cup cooked)

TYPE	PROTEIN (g)	FAT (g)	DIETARY FIBER (g)	IRON (mg)	COMMENT
Amaranth	15	6.9	4.5	11.8	High in protein, iron, and calcium. Native to South America; available in health food stores. Whole kernels sold pearled (polished). Good as side dish or cereal. Flour used in bread, tortillas, cookies, and cereal.
Barley	8	1.0	8.2	2.1	Available as "pot" or "Scotch" barley (whole kernels) or pearl barley (polished). Both good in soups and stews and for side dishes, puddings, and cereal. May lower blood cholesterol.
Buckwheat	12	2.4	11.4	3.8	Not a true grain but a seed. Roasted kernels can be cooked like rice as a side dish (kasha). Flour can be mixed with wheat for bread and pancakes. Distinctive, nutty flavor.
Millet	12	3.9	3.0	3.0	High in phosphorus and B vitamins. Used chiefly as animal feed in U.S. but available in health food stores. Good as side dish or as a substitute for bread stuffings in poultry. Swells enormously in water.
Oats	16	6.3	11.2	4.2	Whole kernels (groats) take an hour to cook. Flattened rolled oats require less time. Oat flour (oatmeal processed in a blender) can be used in bread, pastry, meat loaf, and casseroles. May lower blood cholesterol.
Quinoa (chenopodium)	16	6.9	4.6	6.6	High in protein, calcium, and iron. Good in puddings, soups, and stir-fries. Whole-grain version must be washed and strained. Flour can be used in combination or alone for baking. Native South American grain.
Rye	12	1.7	11.4	4.6	Low-gluten content produces dense bread. Cracked rye makes good cereal. Rolled rye from health food stores can be added to meat loaf and casseroles. Good in soups. Flour mixes well with wheat and/or oats.
Triticale	11	1.8	9.9	2.6	Wheat/rye hybrid; early man-made grain. Comes whole, cracked, and as flour. Flour low in gluten, best combined with wheat for bread making. Commercial brands of triticale bread available in supermarkets.
Whole wheat	10	2.0	9.6	3.5	Comes as whole berries or cracked. Whole berries need 2-3 hours of cooking, cracked about 15 minutes. Both good for cereals, casseroles, and soups. Bulgur (hulled, parboiled wheat) is good for tabbouleh salad and other cold side dishes. Sweet, nutty flavor.

EAT DRINK & BE WARY...
YOUR GUIDE TO EATING LIGHT AND
RIGHT DURING THE HOLIDAYS
Patti Bazel Geil, M.S., R.D.

Thanksgiving signals the beginning of the holiday season and an endless round of parties and special occasions. This year, will visions of sugarplums (and eggnog and candy and cookies...) dance in your head and onto your plate? Or will you hold fast to your healthy eating habits while still celebrating the spirit of the season?

If you are following a particular eating plan, the holiday temptations may appear to be everywhere. Adopt a realistic attitude. Keep in mind that sheer willpower ("I will not eat") is no substitute for self-control ("Ill plan ahead to allow myself to eat sensible.")

Let's imagine you've received your invitation for a wonderful holiday gathering. Preparing your social event survival skills is as improtant as marking the date on your calendar.

Before you go, call your hostess and offer to bring a food item to the party. Besides developing a reputation as a thoughtful guest, you'll be assured there will be at least one dish that will fit your diet plan.

When the day of the festive occasion arrives, pace yourself at breakfast and lunch in anticipation of possible over-eating in the evening. Plan ahead for how much you will eat and tell a good friend for moral support.

Never attend a party on an empty stomach. A healthy, high fiber snack before you leave home will satisfy you and prevent an unplanned attack on the hors d'oeuvre tray.

Once you've arrived on the party scene, remember that there is no such thing as a forbidden food—only those foods that can be eaten less often and those that can be eaten more often. Making a food totally "off-limits" often serves to glamorize it, thus making it more tempting than ever.

Sip on a low calorie, non-alcoholic drink with lots of bubbles (such as club soda or mineral water) to fill you up while you survey the snack situation. Decide in advance what your choices will be. Dont't "cook your holiday goose" by loading your plate. Select a small plate or napkin to make tiny portions look larger. Raw veggies, low cal dips, high fiber crackers, fresh fruit and popcorn are best bets from the buffet. Maybe you could go "halfsies"--take half the portion you normally would so you can still try those irresistible foods and save calories while sharing with your friend or spouse.

Remind yourself that you're at the party to socialize, not to eat. Focus on the people at the party rather than the food that's being served. Choose the food you want to eat and carry on your conversation away from the table. Good small talkers are small eaters. Remember your mother's reprimand "Don't talk with your mouth full" and you'll find it almost impossible to nibble non-stop.

Don't plan to return to the refreshments immediately for a second serving. Enjoy 20 minutes visiting with friends while you wait for your brain to get the message that you're full.

If you feel you've slipped and strayed from your carefully prepared strategy, don't use that as an excuse to give up on your eating plan. Forgive yourself and try again at the next festive occasion.

As party season winds down and the new year begins, reward yourself for maintaining your healthy eating habits with non-food treats: new clothes, a new book or a night at the movies.

And remember: it's not the weeks from Thanksgiving to New Year's, but the weeks from New Year's to Thanksgiving that count the most when you're developing healthy attitudes for a lifetime of living well!

Food Dangers
Migraine Triggers?

Chocolate, aged cheeses and other foods may be the trigger to migraines in one-third to one-half of all sufferers, reports neurologist Seymour Diamond, one of the country's foremost headache experts.

"Many basic researchers doubt that food and drink can cause migraines," says Dr. Diamond, who runs the Diamond Headache Clinic in Chicago. "But clinicians who deal directly with headache victims know otherwise."

He and colleague J. Nathan Blau of the City of London Migraine Clinic surveyed 550 clinicians in the United States and Britain. They uncovered a widespread clinical belief that foods trigger much of the pain among the people, mainly women, who suffer from the one-sided headaches called migraines. 16 million Americans have migraines.

Commonly-cited culprits: chocolate; alcohol, especially red wines; aged cheeses such as Brie, Camembert, cheddar and blue; nuts; citrus fruits; aged, canned, cured and processed meats; dairy products and coffee. The flavor enhancers monosodium glutamate (MSG) and "Marmite," a salty, aged spread popular in Britain and Australia, were also high on the list.

They believe an "internal thermostat," regulated perhaps by hormones, determines whether a person is vulnerable to a certain food at a given time.

If you suffer from migraines, advises Diamond, try avoiding offending foods and eat and sleep at regular times. Keep a headache diary to uncover relations between headaches and diet, and any other factors.

American Health

How to Make Wonderful Meals *Without* Cooking Oil
—Leslie Cerier

Myth: Meals prepared without oil are bland and boring. Actually, not adding oil lets you savor the true flavors and textures. And oil-free foods can be very healthy and low in calories, particularly when you don't include meats, which can be high in saturated fats.

The Alternatives

• STEAMING can be used for vegetables, fish and dried fruits, as well as breads and grains. Steaming gives foods a sweet, light moistness that brings out their true flavors. *Equipment needed:* A bamboo steamer and wok or fry pan...or a stainless-steel basket (avoid aluminum) and a pot big enough to hold it. Bamboo steamers are usually sold in stacking sets, so you can steam a whole meal at once.

Place the bamboo steamer in the wok or fry-pan...or fit the metal steamer into the pot. Add one inch of cold water, arrange the food evenly inside the steamer. Bring the water to a boil, then reduce the heat to a simmer.

Vegetables are done in five to ten minutes, depending upon firmness, size of pieces and desired tenderness. If you are cooking different-textured vegetables together, put the vegetables that take longer to cook (root vegetables such as carrots and turnips) on the bottom of the steamer and the quicker-cooking ones (zucchini, leafy vegetables, broccoli florets, etc.) on top. Experiment with different foods by checking on them during cooking.

Avoid steam burns by using oven mitts and keeping your face away when you remove the pot's lid. Foods can become scorched if all the water boils off, ruining the meal—and the pot. If you are steaming something for a long time, check periodically to be sure there is enough water.

If you use a multi-level bamboo steamer, you can cook several different foods at the same time. Place longer-cooking foods on the bottom level, and when they're partially cooked add the shorter-cooking foods to the upper levels.

Example: place fish filets on the bottom level, carrots on the next and bread or thinly sliced, quick-cooking vegetables—zucchini, cabbage, etc.—on top.

Serve steamed foods, immediately, otherwise, they will continue to cook from internal heat, even when the heat is turned off. To preserve the bright colors of freshly steamed vegetables, rinse them briefly in cold water immediately after they are done.

• BROILING/BRAISING* adds succulence and tenderness to most vegetables and grains. This brings out a salty flavor...*without* adding salt. Cooking time depends on the food.

Boiled apples, tomatoes and other juicy fruits and vegetables make flavorful sauces. For instance, you can easily make applesauce by thinly slicing apples, adding a pinch of salt, covering the pot and letting it simmer until the sauce is the right consistency. Add your favorite spices, like cinnamon or nutmeg, toward the end of the cooking time. Uncover the pot to speed water evaporation. You can make tomato sauce in the same way.

• SAUTÉING' can be done in a wok or skillet. Just omit the oil and proceed as usual. The food will take on the flavor of the spices used.

For a Chinese flavor: Season with ginger, garlic, tamari and mirin (sweet rice wine used for cooking). Add a little water during cooking as needed, to prevent burning the bottom of the pan.

For an Indian flavor: Season with garlic, cumin seeds and a pinch of salt in a few ounces of water. Cook for a minute and then add leeks, onions, carrots, cabbage and string beans.

• NABEMONO, the Japanese method of one-pot cooking, is quick and oil-free. The food has a *very* light, moist, clean flavor.

Use several different kinds of food, including fish or tofu, and vegetables, aiming for a harmonious mixture of colors and flavors. Arrange the pieces decoratively in a cast-iron pan or shallow skillet and add just enough water to cover the vegetables. Cook until the colors are bright and the vegetables are crisp and tender.

Because all ingredients are put in the skillet at once, slow-cooking foods—root vegetables, etc.—must be sliced more thinly than fast-cooking foods—mushrooms, etc.

• BAKING is commonly used for squash, root vegetalbes and casseroles. It's completely oil-free, and especially nice in the winter, when the aromas linger in a warm house. Baking dries food out a bit, so the flavor becomes more concentrated.

• PRESSURE-COOKING is an old-fashioned time-saver that's making a comeback. A gentle salty taste comes through the food. Grains and beans can be pressure-cooked together or separately. Adding vegetables produces great soups and stews.

To braise: Cook the food quickly at a high heat in an uncovered pan until the outside turns brown, then simmer it in a covered pan with a little liquid.
'To sauté: Fry quickly in a pan, stirring frequently.

—BOTTOM LINE PERSONAL

NOTE: A perfect way to serve your steamed or stir fried vegetables is over toasted Nutty Wheat, Sunny Millet, or Hunger Filler Bread. Also, be sure to have fresh and raw vegetables, fruits, sprouts, etc. in salads or by themselves. Fresh squeezed lemon juice adds zest when sprinkled over vegetable sticks or chunks.

389

Energy Drink Brings Home Another Gold

This Spring a young and sprightly 67-year old woman from Fond du Lac, Wisconsin set a new world age-group record in the 400-meter run on her way to winning three gold medals in the Masters Indoor Track Championships at Ohio State University. Her world record setting time was 1:43.9. She won gold medals in the 800-meter and 1500-meter races as well. Our hats off the Carol Peebles for such a fine accomplishment.

Here's what Carol had to say: "I never could have done it without Energy Drink. It has made training much easier and recovery after a hard race much faster. It's never too late to try something new."

If Carol can brush a world record after having had breast cancer, I guess anyone can. Congratulations, Carol!

You and Your Diet

—from The Bottom Line Personal

■ **Adding fiber to your diet** can shrink precancerous polyps in the lower intestine, thus reducing the risk of colon and rectal cancer. These findings are the first to show that ordinary food (a cereal rich in bran) can *reverse* the usual progression to cancer in people.

■ **Why sugar is bad:** It has no nutrients ... depletes stores of vitamins (especially B and C) and minerals (especially magnesium and chromium) ... causes hormone levels to fluctuate, which can cause menstrual problems in women ... sends blood-sugar levels to extremes ... can cause hot flashes in women ... inhibits calcium absorption, which is needed to prevent osteoporosis ... is linked to obesity, digestive problems, tooth decay, diabetes, high cholesterol and urinary-tract infections.

■ **Dates contain no fat,** even though they grow on palm trees. A one-ounce serving (about five dates) contains 115 calories, 271mg of potassium and 3.7 grams of fiber (it's one of the highest-fiber fruits).

To: Natural Ovens
Re: New satisfied customer

Thanks for your quality products. I have been a fortunate consumer of your products since their inception, and I appreciate your philosophy of holding quality and nutrition over gross profits. I wish your company continued success, as I would no doubt suffer an anxiety attack upon entering a grocery store if your products were no longer on the shelves.

With that said... You should be aware of your newest, avid fan. A roommate of mine owns a cat, aptly named "Lumpy." Lumpy is a very reserved cat, who's hobbies include sleeping, eating, and chasing bits of string. Not unlike most cats, Lumpy is a very finicky fellow, and will refuse to eat unless all foreseeable variables such as food temperature, consistency, and moisture level are controlled for his daily repast. (A team of scientists has been contracted to make sure Lumpy's food is presentable to him.) Lumpy is not at all picky about Manitowoc Ovens breads, however. If I return home from the store and fail to place the bread in the refrigerator (the only place safe from the furry guy), Lumpy will use his sharp incisors to gnaw through the two layer package to enjoy a nutritious snack. On one occasion, Lumpy used acrobatic finesse to retrieve the bread from a cupboard, dragging the bread from the cupboard, depositing it on the floor, and digging in. Bon Appetit!!

What is interesting is that Lumpy has no use for refined white bread. [Once, as an experiment, I left a loaf of this sort of white bread] out overnight, well within Lumpy's reach. The bread remained untouched, escaping unscathed. Lumpy has more respect for nutrition than to do *that* to his body.

Although all your breads pass the "Lumpy Test," Nutty Wheat Bread is his favorite. I have to go now, as Lumpy is now tearing the door off the refrigerator.

Thanks again,
P.B.
Milwaukee, WI

RUBBING A BRUISE helps relieve pain and prevent swelling by increasing the blood circulation to the area. *Technique:* Keep fingers in one place and rub in a circular motion. *Don't* rub back and forth over the surface of the skin — the goal is to keep the tissue *beneath* the skin stimulated.
—The Bottom Line Personal

What if you did 5,000 sit-ups a month?

True or false:

Proper sit-ups selectively burn fat deposits around the waist.

The more sit-ups you do, the smaller your waist.

Hooking your feet under a piece of furniture when doing sit-ups helps you isolate your abdominal muscles.

All are false. A few years ago, a study at the University of Massachusetts showed that even men who did 5,000 sit-ups over the course of 27 days had no significant loss of fat in the abdominal area. As we've said before, the whole idea of spot-reducing is a myth. To lose body fat, you must burn more calories than you take in—a deficit of 3,500 calories to lose a pound. This study's subjects burned an average of only 50 calories per five-minute daily session—not enough to trim down. But even if they had burned twice as many calories, the energy would come from fat stores throughout the body, not just from the tummy.

This is not to say that sit-ups are a waste of time. When properly done, they strengthen and tone the three sets of abdominal muscles (the rectus abdominis and the external and internal obliques), which are otherwise hard to exercise. Since strong abdominal muscles provide better support for the back, strengthening these muscles may help prevent or alleviate many back problems. Strong abdominals also give you more power for running, tennis, and other activities that involve the torso.

Sit-up don'ts

• **NO straight legs.** Skip those old-fashioned straight-leg sit-ups, in which you sit up fully while keeping your legs flat on the floor. These can make you overarch and thus strain your lower back. And, anyway, when you sit up all the way, much of the work is done by the hip flexor muscles, not the abdominals.

• **NO hooked feet.** Don't do sit-ups with your feet hooked under a bar or piece of furniture—this lets the legs and hips do most of the work.

• **NO excessive speed and repetitions.** Forget about doing hundreds of rapid sit-ups. When you perform them so quickly, the abdominal muscles don't get a maximal workout—momentum takes over to some extent as you bounce up and down. So rather than increasing the number of sit-ups you do (beyond, say, 50 or so), make them more challenging by doing them more slowly, or try some of the variations described at right.

The better way—the crunch

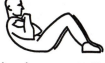

1. Lie on the floor with your knees bent and feet flat on floor.

2. Contract the abdominal muscles while pressing your lower back into the floor, which will cause your upper body to lift up *slowly*.

3. Come up to no more than a 30° to 45° angle.

4. If you're just starting to do sit-ups, keep your arms straight at your side as you sit up. To increase the difficulty of the exercise as you progress, cross your arms over your chest, or place your hands behind your head or near your ears.

5. *Slowly* lower your back to the ground.

6. To prevent arching, always keep your lower back pressed into the floor.

7. Beginners should start with three sets of five sit-ups with a brief rest between sets. Try this three to five times a week. Gradually work up to three sets of 15 sit-ups per session. *Remember, take them slow and easy—this is not a race.*

8. Stop if you feel discomfort in your lower back.

Variations

For a change of pace, try these variations: Lie on the floor, place your legs on a bench (illustration A), and do a crunch as described above. Similarly, place your feet flat against a wall with your legs bent at a right angle. Or try "reverse curls," in which you move your legs, not your torso: keeping your lower back pressed into the floor, your knees bent, and your feet off the floor, slowly bring your knees as close to your chest as possible (illustration B).

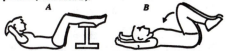

The basic sit-ups work all three abdominal muscle groups, but especially the rectus abdominis. To work the obliques (located toward the sides of the abdominal area) maximally, include a slight twist in any of these exercises. For example, as you sit up, bring your right shoulder (or elbow, if your hands are behind your head) toward your left knee, then reverse.

—BERKELEY WELLNESS LETTER

Smile for the day...

Some people use these rules and then wonder why they are fat instead of fit!

1. If you eat something and no one sees you eat it, it has no calories.

2. If you drink a diet soda with a candy bar, the calories in the candy bar are cancelled out by the diet soda.

3. When you eat with someone else, calories don't count if you don't eat more than they do.

4. Food used for medicinal purposes NEVER counts, such as hot chocolate, brandy, toast, and cheesecake.

5. If you fatten up everyone around you, then you look thinner.

6. Movie related foods do not have additional calories because they are part of the entire entertainment package and not part of one's personal fuel, such as Milk Duds, Buttered Popcorn, Junior Mints, Red Hots, and Tootsie Rolls.

7. Cookie pieces contain no calories. The process of breaking causes calorie leakage.

8. Things licked off of knives and spoons don't count if you are in the process of preparing something. Examples are peanut butter on a knife making a sandwich and ice cream on a spoon making a sundae.

9. Foods that have the same color have the same number of calories. Examples are spinach and pistacio ice cream, mushrooms and white chocolate. NOTE: Chocolate is a universal color and may be substituted for any other food color.

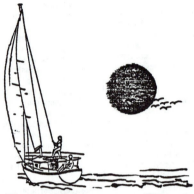

FOR A REFRESHING HOLIDAY...

Manitowoc is a charming city of 32,000 people set on a beautiful strip of Lake Michigan. We have lovely hotels, museums, shopping centers, restaurants, and beaches. While visiting, you can enjoy our sweet, clean air as well as recreational outings like sailing, jet skiing, fishing, hiking, biking, golfing, skiing and snowmobiling. —— It's all here!!

And while you're in the area, visit our beautiful 28,000 square foot bakery, set on an open field just west of Manitowoc. We have free tours, plus samples of course. Tours are given Mondays, Wednesdays, Thursdays and Fridays at 9, 10 and 11 am. We think you'll enjoy seeing how the breads are mixed and baked.

Another feature of our estate is the Natural Ovens Observation Farm. Following each 10:00 bakery tour, guests are invited to visit our farm. There you can see the results of feeding pigs, chickens, and Belgian horses a flax-based diet. You'll be pleased to see how healthy and happy they are. Kids of all ages enjoy seeing the animals.

When you're in the Manitowoc area, stop and see us. We'd love to have you. Our address is 4300 County Trunk CR on the south side of Manitowoc.

THE LATEST WORD

This just in from the September 20, 1990 (p 645-655) issue of the *New England Journal of Medicine.* In a major review article by the editor, Dr. Franklin Epstein and others on the "Mechanism of Disease," they tell how excess arachidonic acid in the absence of sufficient linolenic acid (see chapter 2) leads to excess leukotrienes which they state causes asthma, psoriasis, adult respiratory distress, newborn pulmonary hypertension, allergic rhinites, gout, rheumatoid arthritis and inflammatory bowel disease. The article goes into great details on how the dozens of different pathways and impair the immune system to cause the above diseases.